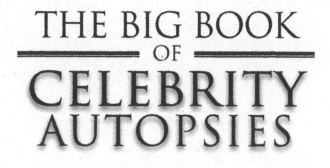

THE BIG BOOK
OF
CELEBRITY
AUTOPSIES

THE BIG BOOK
OF
CELEBRITY
AUTOPSIES

EDITED BY KEVIN VIANI

SKYHORSE PUBLISHING

Skyhorse Publishing books may be purchased in bulk at
special discounts for sales promotion, corporate gifts,
fund-raising, or educational purposes. Special editions
can also be created to specifications. For details, contact
the Special Sales Department, Skyhorse Publishing,
307 West 36th Street, 11th Floor, New York,
NY 10018 or info@skyhorsepublishing.com.

Skyhorse® and Skyhorse Publishing® are registered
trademarks of Skyhorse Publishing, Inc.®,
a Delaware corporation.

Visit our website at www.skyhorsepublishing.com.

10 9 8

Library of Congress Cataloging-in-Publication Data available on file.

ISBN: 978-1-62087-719-7

Printed in the United States of America

Table of Contents

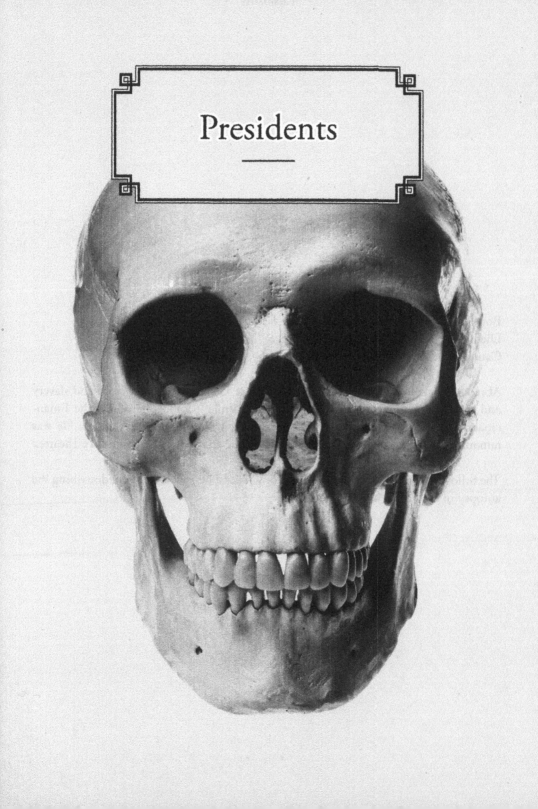

Presidents

Abraham Lincoln

Born: February 12, 1809, Hardin County, Kentucky
Died: April 15, 1865, Washington, DC
Cause of Death: Assassination

Abraham Lincoln, the sixteenth president of the United States, fought to end slavery and reunify the country during the civil war. While in office, he signed the Emancipation Proclamation, abolishing slavery in the United States of America. He was famously assassinated by John Wilkes Booth while attending a play in Ford's Theatre.

The following letter was sent to the Surgeon General by J. J. Woodward describing the autopsy of the president:

Surgeon General's Office

Washington City D.C.
April 15, 1865
Brigadier General J.K. Barnes
Surgeon General U.S.A.

General:
I have the honor to report that in obedience to your orders and aided by Assistant Surgeon E. Curtis, U.S.A., I made in your presence at 12 o'clock this morning an autopsy on the body of President Abraham Lincoln, with the following results: The eyelids and surrounding parts of the face were greatly ecchymosed and the eyes somewhat protuberant from effusion of blood into the orbits.

There was a gunshot wound of the head around which the scalp was greatly thickened by hemorrhage into its tissue. The ball entered through the occipital bone about one inch to the left of the median line and just above the left lateral sinus, which it opened. It then penetrated the dura matter, passed through the left posterior lobe of the cerebrum, entered the left lateral ventricle and lodged in the white matter of the cerebrum just above the anterior portion of the left corpus striatum, where it was found.

The wound in the occipital bone was quite smooth, circular in shape, with bevelled edges. The opening through the internal table being larger than that through the external table. The track of the ball was full of clotted blood and contained several little fragments of bone with small pieces of the ball near its external orifice. The brain around the track was pultaceous and livid from capillary hemorrhage into its substance. The ventricles of the brain were full of clotted blood. A thick clot beneath the dura matter coated the right cerebral lobe.

There was a smaller clot under the dura matter of the left side. But little blood was found at the base of the brain. Both the orbital plates of the frontal bone were fractured and the fragments pushed upwards toward the brain. The dura matter over these fractures was uninjured. The orbits were gorged with blood. I have the honor of being very respectfully your obedient servant.

J.J. Woodward
Assistant Surgeon
U.S.A.

Dr. Edward Curtis was present during the procedure and sent this letter to his mother describing the events:

"The room...contained but little furniture: a large, heavily curtained bed, a sofa or two, bureau, wardrobe, and chairs comprised all there was. Seated around the room were several general officers and some civilians, silent or conversing in whispers, and to one side, stretched upon a rough framework of boards and covered only with sheets and towels, lay - cold and immovable - what but a few hours before was the soul of a great nation. The Surgeon General was walking up and down the room when I arrived and detailed me the history of the case. He said that the president showed most wonderful tenacity of life, and, had not his wound been necessarily mortal, might have survived an injury to which most men would succumb...Dr. Woodward and I proceeded to open the head and remove the brain down to the track of the ball. The latter had entered a little to the left of the median line at the back of the head, had passed almost directly forwards through the center of the brain and lodged. Not finding it readily, we proceeded to remove the entire brain, when, as I was lifting the latter from the cavity of the skull, suddenly the bullet dropped out through my fingers and fell, breaking the solemn silence of the room with its clatter, into an empty basin that was standing beneath. There it lay upon the white china, a little black mass no bigger than the end of my finger - dull, motionless and harmless, yet the cause of such mighty changes in the world's history as we may perhaps never realize.... silently, in one corner of the room, I prepared the brain for weighing. As I looked at the mass of soft gray and white substance that I was carefully washing, it was impossible to realize that it was that mere clay upon whose workings, but the day before, rested the hopes of the nation. I felt more profoundly impressed than ever with the mystery of that unknown something which may be named 'vital spark' as well as anything else, whose absence or presence makes all the immeasurable difference between an inert mass of matter owning obedience to no laws but those covering the physical and chemical forces of the universe, and on the other hand, a living brain by whose silent, subtle machinery a world may be ruled.

The weighing of the brain... gave approximate results only, since there had been some loss of brain substance, in consequence of the wound, during the hours of life after the shooting. But the figures, as they were, seemed to show that the brain weight was not above the ordinary for a man of Lincoln's size."

-Dr. Curtis

Robert King Stone was also present, and he later made these remarks about the autopsy:

Shot. 1 inch left median line traversing left lateral sinus upper edge, through occipital bone toward edge of lateral sinus. Thru occipital bone, touched ledge of lateral sinus, struck posterior lobe traversing it in a horizontal place (passing forwards inclining to the right.) In orifice of wound a scale blood 2 ½ in. in track, pieces of bone – 2 pieces of bone about 4 inches in advance in track of ball . Entered the left ventricle behind, followed the course of ventricle accurately, inching upwards and inwards, ploughing thru the upper part of thalamus nervorum opticorum, other 2 lodged in cerebral matter just above the corpus stratum of the left side. The brain track of ball was in a bubbly disintegrated state.

Both ventricles filled with blood. Whole brain engorged and bloody prints. More matter than wounds. On reviewing, the dura mater was displaced with a large coagulation of blood - lying upon the right hemisphere of the brain. Reviewing the dura mater, no wound in which was found, we found the orbital plates of both sides, the seat of comminuted fracture, the fragments being forced from within, outward. The orbit oculum palpitated membrane and cavity was filled with blood. Origin of which we didn't seek. The right had been notably protruded, later sank back after death. Ecchymoses of the left eye 1st and right eye 2nd

Great oedema of sinus and a little blood extravasated about shot wound, clean cut as if by a punch. 2 feet off orbital plates, very thin.

-Dr. Stone

James A. Garfield

Born: November 19, 1831, Moreland Hills, Ohio
Died: September 19, 1881, Elberon, New Jersey
Cause of Death: Assassination

President Garfield only spent four months in office before he was shot by Charles J. Gaiteau. Garfield survived the gunshot but was in bad health for months as doctors tried to find the bullet. While resting in the White House, Garfield became increasingly ill with what was believed to be an infection. In an effort to give the president some peace and quiet, doctors moved him to a house on the Jersey Shore, where he finally succumbed to his injuries.

The following is the autopsy report preformed by his doctors:

By previous arrangement a *post-mortem* examination of the body of President Garfield was made this afternoon in the presence and with the assistance of Drs. Hamilton, Agnew, Bliss, Barnes, Woodward, Reyburn, Andrew H. Smith, of Elberon, and Acting Assistant Surgeon D. S. Lamb, of the Army Medical Museum, of Washington. The operation was performed by Dr. Lamb. It was found that the ball, after fracturing the right eleventh rib, had passed through the spinal column in front of the spinal cord, fracturing the body of the first lumbar vertebra, driving a number of small fragments of bone into the adjacent soft parts, and lodging below the pancreas, about 2 1/2 inches to the left of the spine and behind the peritoneum, where it had become completely encysted.

The immediate cause of death was secondary hemorrhage from one of the mesenteric arteries adjoining the track of the ball, the blood rupturing the peritoneum and nearly a pint escaping into the abdominal cavity. This hemorrhage is believed to have been the cause of the severe pain in the lower part of the chest complained of just before death. An abscess cavity 6 inches by 4 in dimensions was found in the vicinity of the gall bladder, between the liver and the transverse colon, which were strongly adherent. It did not involve the substance of the liver, and no communication was found between it and the wound.

A long suppurating channel extended from the external wound, between the loin muscles and the right kidney, almost to the right groin. This channel, now known to be due to the burrowing of pus from the wound, was supposed during life to have been the track of the ball.

On an examination of the organs of the chest evidences of severe bronchitis were found on both sides, with broncho-pneumonia of the lower portions of the right lung, and, though to a much less extent, of the left. The lungs contained no abscesses and the heart no clots. The liver was enlarged and fatty, but not from abscesses. Nor were any found in any other organ except the left kidney, which contained near its surface a small abscess about one-third of an inch in diameter.

In reviewing the history of the case in connection with the autopsy it is quite evident that the different suppurating surfaces, and especially the fractured, spongy tissue of the vertebrae, furnish a sufficient explanation of the septic condition which existed.

D. W. BLISS., J. K. BARNES.
J. J. WOODWARD., ROBERT REYBURN.
FRANK H. HAMILTON., D. HAYES AGNEW.
ANDREW H. SMITH., D. S. LAMB.
(SEPTEMBER 20, 1881.)

William McKinley

Born: January 29, 1843, Niles, Ohio
Died: September 14, 1901, Buffalo, New York
Cause of Death: Assassination

President McKinley was the twenty-fifth President of the United States. During his presidency, America won the Spanish American war and increased its trade and influence overseas. He was assassinated by the anarchist Leon Czolgosz after delivering a speech at the Pan American Exposition in Buffalo, New York. McKinley survived for six days after the shooting before his wounds proved too severe.

Special Contribution.

The Official Report on the Case of President McKinley.

SURGICAL HISTORY.

PRESIDENT WILLIAM McKINLEY, was shot, by Leon F. Czolgosz, in the Temple of Music, at the Pan-American Exposition, Buffalo, N.Y., at about 7 minutes past 4 on the afternoon of Friday, September 6, 1901. Two shots were fired. One bullet struck near the upper part of the sternum, and the other in the left hypochondriac region. The President was immediately conveyed to the Emergency Hospital on the exposition grounds by the motor ambulance, where he arrived at 4.18. Dr. G. McK. Hall and Mr. Edward C. Mann, medical student, of the house staff, were in charge of the ambulance, medical student T. F. Ellis being the driver.

On arrival at the hospital, President McKinley was at once placed upon the table in the operating room and undressed. During the removal of his clothing a bullet fell out and was picked up by Mr. Ellis. Dr. Hall placed a temporary antiseptic dressing over the wounds, and Mr. Mann ordered a nurse to administer 0.01 gm. of morphin and 0.002 gm. of strychnin hypodermically.

Dr. Herman Mynter, who had been telephoned from police headquarters to report immediately at the exposition hospital, was the first surgeon to arrive, at 4.45 o'clock. At that time Drs. P. W. Van Peyma and Joseph Fowler, of Buffalo, and Dr. Edward Wallace Lee, of St. Louis, were present. Dr. Mynter brought with him Dr. Eugene Wasdin, of the United States Marine Hospital Service.

Dr. Mynter inspected the President's wounds, and immediately saw their serious nature. He told the President that it would be necessary to operate, and at once set about making preparations, aided by the house staff and nurses, and Dr. Nelson W. Wilson, Sanitary Officer of the Exposition, who at that time assumed charge of the hospital in the absence of Dr. Roswell Park, the Medical Director of the Exposition. The President's pulse on the arrival of Dr. Mynter was 84; he had no particular pain in the abdomen, and no apparent loss of liver dulness. He was evidently slightly under the influence of the morphin.

Dr. Matthew D. Mann arrived at the hospital at 5.10 p.m., having been telephoned for by Mr. John G. Milburn. He was followed, 5 minutes later, by Dr. John Parmenter.

An examination was at once made, followed by a short consultation between Drs. Mann, Mynter and Wasdin, which resulted in the decision to operate at once. The necessity for the operation was explained to President McKinley, and he

gave his full consent. Immediate operation was decided upon because of the danger of possible continued internal hemorrhage and of the escape of gastric or intestinal contents into the peritoneal cavity, and because the President's pulse was getting weaker. Moreover, the daylight was rapidly failing. Dr. Roswell Park, who, by virtue of his office, had he been present would have performed the operation, was at Niagara Falls, and although a special train had been sent for him, it was uncertain when he would arrive.

Dr. Mann was selected to do the operation, with Dr. Mynter as his associate, by the common consent of the physicians present and at the request of Mr. Milburn, president of the Pan-American Exposition, who stated that he had been requested by President McKinley to select his medical attendants. Dr. Mann selected Drs. Lee and Parmenter as assistants.

At 5.20 Dr. Mann directed the administration of ether to President McKinley, and requested Dr. Wasdin to administer it. Ether was chosen as being, on the whole, the safer anesthetic. While the anesthetic was being given the surgeons who were to take part in the operation prepared their hands and arms by thoroughly scrubbing with soap and water, and immersing them in a solution of bichloride of mercury.

The operation began at 5.29. Dr. Mann stood upon the righthand side of the patient, with Dr. Parmenter on his righthand side. Dr. Mynter stood upon the lefthand side of the patient, and on his right was Dr. Lee. To Drs. Parmenter and Lee were assigned the duties of sponging and the care of the instruments. Dr. P. M. Rixey, U. S. N., President McKinley's family physician, having been detailed by the President to accompany Mrs. McKinley to the Milburn home, did not arrive until 5.30, when he gave very efficient service by guiding the rays of the sun to the seat of the operation by aid of a hand-mirror, and later by arranging an electric light. Dr. Roswell Park arrived just as the operation on the stomach was completed, and gave his aid as consultant. Mr. E. C. Mann had charge of the needles, sutures and ligatures. Mr. Simpson, medical student, was at the instrument tray.

The nurses, under the charge of Miss A. C. Walters, superintendent of the hospital, were Miss M. E. Morris and Miss A. D. Barnes, with hands sterilised; Miss Rose Baron, Miss M. A. Shannon and Miss L. C. Dorchester, assistants, and Miss Katherine Simmons attending the anesthetiser.

Besides those immediately engaged in the operation, there were present Drs. P. W. Van Peyma, Joseph Fowler, D. W. Harrington and Charles G. Stockton, of Buffalo, and Dr. W. D. Storer, of Chicago.

THE OPERATION.

President McKinley took the ether well, and was entirely under its influence in 9 minutes after the beginning of the

anesthetisation. The abdomen was carefully shaved and scrubbed with green soap, and then washed with alcohol and ether and the bichlorid solution.

Inspection showed two wounds made by the bullets. The upper one was between the second and third ribs, a little to the right of the sternum. The use of a probe showed that the skin had not been penetrated, but that the bullet had probably struck a button or some object in the clothing which had deflected it. The lower wound made by the other bullet—a 32 caliber—was on a line drawn from the nipple to the umbilicus. It was about half-way between these points, and about 5 cm. to the left of the median line. A probe showed that this wound extended deeply into the abdominal walls, and that the direction was somewhat downward and outward.

An incision was made from the edge of the ribs downward, passing through the bullet wound and nearly parallel with the long axis of the body. A deep layer of fat was opened, and followed by incision of the fascia and muscles to the peritoneum. After cutting through the skin, a piece of cloth, undoubtedly a bit of the President's clothing, was removed from the track of the bullet, a short distance below the skin.

On opening the peritoneum, the finger was introduced and the anterior wall of the stomach palpated. An opening was discovered which would not quite admit the index finger. This opening was located near the greater curvature of the stomach, and about 2 cm. from the attachment of the omentum; its edges were clean-cut and did not appear to be much injured.

The stomach was drawn up into the operation wound, and the perforation very slightly enlarged. The finger was then introduced and the contents of the stomach palpated. This was done to see if the stomach contained food, and also with the hope that possibly the bullet might be in the stomach. The stomach was found to be half full of liquid food, but no evidence of the ball was discovered. In pulling up the stomach a small amount of liquid contents escaped, together with a good deal of gas. The tissues around the wound were carefully irrigated with hot salt solution and dried with gauze pads. The perforation in the anterior stomach wall was then closed with a double row of silk sutures (Czerny-Lembert). The sutures were not interrupted with each stitch, but four stitches were introduced before the ends were tied. The loop was then cut off and the suture continued. About eight stitches were used in each row. The silk used was fine black silk, the needle being a straight, round sewing needle.

In order to examine the posterior wall of the stomach, it was necessary to enlarge the incision, which now reached about 15 cm. in length. The omentum and transverse colon were pulled well out of the abdomen. The omentum was enormously thickened with fat and very rigid. In order to reach the back wall of the stomach, it was necessary to divide about 4 inches of the gastrocolic omentum, the cut ends being tied with strong black

silk in two masses on each side. In this way the stomach could be drawn up in the operation wound, and the bullet wound in its posterior wall reached. This opening was somewhat larger than that in the anterior wall of the stomach, and had frayed and blood-infiltrated edges. Its exact location was impossible to determine, but it appeared to be near the larger curvature.

This opening was closed in the same way as the anterior wound, but with great difficulty, as the opening was down at the bottom of a deep pocket. A short curved surgical needle was necessary here. Little or no gastric contents appeared around this opening, but after it had been closed the parts were carefully irrigated with hot salt solution.

The operation on the stomach being now finished, Dr. Mann introduced his arm so as to palpate carefully all the deep structures behind the stomach. No trace of the bullet or of the further track of the bullet could be found. As the introduction of the hand in this way seemed to have a bad influence on the President's pulse, prolonged search for further injury done by the bullet or for the bullet itself was desisted from. The folds of the intestine which had been below the stomach were inspected for injury, but none was found. The entire gut was not removed from the abdomen for inspection, as the location of the wound seemed to exclude its injury. To have made a satisfactory search for wounds in the President's back, it would have been necessary to have entirely eviscerated him. As he was already suffering from shock, this was not considered justifiable, and might have caused his death on the operating table.

Before closing the abdominal wound, Dr. Mann asked each of the surgeons present, whether he was entirely satisfied that everything had been done which should be done and whether he had any further suggestions to make. Each replied that he was satisfied. The question of drainage was also discussed. Dr. Mynter was in favor of a Mikulicz drain being placed down behind the stomach-wall. Dr. Mann, with the concurrence of the other surgeons, decided against this as being unnecessary.

As the last step in the operation, the tissues around the bullet track in the abdominal wall were trimmed, in order to remove any tissue which might be infected. The abdominal wound was then closed with seven through-and-through silkworm-gut sutures, drawn only moderately tight, the superior layer of the fascia of the rectus muscle being joined with buried catgut. The edges of the skin were brought together by fine catgut sutures. Where the bullet had entered there was slight gaping of the tissues, but it was not thought advisable to close this tightly, as it might allow of some drainage. The wound was then washed with hydrogen dioxide and covered with aristol powder and dressed with sterilised gauze and cotton, which were held in place with adhesive straps. Over all was put an abdominal bandage.

The President bore the operation very well. The time from the beginning of the administration of the anesthetic until its

discontinuance was exactly an hour and 31 minutes; the operation was completed at 6.50 p.m., having lasted from the time of the first incision an hour and 21 minutes. At the beginning of the operation President McKinley's pulse was 84. At 5.38, 0.002 gm. of strychnine was administered hypodermically. At 5.55 the respiration was 32 and the pulse 84—both good in character. At 6.09 the pulse was 88. At 6.20 it was 102, fair in character; respiration, 30. At 6.22, 1.50 gm. of brandy was administered hypodermically. At 6.48 the pulse was 124, the tension good, but quick; respiration, 36. At 7.01, after the bandage was applied, the pulse was 122 and the respiration 32. At 7.17, 0.004 gm. of morphine was administered hypodermically.

At 7.32 the patient was removed from the hospital in the ambulance. Dr. Rixey asked Drs. Park and Wasdin to go in the ambulance, as his duty called him to go at once to inform ·Mrs. McKinley of her husband's condition and to prepare a room for his reception. Drs. Mann and Mynter, with friends of the President, followed in carriages immediately after. President McKinley had not then recovered from the anesthetic. He bore the journey to Mr. Milburn's house exceedingly well, but it was found necessary to give him a small hypodermic injection of morphine during the transit, as he was becoming very restless. On arrival at the house of Mr. Milburn, 1168 Delaware Avenue, he was removed from the ambulance on the stretcher, and carried to a room in the northwest corner of the house, where a hospital bed had been prepared for him.

REMARKS ON THE OPERATION.

BY MATTHEW D. MANN, M. D.

The difficulties of the operation were very great, owing partly to the want of retractors and to the failing light. The setting sun shone directly into the room, but not into the wound. The windows were low and covered with awnings. After Dr. Rixey aided us with a hand mirror, the light was better. Toward the end of the time a movable electric light with reflector was put in use. The greatest difficulty was the great size of President McKinley's abdomen and the amount of fat present. This necessitated working at the bottom of a deep hole, especially when suturing the posterior wall of the stomach.

The operation was rendered possible and greatly facilitated by a good operating table and the other appliances of a hospital, and by the presence of many trained nurses and assistants. Still, the hospital was only equipped for minor emergency work, and had but a moderate supply of instruments. Unfortunately, when called I was not told what I was wanted for, and went to the exposition grounds entirely unprepared. Dr. Mynter had his large pocket case, the contents of which were of great use.

As has already been noted, further search for the bullet was rendered inadvisable by the President's condition. The autopsy shows

that it could not have been found, and that the injuries inflicted by the bullet after it passed through the stomach, were of such a nature as to render impossible and unnecessary any further surgical procedure. A bullet after it ceases to move does little harm. We were often asked why, after the operation, we did not use the .x-ray to find the bullet. There were several reasons for this. In the first place, there were, at no time any signs that the bullet was doing harm. To have used the .x-ray simply to have satisfied our curiosity would not have been warrantable, as it would have greatly disturbed and annoyed the patient, and would have subjected him also to a certain risk. Had there been signs of abscess-formation, then the rays could and would have been used.

My reason for not draining was that there was nothing to drain. There had been no bleeding nor oozing; there was nothing to make any discharge or secretion; the parts were presumably free from infection, and were carefully washed with salt solution. As there was no peritonitis and the abdomen was found post mortem to be sterile, we may safely conclude that no drainage could have been provided which would have accomplished anything. My experience teaches me never to drain unless there is a very decided indication for it, as a drain may do harm as well as good.

In conclusion, I wish to thank all the gentlemen who so kindly and skilfully assisted me. They were all surgeons of large experience in abdominal surgery, and their aid and advice were most valuable. Especially I wish to acknowledge my great obligation to my associate, Dr. Mynter. Not only was he an assistant, but he was much more, and helped me greatly by his skill and, as a consultant, with his good judgment and extensive knowledge of abdominal work. Although called first, he waived his claim, and generously placed the case in my hands, willingly assuming his share of the responsibility.

The anesthetic was most carefully administered by Dr. Wasdin, and the knowledge that he had charge of this very important duty relieved me of any anxiety on that score.

In the eventful week that followed the operation, Dr. Park and Dr. McBurney were towers of strength in helping to decide the many difficult questions which came up.

Dr. Rixey was in constant charge of the sick-room, aided later by Dr. Wasdin, who was detailed for this special duty. Both were unremitting in their care, and faithful to the end.

Dr. Stockton helped us in the last three days with the highest skill and best judgment.

Never, I am sure, under like circumstances, was there a more harmonious or better-agreed band of consultants. That our best endeavors failed was, I believe, no fault of ours; but it must be an ever-living and keen regret to each one of us, that we were not allowed the privilege of saving so noble a man, so attractive a patient, and so useful a life.

THE AFTER-TREATMENT.

When put to bed the President was in fair condition: pulse, 127; temperature, 100.6°; respiration, 30. The nurses on duty were Miss K. R. Simmons and Miss A. D. Barnes, from the Emergency Hospital. Soon after his arrival, at 8.25, he was given morphine, 0.016 gm., hypodermically. There was slight nausea. The pulse soon improved. During the evening the patient slept at intervals, vomiting occasionally, but rallied satisfactorily. A slight discoloration of the dressings was noted at 10.45. There was occasional and slight pain. Ninety c.c. of urine was voided, and an enema of salt solution given and retained.

Second Day, Saturday, September 7.

After midnight the patient slept a good deal; he was free from pain and quite comfortable.

At 6 a.m., the temperature was 102°; pulse, 110; respiration, 24.

Gas in large quantities was expelled from the bowels. A saline enema was given as before. Miss Simmons and Miss Barnes were replaced by Miss Maud Mohan and Miss Jane Connolly. Miss E. Hunt, of San Francisco, Cal., Mrs. McKinley's nurse, also rendered assistance, and Miss Grace Mackenzie, of Baltimore, Md., arrived September 9, and was detailed for regular duty. P. A. Eliot, J. Hodgins and Ernest Vollmeyer, of the U. S. A. Hospital Corps, were detailed as orderlies.

During the forenoon, 0.01 gm. of morphine was administered hypodermically.

At 1.15 p.m., a saline enema of 500 c.c. was given. As the pulse was rising, 0.06 gm. of fluid extract of digitalis was injected hypodermically.

The President rested quietly until 6.30 p.m., when he complained of intense pain in the pit of the stomach, and was given 0.008 gm. morphine sulphate hypodermically. He was very restless, but after being sponged rested again.

At 6.30 p.m., the pulse was 130; temperature, 102.5°; respiration, 29.

During the day the digitalis, morphine and saline enemas were kept up at regular intervals; 4 gm. of somatose was added to the water at 10.30 p.m. At 11.15 p.m. the President passed from the bowels 240 c.c. of a greenish colored fluid and some particles of fecal matter.

The total amount of urine for 24 hours was 270 c.c.

FIRST URINALYSIS, BY DR. H. G. MATZINGER.

Quantity . . . . 30 cc.
Color . . . . dark amber.
Reaction . . . . strongly acid.
Urea . . . . 0.028 gm. per 1 c.c. of urine.
Albumin . . . . a trace.
Phosphates and chlorides . . . . normal.
Sugar . . . . none.
Indican . . . . very small amount.

Microscopic Examination.—The sediment obtained by centrifuge shows a large amount of large and small epithelial cells with some leukocytes and occasional red cells. There is a comparatively large number of hyaline casts, principally small, with some finely granular ones; also an occasional fibrinous one. The amount of sediment is large for the quantity of urine submitted. There were no crystals in the sediment.

Third Day, Sunday, September 8.

During the early morning the President slept a good deal, but was restless, and at times confused and a little chilly. On the whole, he passed a fairly good night.

He expelled a little gas and brown fluid from the rectum. The digitalis was continued, and at 7.45 a.m, 0.002 gm. of strychnine were given hypodermically. At 8.20 a.m. he was clear and bright, with the pulse strong and of good character.

The wound was dressed at 8.30, and found in a very satisfactory condition. There was no indication of peritonitis. Pulse, 132; temperature, 102.8°; respiration, 24.

The dressing on the wound was changed because there was some exudation. The bullet track was syringed out with hydrogen dioxide. There was very little foaming, and there were no signs of pus.

At 10.40 a.m., following an enema of epsom salts, glycerine and water, he had a small stool with gas, and another at noon. He was less restless and slept a good deal.

At noon Dr. Charles McBurney joined the medical staff in consultation, having been summoned by Dr. Rixey.

During the day he continued to improve; he slept 4 or 5 hours and his condition was satisfactory.

At 4.45 p.m., he was given a teaspoonful of water by the mouth; also an enema of sweet oil, soap and water. He passed slightly colored fluid with some little fecal matter and mucus. After this he had a small quantity of water by the mouth, and at 6.20 p.m. a nutritive enema of egg, whisky and water, which was partly retained. Digitalis and strychnine were both given during the evening.

At 9 p.m. the President was resting comfortably. The pulse was 130; temperature, 101.6°; respiration, 30.

Four hundred and twenty c.c. of urine was passed during the day.

SECOND URINALYSIS.

Quantity	450 c.c
Color	amber, slightly turbid
Reaction	strongly acid.
Specific gravity	1.026.
Urea	0.038 gm. per c.c. of urine.
Albumin	mere trace.
Sugar	none.
Indican	abundant.
Sulphates	increased.
Phosphates	somewhat increased.
Chlorides	somewhat increased.

Microscopic Examination.—Microscopic examination of sediment obtained / centrifuge shows fewer organic elements. Some large and small epithelial cells and some leukocytes. Casts are not so abundant as yesterday and are *rincipally* of the small finely granular variety. There is a marked diminution in small renal epithelial cells.

Quite a quantity of large crystals of uric acid and bacteria are present.

Fourth Day, Monday, September 9.

Codeia was substituted for morphia, as the pain was less. Digitalis and strychnine were stopped. Nutritive enemas were given at 3.20 a.m., at 4.30 and 10 p.m. Hot water was taken quite freely by the mouth.

Attempts to get good movement of the bowels were successful at noon, when he had a large, light-brown partly-formed stool. This followed a small dose of calomel and a high enema of oxgall.

On the whole, the President's condition improved steadily during the day. He slept a good deal and was fairly comfortable. There was no pain on pressure over the abdomen.

THIRD URINALYSIS.

Quantity received	540 c c.
Color	amber, slightly turbid.
Specific gravity	1.026,
Albumin	a trace
Indican	not so abundant as yesterday.
Urea	0.047 gm. per c.c. of urine.
Chlorides and phosphates	about normal.
Sulphates	still somewhat high.
Sugar	none.

Microscopic Examination.—Microscopic examination of sediment obtained by centrifuge shows a decrease in the amount of organic elements and an increase of amorphous urates, but fewer crystals of uric acid. Casts are fewer and only the small granular and large hyaline varieties. The proportion of casts is greater. There are very few epithelial cells, mostly of renal type. A large number of cylindroids are found.

Fifth Day, Tuesday, September 10.

Soon after midnight the President had a high enema of soap and water, which was expelled, together with some fecal matter. He took hot water frequently, and slept a good deal.

On awakening he felt very comfortable, and his mind was clear and cheerful. The nutritive enemas were kept up, and water given by the mouth. Had two small stools during the day. The only medicine given was one hypodermic of codeia phosphate, 0.015 gm.

In the evening the dressings were examined, and as there was considerable staining from the discharge, it was thought best to remove four stitches and separate the edges of the wound.

little slough was observed near the bullet track, covering a space nearly an inch wide, the thickness of the flaps. The separation seemed to extend down to the muscle. The surfaces, except those mentioned, looked healthy, but not granulating. It was supposed that the infection of the wound occurred either from the bullet or from the piece of clothing carried into the wound at the time of the shooting. The parts were thoroughly washed with hydrogen dioxide and packed lightly with gauze, and held together with adhesive straps.

Sixth Day, Wednesday, September 11.

The blood count made by Dr. Wasdin in the evening was as follows:

Leukocytes	6,752
Red cells	3,920,000

A little after midnight, Wednesday morning, the patient was given 4 c.c. of beef juice, the first food taken by the stomach. It seemed to be very acceptable. Nutritive enema was given at 2 a.m.; later there was a yellow stool.

From 4 to 8 c.c. of beef juice was given every 1 to 2 hours during the day. The rectum was becoming irritable, and did not retain the nutritive enemas well.

At 10 a.m. the remaining stitches were removed, the wound separated and dressed. It seemed to be doing well. Most of the sloughing tissue had separated.

The patient slept much during the day, and expressed himself as feeling very comfortable. The only medicine administered was one hypodermic of strychnine.

In the evening he was changed to a fresh bed. Nutritive enemas were continued.

Urine was passed much more freely —750 c.c. in 24 hours.

FOURTH URINALYSIS.

Quantity	82 c.c.
Color	amber, clear.
Specific gravity	1.027.
Reaction	strongly acid.
Albumin	a trace.
Indican	abundant.
Urea	0.04 gm. per 1 c.c. of urine.
E. phosphates and chlorides	normal.
Sulphates	still a little high.

Microscopic Examination.—Microscopic examination of sediment obtained by centrifuge, shows a marked diminution in amount of organic elements, but a great increase in uric acid crystals.

There are very few epithelial cells—mostly of renal type.

There are fewer casts —small and large hyaline —some finely granular.

Cylindroids are more abundant.

[From the American Journal of the Medical Sciences, Lea Brothers & Co.]

CHART OF PRESIDENT MC KINLEY'S TEMPERATURE, PULSE AND RESPIRATION.

Seventh Day, Thursday, September 12.

The President slept a good deal during the night, and awoke in the morning feeling better. The beef juice was continued and increased, and a little chicken broth added to the dietary. He also had a little whiskey and water.

At 8.30 a.m. he had chicken broth, a very small piece of toast and a small cup of coffee. He did not care for the toast, and ate scarcely any of it.

The wound was dressed and washed with a weak solution of iodine and then with hydrogen dioxide. He was given 30 c.c. of castor oil at 9.20 a.m.

The President now seemed at his best and his condition to warrant the favorable prognosis given out. The time for peritonitis and sepsis had passed. The bowels had moved and gas passed freely, showing that there was no obstruction. The tongue was clear, and the appetite increasing; and he seemed to be able to digest food. There was no pain nor tenderness in the abdomen, and he was able to turn easily and sleep on his side. The urine was steadily increasing. His spirits were good and his mind clear, while his pulse, though frequent, was strong and of good quality, and the temperature low.

The analysis of the urine gave no uneasiness as the amount of urea was fair; there was no albumin worth considering, and the casts were rapidly diminishing. There were no more of them than are found in a large percentage of cases following a long operation under ether. The excess of indican was taken to mean merely some intestinal indigestion, and to be of no serious import. The only symptom to cause any uneasiness was the frequency of the pulse. Still, anxiety on this score was relieved by knowing that the President had naturally a rapid pulse and that it was easily excited. The open wound was not considered important. It looked healthy, and, although it would take a long time to heal, in itself it was evidently causing no harm nor was it likely to.

Dr. McBurney left Buffalo for his home in the morning, having arranged to return at once if his presence was desired.

Toward noon it was noticed that the character of the pulse was not quite so good. Infusion of digitalis, 8 c.c., was ordered, and strychnine, 0.002 gm.

It was thought probable that there was some intestinal toxemia, as there had been no free movement from the bowels since food had been begun, the oil having failed to act. Gradually the pulse went to 130, and grew weaker.

Dr. Charles G. Stockton was added to the medical staff in consultation. At 7 p.m. the President was given 0.20 gm. of calomel.

At 9.30 p.m. a second dose of 30 c.c. of castor oil was given, followed by a high enema of oxgall. This resulted in a large, dark semifluid stool, which seemed to exhaust him somewhat. Stimulants were given freely. No more beef juice or food was

given. The pulse grew rapidly worse, but at midnight there seemed some improvement, as bulletin 33 shows. At 11 p.m. 420 c.c. of normal salt solution was given simultaneously.

FIFTH URINALYSIS.

Quantity . . . . 132 c.c.
Color . . . . light amber, very turbid.
Specific gravity . . . . 1.025.
Reaction . . . . acid.
Albumin . . . . mere trace, if any.
Indican . . . . less.
Urea . . . . 0.044 gm. per 1 c.c. of urine.
Sulphates . . . . about normal.
E. phosphates . . . . much increased.
Chlorides . . . . normal.

Microscopic Examination —Microscopic examination of sediment obtained by centrifuge, shows fewer organic elements than the last examination. There is less uric acid and a large amount of amorphous phosphates. Renal casts, about as in the last examination, with very few cylindroids.

Eighth Day, Friday, September 13.

At midnight the pulse was fairly good, 132. Strychnine and whiskey were given at intervals, and hypodermics of camphorated oil.

The wound had been dressed regularly in the manner described three times a day. At 9 a.m. the dressing was changed, and a mixture of balsam of Peru and glycerine put in on gauze after the douching.

Stimulants were continued as before, but more freely. Coffee, 45 c.c., and clam broth, 60 c.c., were given; also liquid peptonoids.

At 8.30, 1.50 gm. of adrenalin was given hypodermically, and repeated at 9.40.

At 10 a.m., nearly 2 pints of normal salt solution were given under the skin, and a pint containing adrenalin at 6 p.m. Nitroglycerine and camphor were also injected at various times, together with brandy and strychnine.

Stimulants as detailed above were used freely all day.

3.30 p.m. Pulse growing weaker.
5.00 p.m. Oxygen given and continued for some hours.
6.30 p.m. Last bulletin, No. 39.

At 6.35 p.m., and again at 7.40, morphine was given hypodermically, as he was very restless and seemed to be suffering.

9 00 p.m. Heart sounds very feeble.

The President continued to sink, becoming weaker and weaker.

At 10.00 p.m., the oxygen was discontinued. The heart sounds were very feeble and consciousness lost.

The President died at 2.15 a.m., September 14.

Drs. E. J. Janeway and W. W. Johnston, who, at the request of Dr. Rixey, had been summoned in consultation, arrived too late, but were present at the autopsy. Dr. McBurney also returned on Friday afternoon.

SIXTH URINALYSIS.

Color . . . . amber, turbid, with phosphates.
Quantity . . . . 252 c.c.
Reaction . . . . acid.
Specific gravity . . . . 1.023.
Albumin . . . : . . . . mere trace, if any.
Urea . . . . . : . . . . 0.047 gm. per 1 c.c. urine
Indican . . . . a trace.
E. phosphates . . . . increased.
Chlorides . . . . normal.
Sulphates . . . . a little high.

Microscopic Examination. — Microscopic examination of sediment obtained by centrifuge, before and after clearing, shows no change from yesterday's sample. Casts, hyaline and granular, both large and small, comparatively few. Cylindroids, a few. Crystals, large amount of uric acid, some sodium urate, and in the untreated specimen a large amount of amorphous deposit, principally of phosphates. There are a few epithelial cells, small, granular. Occasional red cells and leukocytes.

REPORT ON THE AUTOPSY.[1]

BY HARVEY R. GAYLORD, M. D.,
Pathologist to the New York State Pathological Laboratory.

Ordinary signs of death: ecchymosis in dependent portions of the body. Rigor mortis well marked. Upon the surface of the chest, to the right of the midsternal line, a spot 1 cm. in diameter, dark-red in color, with a slight crust formation covering it, 5.5 cm. from the suprasternal notch; from the right nipple, 10 cm.; from the line of the right nipple, 8 25 cm. Surrounding this spot, at which point there is an evident dissolution of the continuity of the skin, is a discolored area of oval shape extending upward and to the right. In its greatest length it is 11 cm.; and in its greatest width, 6 cm. It extends upward in the direction of the right shoulder. The skin within this area is discolored, greenish-yellow and mottled.

The surface of the abdomen is covered with a surgical dressing, which extends down to the umbilicus and upward to just below the nipples. The innermost layer of cotton is covered or stained with balsam of Peru and blood. On removing this dressing, a wound parallel to, and somewhat to the left of, the median line, is exposed, inserted in which are two layers of gauze, likewise impregnated with balsam of Peru. The wound is 14.5 cm. in length, and is open down to the abdominal muscles. The layer of abdominal fat is 3.75 cm. in thickness. The appearance of the fat is good, a bright yellow in color. No evidence of necrosis or sloughing. In the left margin of the surgical wound, lying 1 cm. to the right of a line drawn from the umbilicus to the left nipple, 15.5 cm. from the nipple and 16.5 cm. from the umbilicus is a partly healed indentation of the skin, and an excavation of the fat immediately beneath it (this is the site of the entry of the

1. The autopsy was performed by Drs. Gaylord and Matzinger.

bullet), extending down to the peritoneal surface. On making the median incision, starting from the suprasternal notch and extending to a point just below the symphysis, the subcutaneous fat is exposed, which is of bright yellow color and normal appearance, except in an area which corresponds superficially to the area of discoloration described as surrounding the wound upon the chest wall. This area marks the site of a hemorrhage into the subcutaneous fat. The remainder of the subcutaneous fat is firm and measures 4.75 cm. in thickness on the abdominal wall. On opening the sheath of the right rectus muscle, it is seen to be of dark-red color. (Culture taken from ecchymotic tissue under the upper bullet hole and from between the folds of the small intestine. Three tubes from each locality on agar and gelatin)

On opening the abdominal cavity, the parietal surface of the peritoneum is exposed, and is found to be covered with a slight amount of bloody fluid; is perfectly smooth and not injected. The great omentum extends downward to a point midway between the umbilicus and the symphysis. It is thick, firm; its inferior border is discolored by coming in contact with the intestines. Below the umbilicus a few folds of intestines are exposed. These are likewise covered with discolored blood, after the removal of which the peritoneal surface is found to be shiny On the inner aspect of the abdominal wound the omentum is found to be slightly adherent to the parietal peritoneum, and can be readily separated with the hand from the edge of the wound. At this point the omentum is somewhat injected. This adhesion to the omentum is found to extend entirely around the abdominal wound. The parietal peritoneum immediately adjacent to the inner aspect of the abdominal wound is ecchymotic.

On removing the subcutaneous fat and muscles from the thoracic wall, the point which marks the dissolution of continuity of the skin upon the surface, is found to lie directly over the margin of the sternum and to the right side between the second and third ribs. There is no evidence of ecchymosis or injury to the tissues or muscles beneath the subcutaneous fat. On making an incision through the subcutaneous fat, directly through the wound upon the chest, a small cavity is exposed about the size of a pea just beneath the skin which is filled with fluid blood The subcutaneous tissue underlying the area of discoloration on the surface of the chest wall shows hemorrhagic infiltration.

On removing the sternum, the lungs are exposed, and do not extend far forward. A large amount of pericardial fat is exposed. Pleural surface on both sides is smooth. There are no adhesions on either side within the pleural cavities. The diaphragm on the right side extends upward to a point opposite the third rib in the mammary line. No perceptible amount of fluid in either pleural cavity. On opening the pericardial cavity, the surface of the pericardium is found to be smooth and pale. The pericardium contains approximately 6 c.c. of straw-colored, slightly turbid fluid. (Some taken for examination.)

On exposing the heart, it is found covered with a well-developed panniculus. The heart measures, from the base to the apex, on the superficial aspect, 10.5 cm. The right ventricle is apparently empty The heart feels soft and flaccid. On opening the left ventricle, a small amount of dark-red blood is found The muscle of the left ventricular wall is 1.5 cm. in thickness; dark reddish-brown in color; presents a shiny surface. The average thickness of the pericardial fat is 3.5 mm. (Cultures made from the auricle.) The left auricle contains but a small amount of dark currant-colored blood. The mitral valve admits three fingers. The right ventricle, when incised in the anterior line, is found to be extremely soft: the

muscular structure is 2 mm. in thickness The panniculus measures 7 mm. The muscle is dark-red in color; very shiny, and the pericardial fat invades the muscular wall at many points.

On opening the right auricle, it is found to be filled and distended by a large currant-colored clot, which extends into the vessels. The tricuspid orifice admits readily three fingers. The coronary arteries are patulous and soft; no evidence of thickening.

Lungs are gray color and contain a moderate amount of coal-dust pigment. Slight amount of frothy fluid escapes from the bronchi; but the pulmonary tissue is crepitant and free from exudate.

On unfolding the folds of intestine, there is no evidence of adhesion until a point just beneath the mesocolon is reached, when, on removing a fold of small intestine, a few spoonfuls of greenish-gray thick fluid flows into the peritoneal cavity.

On the anterior gastric wall is an area to which a fold of the gastrocolic omentum is lightly adherent. On breaking the adhesion, there is found a wound about midway between the gastric orifices, 3.5 cm. in length, parallel with the greater curvature of the stomach, 1.5 cm. from the line of omental attachment. This wound is held intact by silk sutures. There is no evidence of adhesion at any other point on the anterior wall. The gastric wall surrounding the wound just mentioned for a distance of 2 cm. to 3 cm. is discolored, dark greenish-gray in appearance, and easily torn. On exposing the posterior wall of the stomach from above, along its greater curvature, the omentum is found to be slightly adherent, a line of silk ligatures along the greater curvature of the stomach marking the site where the omentum had been removed. On throwing the omentum downward, the posterior gastric wall is exposed. On the posterior wall, a distance of 2 cm. from the line of omental attachment, is a wound approximately 2 cm long, held intact by silk sutures. The gastric wall surrounding this wound is discolored. On the surface of the mesocolon, which is posterior to the gastric wall at this point, is a corresponding area of discoloration, the portion coming directly in contact with the wound in the gastric wall being of dull gray color. The remainder of the surface of the posterior wall of the stomach is smooth and shiny. Beyond the surgical wound in the posterior wall of the stomach is found an opening in the retroperitoneal fat, large enough to admit two fingers. This opening communicates with a track which extends downward and backward as far as the finger can reach. The tissues surrounding this track are necrotic. On removing the descending portion of the colon, a large irregular cavity is exposed, the walls of which are covered with gray, slimy material, and in which are found fragments of necrotic tissue. Just at the superior margin of the kidney is located a definite opening which forms the bottom of the track traced from the stomach. On stripping the left kidney from its capsule, it is found that the superior portion of the capsule is continuous with the cavity. The weight of the left kidney is 5 oz. 1 gm. The kidney is readily stripped from its capsule; is dark red; the stellate veins are prominent, and along its greater curvature are numerous dark red depressions. On the superior aspect of the kidney is a protrusion of the cortex, dark red in color, and in this protrusion is a laceration 2 cm. long, extending across the superior border, approximately at right angles to the periphery of the kidney and from before backward. On incising the kidney, the cortex and medulla are not easily distinguishable from one another; both are of rose red color, the cortex measuring approximately 6 mm. in thickness. The vessels in the

pyramids of Ferrein are very prominent. Beneath the protruding portion of the surface, the cortex is dark red in color. This discoloration extends downward in pyramidal form into the medulla. The laceration of the surface marks the apex of the protrusion of the kidney substance. Between the spleen and the superior aspect of the kidney is a necrotic tract which extends down and backward, and ends in a blind pocket. The tract which included the superior aspect of the kidney can be traced into the perinephritic fat to a point just above the surface of the muscles of the back.

The necrotic cavity which connects the wound on the posterior wall of the stomach and the opening adjacent to the kidney capsule is walled off by the mesocolon, and is found to involve an area of the pancreas, approximately 45 mm. in diameter and extending about half-through the organ. This organ at its center forms part of the necrotic cavity. Through its body are found numerous minute hemorrhages and areas of gray softening, the size of a pea or smaller. These are less frequent in the head portion of the pancreas.

A careful examination of the track leading down toward the dorsal muscles fails to reveal the presence of any foreign body. After passing into the fat, the direct character of the track ceases; and its direction can be traced no farther. The adjoining fat and the muscles of the back were carefully palpated and incised, without disclosing a wound or the presence of a foreign body. The diaphragm was carefully dissected away, and the posterior portion of the thoracic wall likewise carefully examined. All fat and organs which were removed, including the intestine, were likewise examined and palpated, without result.

The great amount of fat in the abdominal cavity and surrounding the kidney rendered the search extremely difficult.

The right kidney is imbedded in a dense mass of fat; capsule strips freely; it weighs 5 ounces; measures 11.5 cm.; substance is soft; cortex is 6 mm. in thickness; rose-red in color; cut surface slightly dulled. There are a few depressions of the surface, and the stellate veins are prominent.

The liver is dark-red in color; the gall-bladder distended. The organ was not removed.

The autopsy continued for a longer period than was anticipated by those who had charge of the President's body, and we were requested to desist seeking for the bullet and terminate the autopsy. As we were satisfied that nothing could be gained by locating the bullet, which had apparently set up no reaction, search for it was discontinued.

Anatomic Diagnosis.—Gunshot wound of both walls of the stomach and the superior aspect of the left kidney; extensive necrosis of the substance of the pancreas; necrosis of the gastric wall in the neighborhood of both wounds; fatty degeneration, infiltration and brown atrophy of the heart muscle; slight cloudy swelling of the epithelium of the kidneys.

A matter of no inconsiderable embarrassment to us arose in the objection of our removing sufficient portions of the tissues for examination. We were able to secure only two small fragments of the stomach wall; tissue from around the wound upon the chest wall; a portion of fat from the wall of the necrotic cavity; a small piece of each kidney, that of the left kidney including the portion involved by the original wound; and pieces of heart-muscle from the right and left ventricles. The microscopic examination of these tissues follows:

The piece of retroperitoneal fat, where it forms part of the necrotic cavity, is seen on section to be covered with a thick gray deposit, which has an average thickness of from 4 mm. to 6 mm. Beneath this and separating it from the fat, is a well-defined area of hemorrhage from 1 mm. to 2 mm. in thickness. The appearance of this piece of tissue is characteristic of the fat tissue surrounding the entire cavity. A section made perpendicular to the surface and stained with hematoxylin-eosin, shows the following characteristics: Under low power there is no evidence of round-celled infiltration between the fat cells, or of fat necroses. The surface of the tissue which, in the microscopic specimen was covered by a layer of grayish material, proves, under low power, to consist of a partly organised fibrinous deposit. At the base of this deposit is evidence of an extensive hemorrhage, marked by deposits of pigment. The surface of the membrane is of rough and irregular appearance, and contains a large number of round cells with deeply stained nuclei. Under high power the organisation of the membrane may be traced from the base toward the surface. The portion immediately adjacent to the fat tissue consists of a network of fibrin enclosing large numbers of partly preserved red blood corpuscles. In many areas the red blood corpuscles are broken down and extensive deposits of pigment are found. Extending into the fibrin structure of the membrane are numerous typical fibroblasts and round cells. In some regions pigment is evidently deposited in the bodies of large branching and spindle cells. Here and there, included in the membrane, are the remains of fat cells, and toward the surface of the membrane a large number of round cells scattered through the interstices of the membrane. There are but few polymorphonuclear leukocytes. Here and there in the membrane are fragments of isolated fibrous connective tissue with irregular contours and an appearance suggesting that they are fragments of tissue which have been displaced by violence and included in the fibrin deposit. The fibrin in the superficial layers of the membrane is formed in hyaline clumps. The organisation along the base of the deposit is comparatively uniform.

Sections stained with methylen blue, carbol-thionin and Gram's method were carefully examined for the presence of bacteria, with negative results. Even upon the surface of the membrane there are no evidences of bacteria.

The section of the left kidney, including the triangular area of hemorrhage described in the macroscopic specimen, reveals the following appearances: (Section hardened in formalin, stained with hematoxylin-eosin.) Examined macroscopically, section represents a portion of a kidney cortex made perpendicular to the surface of the cortex, and including an area of hemorrhage into the substance of the cortex 1 cm. in length, measured from the capsular surface downward, and presenting a width of from 5 mm. to 6 mm. The capsular surface has apparently been torn.

Under low power the margins of the preparation are found to consist of well preserved kidney structure. There is a slight amount of thickening of the interstitial tissue, and occasional groups of tubules are affected by beginning cloudy swelling. The glomeruli are large and present a perfectly normal appearance. As we approach toward the center of the preparation, occasional glomeruli are met with in which the capillary loops are engorged and the adjacent tubules contain red blood-corpuscles. A short distance farther, the kidney structure becomes entirely necrotic. Here and there the remains of tubules may be made out, and these are infiltrated with cells. The necrotic area presents a rough, net-like structure. As we approach toward the surface of the kidney, we find that the necrosis

becomes more marked. There is the merest suggestion of kidney structure, its place being taken by disintegrated red blood-cells and leukocytes, embedded in a well-defined fibrinous network. There is great distortion of the kidney structure about the periphery of the necrotic area. In this region a considerable amount of pigment is also found in the necrotic tissues.

Under high power, the characteristics of the necrotic tissues may be better observed. The kidney structure is broken up and torn into irregular fragments, infiltrated by red blood corpuscles and leukocytes. In the portion of the necrotic mass beneath the capsule, the kidney structure is practically obliterated and is replaced by a network of fibrin, which includes large numbers of red blood cells and leukocytes. Scattered through the entire necrotic area are frequent deposits of pigment. In the deeper portions of the necrotic area, the margins of the fibrin deposit are invaded by fibroblasts from the connective tissue structure of the kidney. The organisation in these areas is, however, slight.

Sections stained with methylen blue and Gram's method and carefully examined under oil immersion, fail to reveal the presence of any organisms. In preparations stained with methylen blue, the deposits of pigment may be readily observed. Section of the same tissue hardened in Hermann's solution and examined for fat, shows the presence of numerous fat droplets within the epithelium of the tubules which are adjacent to the area of necrosis. In the portions of the preparation more widely distant from the area of necrosis no fat is present.

Section of the right kidney hardened in formalin and stained with hematoxylin-eosin reveals the presence of areas in which slight parenchymatous degeneration of the epithelium in the uriniferous tubules may be noted. These areas are not extensive and are confined to single groups of tubules. The interstitial connective tissue of the organ seems to be slightly increased in amount, but there is no well-defined round-celled infiltration. An occassional hyaline glomerulus is to be met with in these cases surrounded by increased connective tissue The epithelium of the kidney tubules, aside from those in which the parenchymatous degeneration is present, is well preserved. The nuclei are well stained; protoplasm, finely granular.

A fragment of the stomach wall taken from the immediate neighborhood of the anterior wound is in a condition of complete necrosis. The nuclei of the cells are scarcely demonstrable. The epithelial surface is recognised with difficulty. At its base are apparently a few round cells. Examination of the blood vessels reveals nothing characteristic. There is apparently no evidence of thrombosis A section made through the gastric wall at some distance from the wound reveals the well-preserved muscular structure of the gastric wall, which presents no characteristic alterations. Superficial portions of the epithelium have apparently been affected by post-mortem digestion. However, in one portion of the preparation, the epithelium is intact, and shows distinct evidence of marked round-celled infiltration between the glandular structures. The blood vessels contained blood-corpuscles with the usual number of leukocytes.

The fragments of heart-muscle which were removed from the right and left ventricular walls, were examined in the fresh state, and exhibited a well-defined fatty degeneration of the muscle fibers, and in the case of the right ventricular wall, an extensive infiltration between the muscle fibers, of fat, was apparent. Sections from these fragments of muscle hardened in Hermann's solution, are taken for examination. A fragment of muscle from the right ventricular wall was removed at a point where the fat penetrated deeply into the muscular structure, the

ventricular wall at this point showing an average thickness of 2.5 mm. Under low power, the muscle fibers are separated into bundles by masses and rows of deeply stained fat cells. The muscle fibers are seen to contain groups of dark brown granules lying in the long axes of the cells. Under high power, these are resolved into extensive groups of dark brown pigment arranged around the nuclei. The muscle fibers are slender, the cross and longitudinal striation is well defined. Examined near the margin of the preparation, where the osmic-acid fixation has been successful, all of the muscle fibers are found to contain minute black spherical bodies, extending diffusely through all the muscle fibers about the entire margin of the preparation. These fine fat droplets are present in sufficient amount to speak of an extensive diffuse fatty degeneration of the muscle fibers. Where the large fat cells have separated the muscle fibers, these are found to be more atrophic than those in the central portions of the larger bundles.

The examination of the section through the healed bullet wound on the chest walls reveals nothing of importance. The dissolution of continuity is filled in by granulation-tissue, and there is evidence of beginning restoration of the epithelium from the margins. Stains for bacteria give negative results.

In summing up the macroscopic and microscopic findings of the autopsy, the following may be stated: The original injuries to the stomach wall had been repaired by suture, and this repair seems to have been effective. The stitches were in place, and the openings in the stomach-wall effectually closed. Firm adhesions were formed both upon the anterior and posterior walls of the stomach, which reinforced these sutures. The necroses surrounding the wounds in the stomach do not seem to be the result of any well-defined cause. It is highly probable that they were practically terminal in their nature, and that the condition developed as a result of lowered vitality. In this connection there is no evidence to indicate that the removal of the omentum from the greater curvature and the close proximity of both of these wounds to this point, had any effect in bringing about the necrosis of the gastric wall, although circulatory disturbances may have been a factor. The fact that the necrotic tissue had not been affected by digestion strongly indicates that the necrosis was developed but shortly before death. The excavation in the fat behind the stomach must be largely attributed to the action of the missile. This may have been the result of unusual rotation of a nearly spent ball, or the result of simple concussion from the ball passing into a mass of soft tissues. Such effects are not unknown. The fact that the ball grazed the superior aspect of the left kidney, shown by the microscopic investigation of that organ, indicates the direction of the missile, which passed in a line from the inferior border of the stomach to the tract in the fat immediately posterior to the kidney. There was evidence that the left adrenal gland was injured.

The injury to the pancreas must be attributed to indirect, rather than direct, action of the missile. The fact that the wall of the cavity is lined by fibrin, well advanced in organisation, indicates that the injury to the tissues was produced at the time

of the shooting. The absence of bacteria from the tissues, indicates that the wound was not infected at the time of the shooting, and that the closure of the posterior gastric wound was effectual. The necrosis of the pancreas seems to us of great importance. The fact that there were no fat necroses in the neighborhood of this organ, indicates that there was no leakage of pancreatic fluid into the surrounding tissues. It is possible that there was a leakage of pancreatic fluid into the cavity behind the stomach, as the contents of this cavity consisted of a thick, grayish fluid, containing fragments of connective tissue. In this case the wall of fibrin would have been sufficient to prevent the pancreatic fluid from coming in contact with the adjacent fat. The extensive necrosis of the pancreas would seem to be an important factor in the cause of death, although it has never been definitely shown how much destruction of this organ is necessary to produce death. There are experiments upon animals upon record, in which the animals seem to have died as a result of not very extensive lesions of this organ. One experiment of this nature reported by Flexner (*Journal of Experimental Medicine*, Vol. II.) is of interest. The fact that concussion and slight injuries of the pancreas may be a factor in the development of necrosis is indicated by the researches of Chiari (*Zeitschrift fur Heilkunde*, Vol. XVII., 1896, and *Prager Med. Wochenschr.*, 1900, No. 14), who has observed (although a comparatively rare condition) extensive areas of softening and necrosis of the pancreas, especially of the posterior central portion which lies directly over the bodies of the vertebra, where the organ is most exposed to pressure or the effects of concussion. The wound in the kidney is of slight importance, except as indicating the direction taken by the missile. The changes in the heart, as shown by the macroscopic inspection and the microscopic examination, indicate that the condition of this organ was an important factor. The extensive brown atrophy and diffuse fatty degeneration of the muscle, but especially the extent to which the pericardial fat had invaded the atrophic muscle fibers of the right ventricular wall, sufficiently explain the rapid pulse and lack of response of this organ to stimulation during life.

REPORT ON THE BACTERIOLOGIC EXAMINATION.

BY HERMAN G. MATZINGER, M. D.,
Bacteriologist to the New York State Pathological Laboratory.

It is obvious that the short space of time which has elapsed since the death of the President has hardly been sufficent to prepare a complete and thorough bacteriologic report. This report contains all the observations which have been made up to this time:

On September 11, during the life of the President, cultures were made by Dr. Wasdin from the base of the abdominal wound and from dressings removed at

the same time. These were submitted to me for examination, and showed the presence of the ordinary pus organisms: Staphylococcus pyogenes aureus and S. cereus albus, with a gas-forming bacillus which, in pure anerobic culture on glucose gelatin, forms small, pearly, translucent colonies, with no liquefaction. In litmus milk it produces acid, but no coagulation. Morphologically, it is apparently a capsulated, short bacillus, which takes stains poorly, and which does not stain by Gram's method. Inoculated into the ear vein of a rabbit, which was killed immediately afterward, it produced, after twenty-four hours in the body of the rabbit, a marked accumulation of gas in the organs, and again grew out in pure culture. As yet the organism is not fully identified.

None of these cultures showed streptococci. A bacterium which appears to be one of the proteus group was, however, isolated which does not stain by Gram, and appears in varying forms, sometimes small oval, and again quite rod-shaped and in short chains. Sometimes it is surrounded with a slimy covering, which remains clear like a capsule when the organism is stained. On slanting agar, it produces a whitish, slimy growth, which gradually runs to the bottom of the slant and produces an odor of decomposition. On gelatin, it grows very slowly with slight and slow indication of liquefaction. In litmus milk, it produces acid and rapid coagulation.

At the time of the autopsy, September 14, inoculations were made by myself. From the base of the wound, there was again obtained a number of pus organisms, principally a white staphylococcus and the bacterium described above, but no streptococci. Cultures made from the peritoneal surface of the intestines were entirely negative. Cultures made from the under surface of the omentum near the colon, were entirely negative, both with and without oxygen. Cultures from the blood of the right auricle were likewise negative. A very careful and extensive search for microörganism in the contents of the necrotic cavity, behind the stomach, reveals nothing but a short, stumpy bacterium, which, as far as the work has been carried at present appears to belong to the proteus group, and is very like proteus hominis capsulatus, described by Bordoni and Uffreduzzi.

Morphologically, it is not uniform, and sometimes appears almost encapsulated, being surrounded by material that does not stain; is quite refractory to Gram, and produces an odor of decomposition as it grows. It does not liquefy gelatin rapidly and grows slowly, as a glistening white elevated surface growth which slowly sinks; but on agar in the thermostat it grows very rapidly, as a moist, grayish-white, translucent mass. Colonies on gelatin plates have a clean circumference, are granular and quite refractive. In litmus milk it produces acid and rapid coagulation. Animal experiments are still incomplete and cannot be published at this time.

It must be stated that there is occasion for suspecting that this may be a contamination, either from the outer wound or elsewhere, because, quite unavoidably, the technic in obtaining the material and cultures from the necrotic cavity was not absolutely correct.

Cultures made from the small area of broken-down tissue under the chest wound at the time of the autopsy, grew what appears to be staphylococcus epidermidis albus, described by Dr. Welch.

The slimy, gray, necrotic material from the cavity above the transverse mesocolon behind the stomach, was carefully examined microscopically, with the result that very few microörganisms were found in the fresh state, and no recognisable tissue elements of any kind, no leukocytes or pus-corpuscles, but an abundance of

crystals which appeared more like fatty acid than fat crystals. It contained no free hydrochloric acid, and was alkaline in reaction. Experiments as to its digestive power were negative. About 2 c.c. of this material was injected into the space behind the stomach of a dog (still living), with no results except quite an elevated temperature for three or four days. Other animal experiments are still incomplete.

It might be well to state here that the bacteriologic examination of the chambers and barrel of the weapon used, as well as the empty shells and cartridges, ordered by the District Attorney, was entirely negative, except that from a loaded cartridge there was grown an ordinary staphylococcus and a mold. The chemical examination of the balance of the loaded cartridges, made by Dr. Hill, chemist, was also negative.

The absence of known pathogenic bacteria, particularly in the necrotic cavity, warrants the conclusion that bacterial infection was not a factor in the production of the conditions found at the autopsy.

The foregoing report has received the approval of, and is issued by, the undersigned, the medical staff attending the late President, William McKinley.

P. M. RIXEY,
MATTHEW D. MANN,
HERMAN MYNTER,
ROSWELL PARK,
EUGENE WASDIN,
CHARLES McBURNEY,
CHARLES G. STOCKTON.

BUFFALO, October 12, 1901.

NOTE BY THE EDITOR—The report of the medical staff in attendance upon President McKinley is printed in full, with the exception of the bulletins. These were all printed in the October issue of the JOURNAL and may be referred to with interest in relation to this report.

John F. Kennedy

Born: May 29, 1917, Brookline, Massachusetts
Died: November 22, 1963, Dallas, Texas
Cause of Death: Assassination

Considered one of the most popular presidents in US history, John F. Kennedy was the first president born in the twentieth century. While in office, he laid the groundwork for the space race and putting a man on the moon. He started the Peace Corps and was a champion of civil rights. He was assassinated by Lee Harvey Oswald while traveling in his motorcade in Dallas, Texas.

The Assassination of John F. Kennedy

Warren Report
Appendix IX - Autopsy Report and Supplemental Report
Clinical Record - Autopsy Protocol

Date 11/22/63 1300 (CST)

Prosecter: CDR J.J. Humes, MC, USA (497831)

Assistant: CDR "J" Thornton Boswell, MC, USN, (439878);
LCOL, Pierre A. Finck, MC, USA (04 043 322)

Full Autopsy

Ht. - 72 1/2 inches Wt. - 170 pounds Eyes - blue Hair - Reddish brown

Pathological diagnosis: Cause of Death: Gunshot wound, head.

Signature: J.J. Humes, CDS, MC, USN

Military organization: President, United States

Age: 46 Sex: Male Race: Caucasian

Autopsy No. A63-272

Patient's Identification: Kennedy, John F., Naval Medical School

Clinical Summary

According to available information the deceased, President John F. Kennedy, was riding in an open car in a motorcade during an official visit to Dallas, Texas on 22 November 1963. The President was sitting in the right rear seat with Mrs. Kennedy seated on the same seat to his left. Sitting directly in front of the President was Governor John B. Connally of Texas and directly in front of Mrs. Kennedy sat Mrs. Connally. The vehicle was moving at a slow rate of speed down an incline into an underpass that leads to a freeway route to the Dallas Trade Mart where the President was to deliver an address.

Three shots were heard and the President fell forward bleeding from the head. (Governor Connally was seriously wounded by the same gunfire.) According to newspaper reports ("Washington Post" November 23, 1963) Bob Jackson, a Dallas "Times Herald" Photographer, said he looked around as he heard the shots and saw a rifle barrel disappearing into a window on an upper floor of the nearby Texas School Book Depository Building.

Shortly following the wounding of the two men the car was driven to Parkland Hospital in Dallas. In the emergency room of that hospital the President was attended by Dr. Malcolm Perry. Telephone communication with Dr. Perry on November 23, 1963 develops the following information relative to the observations made by Dr. Perry and procedures performed there prior to death.

Dr. Perry noted the massive wound of the head and a second much smaller wound of the low anterior neck in approximately the midline. A tracheostomy was performed by extending the latter wound. At this point bloody air was noted bubbling from the wound and an injury to the right lateral wall of the trachea was observed. Incisions were made in the upper anterior chest wall bilaterally to combat possible subcutaneous emphysema. Intravenous infusions of blood and saline were begun and oxygen was administered. Despite these measures cardiac arrest occurred and closed chest cardiac massage failed to re-establish cardiac action. The President was pronounced dead approximately thirty to forty minutes after receiving his wounds.

The remains were transported via the Presidential plane to Washington, D.C. and subsequently to the Naval Medical School, National Naval Medical Center, Bethesda, Maryland for postmortem examination.

General Description of the Body

The body is that of a muscular, well-developed and well nourished adult Caucasian male measuring 72 1/2 inches and weighing approximately 170 pounds. There is beginning rigor mortis, minimal dependent livor mortis of the dorsum, and early algor mortis. The hair is reddish brown and abundant, the eyes are blue, the right pupil measuring 8 mm. in diameter, the left 4 mm. There is edema and ecchymosis of the inner canthus region of the left eyelid measuring approximately 1.5 cm. in greatest diameter. There is edema and ecchymosis diffusely over the right supra-orbital ridge with abnormal mobility of the underlying bone. (The remainder of the scalp will be described with the skull.) There is clotted blood on the external ears but otherwise the ears, nares, and mouth are essentially unremarkable. The teeth are in excellent repair and there is some pallor of the oral mucous membrane.

Situated on the upper right posterior thorax just above the upper border of the scapula there is a 7 x 4 millimeter oval wound. This wound is measured to be 14 cm. from the tip of the right acromion process and 14 cm. below the tip of the right mastoid process.

Situated in the low anterior neck at approximately the level of the third and fourth tracheal rings is a 6.5 cm. long transverse wound with widely gaping irregular edges. (The depth and character of these wounds will be further described below.)

Situated on the anterior chest wall in the nipple line are bilateral 2 cm. long recent transverse surgical incisions into the subcutaneous tissue. The one on the left is situated 11 cm. cephalad to the nipple and the one on the right 8 cm. cephalad to the nipple. There is no hemorrhage or ecchymosis associated with these wounds. A similar clean wound measuring 2 cm. in length is situated on the antero-lateral aspect of the left mid arm. Situated on the antero-lateral aspect of each ankle is a recent 2 cm. transverse incision into the subcutaneous tissue.

There is an old well healed 8 cm. McBurney abdominal incision. Over the lumbar spine in the midline is an old, well healed 15 cm. scar. Situated on the upper antero-lateral aspect of the right thigh is an old, well healed 8 cm. scar.

Missile Wounds

1. There is a large irregular defect of the scalp and skull on the right involving chiefly the parietal bone but extending somewhat into the temporal and occipital regions. In this region there is an actual absence of scalp and bone producing a defect which measures approximately 13 cm. in greatest diameter.

   From the irregular margins of the above scalp defect tears extend in stellate fashion into the more or less intact scalp as follows:

   a. From the right inferior temporo-parietal margin anterior to the right ear to a point slightly above the tragus.
   b. From the anterior parietal margin anteriorly on the forehead to approximately 4 cm. above the right orbital ridge.
   c. From the left margin of the main defect across the midline antero-laterally for a distance of approximately 8 cm.
   d. From the same starting point as c. 10 cm. postero-laterally.

   Situated in the posterior scalp approximately 2.5 cm. laterally to the right and slightly above the external occipital protuberance is a lacerated wound measuring 15 x 6 mm. In the underlying bone is a corresponding wound through the skull which exhibits beveling of the margins of the bone when viewed from the inner aspect of the skull.

   Clearly visible in the above described large skull defect and exuding from it is lacerated brain tissue which on close inspection proves to represent the major

portion of the right cerebral hemisphere. At this point it is noted that the falx cerebri is extensively lacerated with disruption of the superior saggital sinus.

Upon reflecting the scalp multiple complete fracture lines are seen to radiate from both the large defect at the vertex and the smaller wound at the occiput. These vary greatly in length and direction, the longest measuring approximately 19 cm. These result in the production of numerous fragments which vary in size from a few millimeters to 10 cm. in greatest diameter.

The complexity of these fractures and the fragments thus produced tax satisfactory verbal description and are better appreciated in photographs and roentgenograms which are prepared.

The brain is removed and preserved for further study following formalin fixation.

Received as separate specimens from Dallas, Texas are three fragments of skull bone which in aggregate roughly approximate the dimensions of the large defect described above. At one angle of the largest of these fragments is a portion of the perimeter of a roughly circular wound presumably of exit which exhibits beveling of the outer aspect of the bone and is estimated to measure approximately 2.5 to 3.0 cm. in diameter. Roentgenograms of this fragment reveal minute particles of metal in the bone at this margin. Roentgenograms of the skull reveal multiple minute metallic fragments along a line corresponding with a line joining the above described small occipital wound and the right supra-orbital ridge. From the surface of the disrupted right cerebral cortex two small irregularly shaped fragments of metal are recovered. These measure 7 x 2 mm. and 3 x 1 mm. These are placed in the custody of Agents Francis X. O'Neill, Jr. and James W. Sibert, of the Federal Bureau of Investigation, who executed a receipt therefor (attached).

2. The second wound presumably of entry is that described above in the upper right posterior thorax. Beneath the skin there is ecchymosis of subcutaneous tissue and musculature. The missile path through the fascia and musculature cannot be easily proved. The wound presumably of exit was that described by Dr. Malcolm Perry of Dallas in the low anterior cervical region. When observed by Dr. Perry the wound measured "a few millimeters in diameter", however it was extended as a tracheostomy incision and thus its character is distorted at the time of autopsy. However there is considerable eccymosis of the strap muscles of the right side of the neck and of the fascia about the trachea adjacent to the line of the tracheostomy wound. The third point of reference in connecting these two wounds is in the apex (supra-clavicular portion) of the right pleural cavity. In this region there is contusion of the parietal

pleura and of the extreme apical portion of the right upper lobe of the lung. In both instances the diameter of contusion and ecchymosis at the point of maximal involvement measures 5 cm. Both the visceral and parietal pleura are intact overlying these areas of trauma.

Incisions
The scalp wounds are extended in the coronal plane to examine the cranial content and the customary (Y) shaped incision is used to examine the body cavities.

Thoracic Cavity
The bony cage is unremarkable. The thoracic organs are in their normal positions are relationships and there is no increase in free pleural fluid. The above described area of contusion in the apical portion of the right pleural cavity is noted.

Lungs
The lungs are of essentially similar appearance the right weighing 320 Gm., the left 290 Gm. The lungs are well aerated with smooth glistening pleural surfaces and gray-pink color. A 5 cm. diameter area of purplish red discoloration and increased firmness to palpation is situated in the apical portion of the right upper lobe. This corresponds to the similar area described in the overlying parietal pleura. Incision in this region reveals recent hemorrhage into pulmonary parenchyma.

Heart
The pericardial cavity is smooth walled and contains approximately 10 cc. of straw-colored fluid. The heart is of essentially normal external contour and weighs 350 Gm. The pulmonary artery is opened in situ and no abnormalities are noted. The cardiac chambers contain moderate amounts of postmortem clotted blood. There are no gross abnormalities of the leaflets of any of the cardiac valves. The following are the circumferences of the cardiac valves: aortic 7.5 cm., pulmonic 7 cm., tricuspid 12 cm., mitral 11 cm. The myocardium is firm and reddish brown. The left ventricular myocardium averages 1.2 cm. in thickness, the right ventricular myocardium 0.4 cm. The coronary arteries are dissected and are of normal distribution and smooth walled and elastic throughout.

Abdominal Cavity
The abdominal organs are in their normal positions and relationships and there is no increase in free peritoneal fluid. The vermiform appendix is surgically absent

and there are a few adhesions joining the region of the cecum to the ventral abdominal wall at the above described old abdominal incisional scar.

Skeletal System
Aside from the above described skull wounds there are no significant gross skeletal abnormalities.

Photography
Black and white and color photographs depicting significant findings are exposed but not developed. These photographs were placed in the custody of Agent Roy E. Kellerman of the U.S. Secret Service, who executed a receipt therefore (attached).

Roentgenograms
Roentgenograms are made of the entire body and of the separately submitted three fragments of skull bone. These are developed are were placed in the custody of Agent Roy H. Kellerman of the U.S. Secret Service, who executed a receipt therefor (attached).

Summary
Based on the above observations it is our opinion that the deceased died as a result of two perforating gunshot wounds inflicted by high velocity projectiles fired by a person or persons unknown. The projectiles were fired from a point behind and somewhat above the level of the deceased. The observations and available information do not permit a satisfactory estimate as to the sequence of the two wounds.

The fatal missile entered the skull above and to the right of the external occipital protuberance. A portion of the projectile traversed the cranial cavity in a posterior-anterior direction (see lateral skull roentgenograms) depositing minute particles along its path. A portion of the projectile made its exit through the parietal bone on the right carrying with it portions of cerebrum, skull and scalp. The two wounds of the skull combined with the force of the missile produced extensive fragmentation of the skull, laceration of the superior saggital sinus, and of the right cerebral hemisphere.

The other missile entered the right superior posterior thorax above the scapula and traversed the soft tissues of the supra-scapular and the supra-clavicular portions of the base of the right side of the neck. This missile produced contusions of the right apical parietal pleura and of the apical portion of the right upper lobe of the lung. The missile contused the strap muscles of the right side of the

neck, damaged the trachea and made its exit through the anterior surface of the neck. As far as can be ascertained this missile struck no bony structures in its path through the body.

In addition, it is our opinion that the wound of the skull produced such extensive damage to the brain as to preclude the possibility of the deceased surviving this injury.

A supplementary report will be submitted following more detailed examination of the brain and of microscopic sections. However, it is not anticipated that these examinations will materially alter the findings.

/s/
J. J. HUMES
CDR, MC, USN (497831)
/s/
"J" THORNTON BOSWELL
CDR, MC, USN (489878)
/s/
PIERRE A. FINCK
LT COL, MC, USA
(04-043-322)

Supplementary Report of Autopsy Number A63-272
President John F. Kennedy

Pathological Examination Report No. A63-272
Gross Description of the Brain

Following formalin fixation the brain weighs 1500 gms. The right cerebral hemisphere is found to be markedly disrupted. There is a longitudinal laceration of the right hemisphere which is para-sagittal in position approximately 2.5 cm. to the right of the of the midline which extends from the tip of the occipital lobe posteriorly to the tip of the frontal lobe anteriorly. The base of the laceration is situated approximately 4.5 cm. below the vertex in the white matter. There is considerable loss of cortical substance above the base of the laceration, particularly in the parietal lobe. The margins of this laceration are at all points jagged and irregular, with additional lacerations extending in varying directions and for varying distances from the main laceration. In addition, there is a laceration of the corpus callosum extending from the genu to the tail. Exposed in this latter laceration are the interiors of the right lateral and third ventricles.

When viewed from the vertex the left cerebral hemisphere is intact. There is marked engorgement of meningeal blood vessels of the left temporal and frontal regions with considerable associated sub-arachnoid hemorrhage. The gyri and sulci over the left hemisphere are of essentially normal size and distribution. Those on the right are too fragmented and distorted for satisfactory description.

When viewed from the basilar aspect the disruption of the right cortex is again obvious. There is a longitudinal laceration of the mid-brain through the floor of the third ventricle just behind the optic chiasm and the mammillary bodies. This laceration partially communicates with an oblique 1.5 cm. tear through the left cerebral peduncle. There are irregular superficial lacerations over the basilar aspects of the left temporal and frontal lobes.

In the interest of preserving the specimen coronal sections are not made. The following sections are taken for microscopic examination:

a. From the margin of the laceration in the right parietal lobe.
b. From the margin of the laceration in the corpus callosum.
c. From the anterior portion of the laceration in the right frontal lobe.
d. From the contused left fronto-parietal cortex.
e. From the line of transection of the spinal cord.

f. From the right cerebellar cortex.

g. From the superficial laceration of the basilar aspect of the left temporal lobe.

During the course of this examination seven (7) black and white and six (6) color 4x5 inch negatives are exposed but not developed (the cassettes containing these negatives have been delivered by hand to Rear Admiral George W. Burkley, MC, USN, White House Physician).

Microscopic Examination
Brain

Multiple sections from representative areas as noted above are examined. All sections are essentially similar and show extensive disruption of brain tissue with associated hemorrhage. In none of the sections examined are there significant abnormalities other than those directly related to the recent trauma.

Heart

Sections show a moderate amount of sub-epicardial fat. The coronary arteries, myocardial fibers, and endocardium are unremarkable.

Lungs

Sections through the grossly described area of contusion in the right upper lobe exhibit disruption of alveolar walls and recent hemorrhage into alveoli. Sections are otherwise essentially unremarkable.

Liver

Sections show the normal hepatic architecture to be well preserved. The parenchymal cells exhibit markedly granular cytoplasm indicating high glycogen content which is characteristic of the "liver biopsy pattern" of sudden death.

Spleen

Sections show no significant abnormalities.

Kidneys

Sections show no significant abnormalities aside from dilatation and engorgement of blood vessels of all calibers.

Skin Wounds

Sections through the wounds in the occipital and upper right posterior thoracic regions are essentially similar. In each there is loss of continuity of the epidermis

with coagulation necrosis of the tissues at the wound margins. The scalp wound exhibits several small fragments of bone at its margins in the subcutaneous tissue.

Final Summary
This supplementary report covers in more detail the extensive degree of cerebral trauma in this case. However neither this portion of the examination nor the microscopic examinations alter the previously submitted report or add significant details to the cause of death.

/s/
J. J. HUMES
CDR, MC, USN, 497831

Date: 6 December 1963
From: Commanding Officer, U. S. Naval Medical School
To: The White House Physician
Via: Commanding Officer, National Naval Medical Center
Subj: Supplementary report of Naval Medical School autopsy No. A63-272, John F. Kennedy; forwarding of

1. All copies of the above subject final supplementary report are forwarded herewith.
/s/
J. H. STOVER, JR.

6 December 1963
First Endorsement
From: Commanding Officer, National Naval Medical Center
To: The White House Physician
1. Forwarded.
/s/
1.B. GALLOWAY

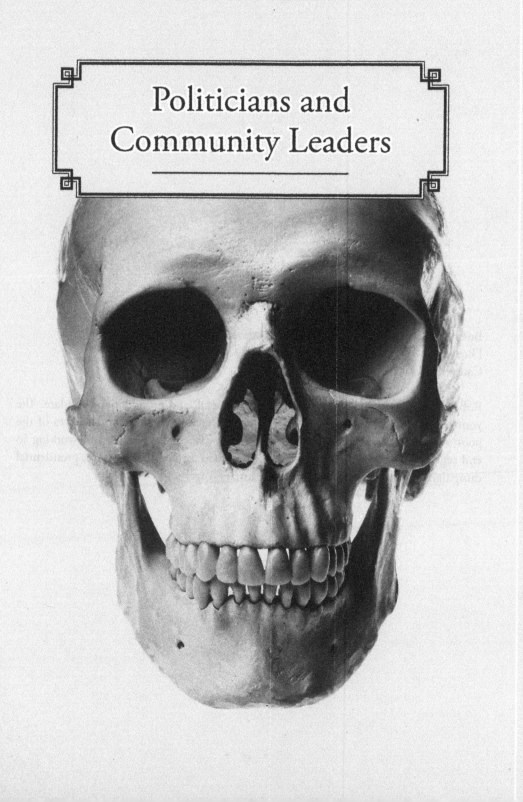

Politicians and
Community Leaders

Robert F. Kennedy

Born: November 20, 1925, Brookline, Massachusetts
Died: June 6, 1968, Los Angeles, California
Cause of Death: Assassination

Robert F. Kennedy was a Senator, Attorney General, and presidential candidate. The youngest brother of President John F. Kennedy he worked to better the lives of the poor and disenfranchised, aligning himself with civil rights leaders and working to end segregation. He was assassinated by Palestinian Sirhan Sirhan after a presidential campaign event at the Ambassador Hotel in Los Angeles.

ROUGH DRAFT   1   Senator ..obert F. Kennedy
                                        #68-5731

2nd rough draft,
edited 6/21/68 - JEH

"Dr. Holloway with dictation on the first composite gross protocol
for case 68-5731."

                     re-edited 7/18/68 by TTW and JEH.
                     re-edited 9/20/68 by JEH.

ANATOMICAL SUMMARY

GUNSHOT WOUND NO. 1 (FATAL GUNSHOT WOUND)

     ENTRY: Right mastoid region.

     COURSE: Skin of right mastoid region, right mastoid, petrous
                 portion of right temporal bone, right temporal lobe,
                 right cerebellum, and brain stem.

     EXIT: None.

     DIRECTION: Right to left, slightly back to front upward.

     BULLET RECOVERY: Fragments (see text).

GUNSHOT WOUND NO. 2, THROUGH-AND-THROUGH.

     ENTRY: Right axillary region.

     COURSE: Soft tissue of right axilla and right infraclavicular
                 region.

     EXIT: Right infraclavicular region.

     DIRECTION: Right to left, back to front upward.

     BULLET RECOVERY: None.

GUNSHOT WOUND NO. 3.

     ENTRY: Right axillary region (just below Gunshot Wound No. 2
                 entry).

     COURSE: Soft tissue of right axilla, soft tissue of right
                 upper back to the level of the 6th cervical vertebra
                 just beneath the skin.

     EXIT: None.

ROUGH DRAFT   2   #68-5731
                                               SENATOR ROBERT F. KENNEDY
                                               JUNE 6, 1968

    DIRECTION: Right to left, back to front, upward.

    BULLET RECOVERY: .22 caliber bullet from the soft tissue
                       of paracervical region at level of 6th
                       cervical vertebra at 8:40 A.M. June 6,
                       1968.

GUNSHOT WOUND NO. 1:

The wound of entry, as designated by Maxwell M. Andler, Jr, M.D.,
Neurosurgeon attending the autopsy, and more or less evident by
inspection of the apposed craniotomy incision, is centered 5
inches (12.7 cm) from the vertex, about 3/4 inch (1.9 cm) posterior
to the center of the right external auditory meatus, about 3/4 inch
(1.9 cm) superior to the Reid line, and 2-1/2 inches (6.4 cm)
anterior to a coronal plane passing through the occipital protuberance
at its scalp-covered aspect. The defect appears to have been about
3/16 inch (0.5 cm) in diameter at the skin surface. The surgical
incision passing through the area of the wound of entry has been
fashioned in a semilunar configuration with the concavity directed
inferiorly and posteriorly. The incision has been intactly sutured
by metallic and other material. The arc length is about 4 inches
(10 cm).

Further detailed description of the area is given in the Neuropathology portion of this report.

Varyingly moderate degrees of very recent hemorrhage are noted
in the soft tissue inferior to the right mastoid region, extending
medially, as well. There is no hematoma in the soft tissue.

In conjunction with the wound of entry, the right external ear
shows, on the posterior aspect of the helix, an irregularly
fusiform zone of dark red and gray stippling about one inch
(2.5 cm) in greatest dimension, along the posterior cartilaginous
border and over a maximum width of about 1/4 inch (0.6 cm) at
the midportion of the stippled zone. This widest zone of
stippling is approximately along a radius originating from the
wound of entry in the right mastoid region. Moderate edema
and variable ecchymosis is present in the associated portions
of right external ear as well.

GUNSHOT WOUND NO. 2:

This is a through-and-through wound of the right axillary, medial
shoulder, and anterior superior chest areas, excluding the thorax
proper. The wound of entry is centered 12-1/2 inches (13.6 cm)
from the vertex, 9 inches (22.9 cm) to the right of midline, and

ROUGH DRAFT   3   #68-5731
                               SENATOR ROBERT P. KENNEDY
                               JUNE 6, 1968

3-3/4 inches (8.3 cm) from the back (anterior to a coronal plane
passing through the surface of the skin at the scapula region).
There is a regularly elliptical defect 3/16 x 1/8 inch over-all
(about 0.5 x 0.3 cm) with thin rim of abrasion. There is no
apparent charring or powder residue in the adjacent and subjacent
tissue. The subcutaneous fatty tissue is hemorrhagic.

The wound path is through soft tissue, medially to the left,
superiorly and somewhat anteriorly. Bony structures, major
blood vessels and the brachial plexus have been spared.

The exit wound is centered 9-3/4 inches (about 24.5 cm) from the
vertex and about 5 inches (about 12.5 cm) to the right of midline
anteriorly in the infraclavicular region. There is a nearly
circular defect slightly less than 1/4 inch x 3/16 inch overall
(0.6 x 0.5 cm).

Orientation of the wounds of entry and exit is such that their
major axes at the skin surfaces coincide with the central axis of
a probe passed along the entirety of the wound path. No evidence
of deflection of trajectory is found.

GUNSHOT WOUND NO. 3:

The wound of entry is centered 14 inches (35.6 cm) from the vertex
and 8-1/2 inches (21.6 cm) to the right of midline, 2 inches (5 cm)
from the back anterior to a plane passing through the skin surface
overlying the scapula, and 1/2 inch (1.2 cm) posterior to the
mid-axillary line. There is a nearly circular defect 3/16 inch by
slightly more than 1/8 inch overall (0.5 x 0.4 cm). There is a
thin marginal abrasion rim without evidence of charring or apparent
residue in the adjacent skin or subjacent soft tissue. The subcutaneous fatty tissue is hemorrhagic.

The wound path is directed medially to the left, superiorly and
posteriorly through soft tissue of the medial portion of the axilla
and soft tissue of the upper back, terminating at a point at the
level of the 6th thoracic vertebra as close as about 1/2 inch
(1.2 cm) to the right of midline.

Bullet Recovery: A bullet of .22 caliber with lubaloy covering is
recovered at the terminus of the wound path just described, at
8:40 A.M. June 6, 1968. There is a unilateral, transverse
deformation, the contour of which is indicated on an accompanying
diagram. The initials, TN, and the numbers 31 are placed on the
base of the bullet for future identification. The usual Evidence
envaolpe is prepared. The bullet, so marked and so enclosed as
evidence, is given to Sergeant W. Jordan, No. 7167, Rampart
Detectives, Los Angeles Police Department, at 8:49 A.M. this date
for further studies.

ROUGH DRAFT   4   #68-573
                                              SENATOR ROBERT F. KENNEDY
                                              JUNE 6, 1968

An irregularly bordered and somewhat elliptical zone of
variably mottled recent ecchymosis is present in the superior-
medial axillary skin on the right, in the zones of wounds of
entry No. 2 and No. 3, especially the former. The ecchymosis
measures 3-1/2 x 1-1/2 inches (9 x 3.8 cm) overall with the
right upper extremity extended completely upward(longitudinally).

EXAMINATION OF CLOTHING AT TIME OF AUTOPSY:

1) There is a dark blue, fine worsted-type suit coat bearing
the label "Georgetown University Shop - Georgetown, D.C". The
coat has been cut and/or torn at the left yoke and left sleeve
area. The right sleeve is intact. There is variable blood
staining over the right shoulder region and on the right lapel.
Two apparent bullet holes are identified in the right axillary
region, slightly over 1 inch (2.5 cm) and slightly over 1-1/4
inch (3.2 cm) from the underseam area, respectively, and
corresponding with wounds described on the body elsewhere in
this report. Also noted at the top of the right shoulder region,
centered about 1-1/4 inches from the shoulder seam and about 5/8
inch (1.6 cm) posterior to the yoke seam superiorly is an irregular
rent of the fabric, somewhat less than 1/4 inch (3.2 cm) in diameter
and definitely everting superficially and upward. The 3 front
buttons of the garment are intact.

Subsequent examination of the coat showed the presence of a
superficial through-and-through bullet path through the upper
right shoulder area, passing through the suit fabric proper,
but not the lining.

2) There is a pair of trousers of matching material with a
very dark brown leather belt with rectangular metal buckle and
showing the gold-stamped label "Custom Leather, Reversible, 32".
The zipper is intact. Thre is a minimal amount of apparent blood
staining over the anterior portions of the trouser legs.

3) There is a white cotton shirt with the label "K WRAGGE, 48
West 46th Street, New York". The laundry mark initials "RFK"
are present on the neck band. The left portion of the shirt has
been disrupted in approximately the same manner as the suit coat
and is similarly absent. The right cuff is intact and is of
semi-French design. A chain-connected yellow metal cufflink with
plain oval design is in place. A corresponding left cufflink is
not among the items submitted. Apparent bullet holes are identified
as corresponding to those in the previously described area of suit
coat.

4) There is a tie of apparent silk rep, navy blue with an
approximately 3/16 inch (0.5 cm) grey diagonal stripe. The
label is "Chase and Collier, McLean, Virginia". The maker is
RIVETZ.

ROUGH DRAFT   5   #68-5731
                                SENATOR ROBERT F. KENNEDY
                                JUNE 6, 1968

5)   There is a pair of navy blue, nearly calf length socks of mixed cashmere and apparently nylon fiber, the fiber content stencil labeling still being nearly discernible on the foot portions.

6)   There is a pair of white broadcloth boxer type shorts with two labels: "Sunsheen Broadcloth V'Cloth - 34; and "Custom fashioned for Lewis and Thos. Saltz, Washington". There is a small amount of blood stain at the anterior crotch, along with pale straw colored discoloration to the left of the fly. A few patches of dry blood are present on the back as well.

7)   There is a trapezoidally folded cotton handkerchief showing, on what appears to be the presenting (anterior) surface, several scattered dark red and somewhat brown spots ranging from a fraction of a millimeter to about 4 mm (less than 3/16 inch) in greatest dimension.

8)   No shoes are submitted for examination.

The above listed items are saved for further and more detailed study by others.

GENERAL EXTERNAL EXAMINATION:

The non-embalmed body, measuring 70-1/2 inches (179 cm) in length and weighing about 165 pounds (74.5 kg), is that of a well-developed, well-nourished and muscular Caucasian male appearing about the recorded age of 42 years. The extremities are generally symmetrical bilaterally, showing no obvious structural abnormality.

The head shows extensive bandaging, somewhat blood-stained in the posterior aspect. Dressings are also present in the right clavicular region, the right axilla, and the right ankle regions. Also present over the right inguino-femoral region are apparently elastoplast dressings. A recent tracheostomy has been performed at a comparatively low level. A clear plastic tracheostomy tube fitted with an inflatable cuff is in place. The area also shows a gauze dressing.

Lividity is well developed in the posterior aspect of the body, mainly at the upper shoulder and midback regions with approximately equal distribution bilaterally. The lividity blanches definitely on finger pressure.

Rigor mortis is not detected in the extremities or in the neck.

Rigor was noted to be developing in the arms and legs by the time of conclusion of the autopsy.

ROUGH DRAFT   6   #68-5731
                                           SENATOR ROBERT F. KENNEDY
                                           JUNE 6, 1968

A complete examination of the external surfaces of the body
is udnertaken following removal of all dressings.

The head contour is generally symmetrical, due allowance
being made for the soft-tissue edema and hemorrhage in the
right post-auricular region in general. The hair is graying
light brown and of male distribution. Calvity lines are well
delineated on the scalp. Portions of the right half of the
scalp have clipped and/or shaved. Hair in the inguinal and
femoral regions has also been shaved in part. Hair texture is
medium.

There is an irregularly bordered area of comparatively recent
yet pale ecchymosis centered about one inch (2.5 cm) above
the midportion of the right eyebrow. Marked ecchymosis with
moderate edema is present in the right periorbital region
but mainly of the upper eyelid. No abnormality is noted in the
left periorbital tissue externally. No hemorrhage or generalized
congestion is seen in the conjunctival or scleral membranes. The
nose is symmetrical, showing no evidence of fracture or hemorrhage.
The glabella shows no evidence of trauma.

Eye color is hazel. Pupillary diameters are equal at about
5 mm (3/16 in).

The buccal mucosa and the tongue show no lesion.

Chest diameters are within normal limits and there is bilateral
symmetry. The breasts are those of a normal adult male. The
abdomen is scaphoid. No abdominal scar is identified. There
is an old low medial inguinal scar on the right.

Texture and configuration of the nails are within normal limits,
and no focal lesions are noted. There is no peripheral edema.

The skin in general shows a smooth texture and no additional
significant focal lesion. There is abundant sun tan, especially
at the neck region where its contrast with the areas shaved for
surgical preparation on the right can be noted. No evidence of
powder burn, tattoo, or stippling is found in the area surrounding
the wound of entry of Gunshot Wound No. 1, in an arbitrary circular
zone to include the above-described stippling on the right ear,
or beyond.

No structural abnormality is noted on the back.

There is a diagonally disposed recent surgical incision about
3 inches (7.5 cm) in length in the right anterolateral femoral
region. This incision has been intactly sutured. There is an
associated plastic tubing of small diameter, centered about
1/2 inch (12 mm) from the infero-medial margin of the incision.

ROUGH DRAFT   7   #68-5731
SENATOR ROBERT F. KENNEDY
JUNE 6, 1968

Also noted in a comparable location on the left are several
hypodermic puncture marks. These just-mentioned areas show
the presence of red-orange dye.

There are recent cutdowns at the right ankle and the lateral
right knee with thin polyethylene tubes in place. No extravasation is noted.

The external genitalia are those of a normal circumcised adult
male.

CAVITIES:

Primary incision is first made as far as the two upper incisions,
allowing upward reflection of skin and soft tissue to afford
access for carotid angiography before the head is opened.
Following completion of these roentgenographic studies, the
traditional Y incision is continued. The peritoneal surfaces
are smooth and glistening. No free fluid is found in the
abdominal cavity. There are no adhesions. Abdominal organs
are in their usual relative positions.

The pleural surfaces are smooth. There is no pleural effusion.

The pericardium is intact and encloses a small amount of transparent straw-colored liquid.

CARDIOVASCULAR SYSTEM:

The heart weighs 360 gm and presents smooth epicardial surfaces.
There is moderate right atrial dilatation. The contour otherwise is within normal limits. Cut surfaces of myocardium show
a uniform gray-red muscle fiber texture with no focal lesion.
The endocardial surfaces are smooth. About 50 ml of dark red
postmortem clot is present in the chambers collectively. No
cardiac anomaly is demonstrated. The thickness of the left
ventricular wall is up to 1.3 cm, and that of the right 0.3 cm.
Valve circumferences are: Tricuspid - 13, pulmonic - 8.5,
mitral - 10.5, and aortic - 7 cm. There are no focal lesions.
The coronary arterial tree arises in the usual sites and distri-
butes normally. The coronary arteries are thin-walled and pliable,
showing widely patent lumina. The aorta has a normal configuration
and varies from 3.3 to 5.2 cm in circumference. The intinal surface
of the aorta shows small and comparatively pale yellow atheromatous
areas totaling no more than 10% of the area studied.

The lining of the inferior vena cava is smooth throughout. The
distal end of the intravenous polyethylene catheter is noted at
the level of the 2nd lumbar vertebra and shows no evidence of
thrombosis at the tip. Free flow is also demonstrated.

ROUGH DRAFT 8 #68-573
SENATOR ROBERT F. KENNEDY
JUNE 6, 1968

Other vessels studied are not remarkable, save where special
descriptions are given elsewhere in this report.

RESPIRATORY SYSTEM:

The right lung weighs 490 gm; the left, 330 gm. There is
a moderate amount of wrinkling of the external surfaces,
suggestive of atelectasis. Dusky discoloration is noted
in the hypostatic portions bilaterally. The outer surfaces
of the lungs are intrinsically smooth. Cut surfaces of the
lungs disclose a few scattered areas of atelectasis, especially,
in the left lower lobe. There is mild edema throughout. Hypostatic congestion is noted in an estimated 30% of the total
lung volume, approximately equally distributed bilaterally.
In these hypostatic areas there is probably patchy hemorrhage
of the matrix as well. No areas of consolidation are identified. Non-congested portions of the lungs are comparatively
pale tan in color. Anthracotic pigmentation is not excessive
for the age of the subject.

A small amount of slightly pink frothy mucoid material is
present in the bronchial tree, but no exudate. There is no
evidence of aspiration of gastric content.

The hilar lymph nodes show no abnormality.

NECK ORGANS:

The pharyngeal and laryngeal mucosa shows no focal lesion.
There are a few petechial hemorrhages of the epiglottis.
Intrinsic musculature and soft tissue of the larynx shows no
hemorrhage or other evidence of trauma. The vocal cords do
not appear edematous, nor is there evidence of generalized
submucosal edema. The hyoid bone is intact.

The trachea is in midline. The plastic tracheostomy tube
previously mentioned shows no obstruction of its airway and
no exudates or hemorrhagic material. The mucosa lining the
trachea is moderately injected at the general level of the
tracheostomy, again with no obvious exudate.

The thymus shows the usual atrophy and is comparatively fatty
but not otherwise remarkable.

HEPATOBILIARY SYSTEM:

The liver weighs 1810 gm and has a smooth intact capsule. The
edges are sharp. Cut surfaces of the liver show no focal lesion

ROUGH DRAFT   9   #68-5731
                                    SENATOR ROBERT F. KENNEDY
                                    JUNE 6, 1968

in the comparatively dark brown matrix. Little blood wells
up from freshly cut surfaces. A number of normal sized portal
veins present themselves. There is no evidence of fibrosis.
No fatty sheen is seen on the cut surfaces.

The gallbladder has a wall of average thickness and a smooth
serosal surface. The organ is distended by the presence of
more than 25 ml of green-black bile of intermediate viscosity.
There are no calculi. The extrahepatic biliary system is patent.

HEMIC AND LYMPHATIC SYSTEM:

The 150 gm spleen is moderately firm and has a smooth intact
capsule. Multiple cut surfaces of the spleen show no focal
lesion in the dark gray-red matrix. The capsule shows no areas
of thickening. The malpighian bodies are distinct. No accessory
spleen is identified.

There is no evidence of marked departure from normal blood
volume. In areas where postmortem clot is found, this is of
uniformly normal degree and texture. No evidence of any
hemorrhagic diathesis is noted.

The abdominal lymph nodes, mainly the para-aortic, show moderate
enlargement (up to three times the normal size) but no induration
or focal change. Other lymph nodes studied are not remarkable.

PANCREAS:

Configuration and size are within normal limits. Multiple cut
surfaces show no evidence of an acute inflammatory change,
fatty necrosis, scarring, or hemorrhage.

UROGENITAL SYSTEM:

The right kidney weighs 180 gm and has a smooth capsule which
strips readily. Cut surfaces disclose normal corticomedullary
ratios, with an average cortical thickness of about 6 mm,
compared with 1.0 cm of the medulla. There are no focal lesions.
A moderate amount of engorgement is noted.

The left kidney weighs 175 gm and has a generally smooth capsule
which can be stripped readily. Also present, however, is a
retention cyst about 2.5 cm in greatest dimension but showing,
on subsequent study, a principal volume delineated by a space
2.0 x 1.8 x 1.5 cm. Thin watery liquid is enclosed. About
3.0 cm from one pole of the left kidney and 2.0 cm from the pelvis,

ROUGH DRAFT 10 #68-513
SENATOR ROBERT F. KENNEDY
JUNE 6, 1968

is a well-circumscribed and slightly raised subcapsular nodule having a uniform yellow matrix and measuring 1.0 x 0.9 x 0.9 cm overall. The cut surface of this yellow nodule protrudes slightly. The lesion is about 6.0 cm from the just-described retention cyst. Intervening matrix of the left kidney shows no focal change. The renal pelves of both kidneys and both ureters show no induration, dilatation, or exudates. Ureteral implantation is noted to be normal in the urinary bladder. About 8 ml of faintly amber-pink cloudy urine is contained. There is no focal lesion of the urothelial lining. There are no urinary calculi.

The prostate is symmetrical with a transverse diameter of 3.5 cm. Cut surfaces show no distinct nodular areas and no focal lesion. there are scattered areas of vascular engorgement near the origin of the prostatic urethra. A slightly gritty texture is found on the cut surfaces of the prostate. Scattered discrete calculi up to 2 mm in diameter are found.

The seminal vesicles are of normal configuration and contain a small amount of green-gray mucoid material.

Both testes are present in the scrotal sac and are of normal size and consistence. Tubular stringing is readily accomplished. No evidence of hydrocele is present.

DIGESTIVE SYSTEM:

The esophagus is lined by smooth pale-gray epithelium following the usual longitudinal folds. No focal lesion is found. The stomach has a wall of average thickness and a smooth serosal surface. There is mild gaseous dilatation. No evidence of hemorrhage or ulceration is found in the gastric mucosa. Within the lumen is about 500 ml of cloudy gray watery mucoid material in which no discrete food fragments are found. A small amount of hemorrhagic material is inadvertently admitted into the gastric content as the latter is secured for possible toxicological studies. The duodenum, small intestine, and colon show no gross abnormalities of mucosal or serosal elements. The mesenteric lymph nodes are not remarkable.

ENDOCRINE ORGANS:

The pituitary is intrinsically symmetrical and within the normal limits of size, as is the sella turcica.

The thyroid is symmetrical and not enlarged; cut surfaces of the brown-red colloid matrix shows no focal change.

ROUGH DRAFT   11   #68-57.
                                         SENATOR ROBERT F. KENNEDY
                                         JUNE 6, 1968

The adrenals total 13.5 gm and are of normal configuration.
Multiple cut surfaces show no focal lesion. The thickness of
the cortex is little more than one millimeter. The medullary
tissue is not remarkable.

MUSCULOSKELETAL SYSTEM:

The bony framework is well developed and well retained. No
evidence of a diffuse osseous lesion is found. The fracture
of the right orbital plate and of other components of the base
of the skull are described in detail elsewhere in this report,
mainly the Neuropathology section. No additional evidence of
recent fracture or other focal trauma is demonstrated in the
skeleton.

The clinically described and radiologically documented old
fractures are not dissected.

The vertebral marrow is a uniform brown-red, showing no focal
change.

Cut surfaces of muscles studied, in areas apart from the trauma,
show no abnormality.

HEAD AND NERVOUS SYSTEM:

Additional features revealed by reflection of the scalp include
a fairly well demarcated area of non-recent hemorrhagic discoloration, about 1.5 cm in greatest dimension, in the left
parietal-occipital region. No associated galeal hemorrhage is
demonstrated.

A complete description of the brain in situ and following removal,
before and after fixation, will be found elsewhere in this report.

The cerebrospinal fluid is blood tinged.

Abundant and freshly clotted but drying blood is found at the
right external auditory canal, extending outward to the lateral
interstices of the external ear. No evidence of hemorrhage is
found at the left ear.

The spinal cord is taken for further evaluation by the Neuropathologist. At time of removal of the cord, a small amount of
cervical epidural hemorrhage is noted. There is no evidence, on
preliminary inspection, of avulsion of roots leading to the right
brachial plexus.

ROUGH DRAFT   12   #68-5731
                                        SENATOR ROBERT F. KENNEDY
                                        JUNE 6, 1968

Those portions of peripheral nervous system exposed by the extent
of dissection indicated above in general show no abnormality.

SPECIMENS SUBMITTED:

Organs and body fluids enumerated elsewhere in this report, for
the purpose of toxicological examinations.

Tissue sections for microscopic examination as denoted in other
portions of this report.

Other specimens for special studies as described in accompanying
reports.

COMPLETION OF AUTOPSY:

The above-described dissections, postmortem radiographic studies,
the autopsy photographs, and the placing of retained specimens in
suitably labeled containers, were all completed by 9:15 A.M., this
date. The body was then released to the embalmers who had arrived
to perform their functions.

THOMAS T. NOGUCHI, M.D.
CHIEF MEDICAL EXAMINER-CORONER

JOHN E. HOLLOWAY, M.D.
DEPUTY MEDICAL EXAMINER

ABRAHAM T. LU, M.D.
DEPUTY MEDICAL EXAMINER

JEH::AMJ::C
9/25/68

Martin Luther King, Jr.

Born: January 15, 1929, Atlanta, Georgia
Died: April 4, 1968, Memphis, Tennessee
Cause of Death: Assassination

The Reverend Dr. Martin Luther King, Jr. was one of the most prominent leaders of the civil rights movement and the recipient of the Nobel Peace Prize in 1964 for his call to combat racial inequality through nonviolence. Dr. King led the march on Washington where he delivered his famous "I have a dream" speech. He led various civil rights movements including bus boycotts, opposition to the Vietnam War, and the Poor People's Campaign. He was assassinated while in Memphis to support the sanitation workers strike. Escaped convict James Earl Ray confessed to the assassination; however, he later recanted his confession, saying the murder was the result of a conspiracy. The jury of a 1999 civil trial found a man called Loyd Jowers to be complicit in a conspiracy to assassinate King.

TENNESSEE DEPARTMENT OF PUBLIC HEALTH

OFFICE OF THE CHIEF MEDICAL EXAMINER
915 Madison Avenue
Memphis, Tennessee 38103

CASE NO. A68-252

COUNTY Shelby

AUTOPSY REPORT

NAME OF DECEDENT   Martin Luther King, Jr.   RACE N   SEX M   AGE 39

HOME ADDRESS   Atlanta, Georgia

COUNTY MEDICAL EXAMINER   J. T. Francisco, M.D.

    ADDRESS   Memphis, Tennessee

DISTRICT ATTORNEY GENERAL   Phil A. Canale

    ADDRESS   Memphis, Tennessee

ANATOMICAL DIAGNOSIS   Gunshot wound to body and face with:
    Fracture of mandible
    Laceration vertebral artery, jugular vein and sub-
        clavian artery, right.
    Laceration of spinal cord (lower cervical, upper
                            thoracic).
    Intrapulmonary hematoma, apex, right upper lobe

CAUSE OF DEATH   Gunshot wound to spinal column, lower cervical, upper
    thoracic

NARRATIVE OF FINDINGS   Death was the result of a gunshot wound to the
    chin and neck with a total transection of the lower cervical and
    upper thoracic spinal cord and other structures in the neck. The
    direction of the wounding was from front to back, above downward and
    from right to left. The severing of the spinal cord at this level
    and to this extent was a wound that was fatal very shortly after its
    occurrence.

        The purpose of this report is to provide a certified opinion to the County Medical
    Examiner and the District Attorney General. The facts and findings to support these con-
    clusions are filed with the office of the State Medical Examiner.

DATE   April 11, 1968   SIGNATURE   _____ M.D.
                            J. T. Francisco
        ADDRESS   915 Madison Avenue-Memphis, Tennessee

TENNESSEE DEPARTMENT OF PUBLIC HEALTH - 168

Form 366

THE CITY OF MEMPHIS HOSPITALS
AUTOPSY PROTOCOL

Autopsy No. A68-252   Service Med. Ex.   Hospital No.

Name Martin Luther King, Jr.   Age 39   Race Negro   Sex Male

Unknown—Approximately

Date of Admission   DOA   Date and Hour of Death 4-4-68   P.M.

Date and Hour of Autopsy   4-4-68   10:45 P.M.

Pathologist Drs.Sprunt and Francisco   Assistant

Checked by   Date Completed   4-11-68

FINAL PATHOLOGICAL DIAGNOSIS

PRIMARY SERIES:

   I. Distant gunshot wound to body and face
      A. Fracture of right mandible
      B. Laceration of vertebral artery, jugular vein and subclavian artery, right
      C. Fracture of spine (T-1, C-7)
      D. Laceration of spinal cord (lower cervical, upper thoracic)
      E. Submucosal hemorrhage, larynx
      F. Intrapulmonary hematoma, apex right upper lobe

SECONDARY SERIES:

   1. Remote scars as described
   2. Pleural adhesions
   3. Fatty change liver, moderate
   4. Arteriosclerosis, moderate
   5. Venous cut-downs
   6. Tracheostomy

LABORATORY FINDINGS:

  Blood Alcohol - 0.01%

A60-252

EXTERNAL EXAMINATION OF THE BODY

This is a well developed, well nourished Negro male measuring 69 1/2 inches in length and weighing approximately 140 pounds. The hair is black, the eyes are brown. There is a line mustache present.

EXTERNAL MARKS AND SCARS

There is a remote midline scar present in the center of the chest and a remote scar present extending to the right axilla measuring 6 inches in length. There is a sutured vertical surgical incision present at the base of the neck. A sutured incision is present in the right chest at the anterior axillary line. Three needle punctures are present in the precordium, having no hemorrhage present surrounding the area. There are blood splatters present on the palm and dorsum of the right hand. A remote scar is present in the right lateral chest. Sutured incisions are present in the left ante cubital fossa, one that is obliquely directed measuring 2 inches in length, one that is horizontally directed measuring 1 inch in length. There are two sutured incisions present on the medial aspect of the left ankle. The superior incision measuring 2 inches in length, the inferior incision measuring 1/4 inch in length. There is an extensive excavating lesion affecting the right side of the face beginning at a point 1 inch lateral to the right corner of the mouth and 1/2 inch inferior to the right corner of the mouth that measures approximately 3 inches in length. At the superior aspect of this gaping wound there is an abrasion collar that measures 1/8 of an inch in maximum thickness, having brownish discoloration present at the superior margin. Adjacent to this area there is extensive laceration of the soft tissues of the face with a fracturing of the right side of the mandible. A re-approximation of the tissues reveals the laceration to extend to the base of the neck and into the base of the neck with intervening skin unaffected in this area. The second penetrating wound at the base of the neck in the superior aspect of the chest measures 3 inches in length. The missile path is through the external jugular vein and vertebral artery. There is a penetration into the lateral aspect of the base of the neck into the upper thoracic and lower cervical cord totally severing the lower cervical and upper thoracic cord passing through the spinal column at the level of C7 and T1 into the posterior aspect of the back. The bullet is removed from the posterior aspect of the back, 56 inches superior to the right heel and 55 1/2 inches superior to the left heel, 3 inches to the left of the midline of the spine in the medial aspect of the left scapula. The entrance wound is 61 1/2 inches superior to the right heel and 59 inches superior to the right heel with the head turned and positioned so that the wound in the face corresponds with the path of the missile into the neck and spine. The total thickness from the entrance wound to the posterior aspect of the back is 6 1/2 inches in thickness. The angle of the penetrating wound is approximately 45° from a sagittal plane at an angle from right to left inferiorly and anterior to posteriorly at about a 30° angle with a coronal plane.

SECTION

The abdominal panniculus measures an inch in maximum thickness. The skeletal muscles are red and fibrillary. There is scarring present over the right anterior-superior chest with pleural adhesions present in this area.

continued...........

BODY CAVITIES

There is approximately 25cc. of blood present within the right thoracic cavity and some subpleural hemorrhage that is present affecting the right and the left in the posterior apex. The missile did not enter the right pleural cavity.

GROSS DESCRIPTION OF THE ORGANS

HEART: The heart weighs 450 grams. The myocardium is pale brown. The valvular surfaces reveal no significant changes. There is focal yellowing of the subendocardial areas affecting the left aspect of the interventricular septum. The right ventricle measures 5mm. in maximum thickness. The left ventricle measures 20mm. in maximum thickness. The coronary ostia originate in normal position and have a normal distribution over the epicardial surface. There is minimal intimal proliferation present. Focal yellow plaquing is present in the ascending aspect of the aortic arch but ulceration is not present. There is no significant dilatation affecting the chambers of the heart.

AORTA: Focal yellow plaques are present throughout the aorta but ulceration and calcification is not present. The great vessels originate normally. There is perivascular hemorrhage affecting the right carotid artery but no penetration of the wall. The right subclavian artery is lacerated.

ESOPHAGUS: Partially digested food fragments are present throughout the esophagus.

TRACHEA: Hemorrhagic mucoid material is present throughout the upper trachea.

LUNGS: The right lung weighs 360 grams. The left lung weighs 325 grams. There is diffuse congestion, consolidation and hemorrhage affecting the right upper lobe of the lung. Frothy fluid is expressable from the sectioned surface. There is minimal wrinkling of the pleura diffusely throughout the pulmonary parenchyma.

BRAIN: The brain weighs 1400 grams. There is some flattening of the gyri and narrowing of the sulci. The cerebral vessels are symmetrical. There is no subdural, epidural, or extradural hemorrhage present. There is no significant flattening throughout the cerebral vessels.

KIDNEYS: The kidneys weigh 175 grams on the left and 150 grams on the right. The capsular surface is smooth. The parenchyma is of normal coloration. The corticalmedullary junction is prominent.

continued......

Page 3.....
ACE-252

PANCREAS:
The pancreatic parenchyma is well preserved. The lobular pattern is preserved. There is no fatty infiltration present. The parenchyma is yellowish-grey.

LARYNX:
There is diffuse hemorrhage present throughout the superior larynx along with submucosal hemorrhage that is present within the intra-laryngeal areas. There is a tracheostomy perforation that is superior to the thyroid penetrating to the right of the pyramidal lobe.

THYROID:
No significant changes.

SPLEEN:
The spleen weighs 80 grams. The capsule is wrinkled. There is no capsular thickening present. The follicles are not prominent.

STOMACH:
The stomach contains approximately 10cc. of partially digested food fragments. There is no ulceration present.

DUODENUM:
No significant changes.

GALLBLADDER:
The gallbladder contains approximately 5cc. of light green bile. No stones are present.

LIVER:
The liver weighs 1600 grams. The parenchyma is pale yellowish-brown. The lobular pattern is accentuated. The parenchyma is quite soft.

BLADDER:
There is approximately 25cc. of cloudy yellow urine present.

PROSTATE:
No significant gross abnormalities are present.

COLON:
The appendix is present. The colonic contents is normal.

SMALL INTESTINE:
There is alternately liquid and gaseous distention present throughout the small intestine.

ADRENALS:
The adrenals are in normal position and weigh 8 grams together. The cortex is bright yellow. The medulla is grey.

Special Chart 11

Autopsy No.________

A68-252

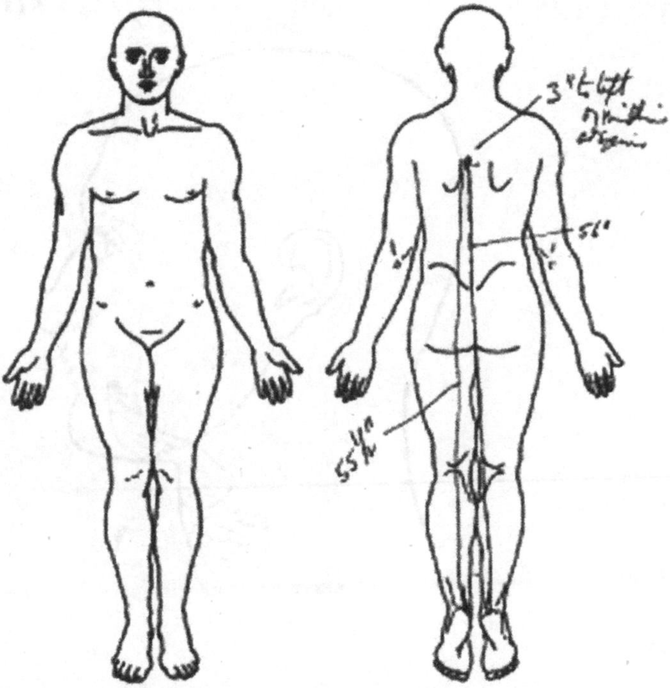

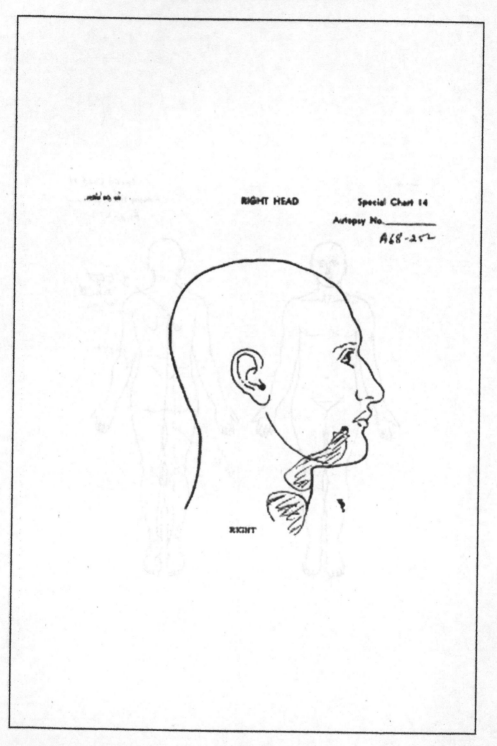

RIGHT HEAD   Special Chart 14

Autopsy No.

A68-252

RIGHT

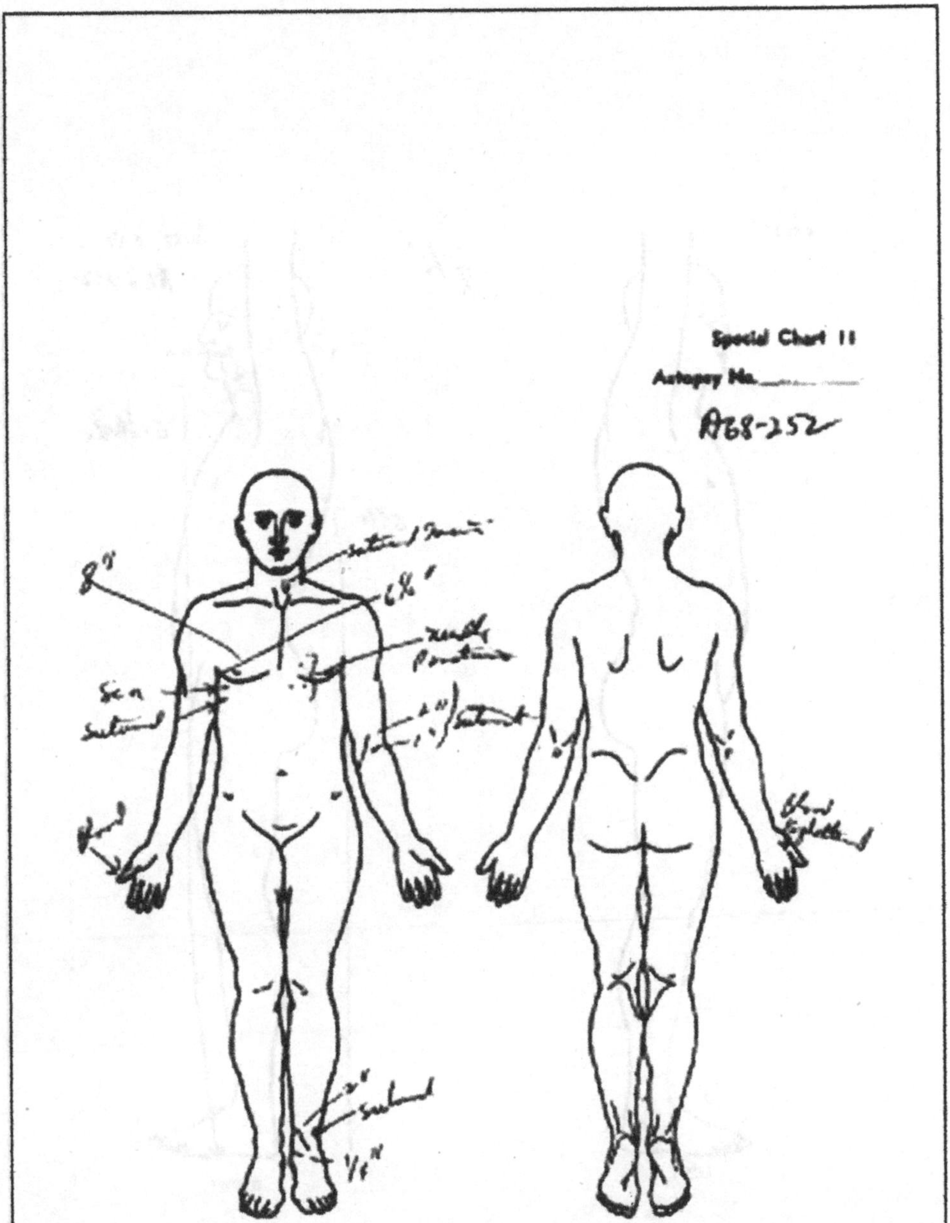
Special Chart 11
Autopsy No.
A68-252

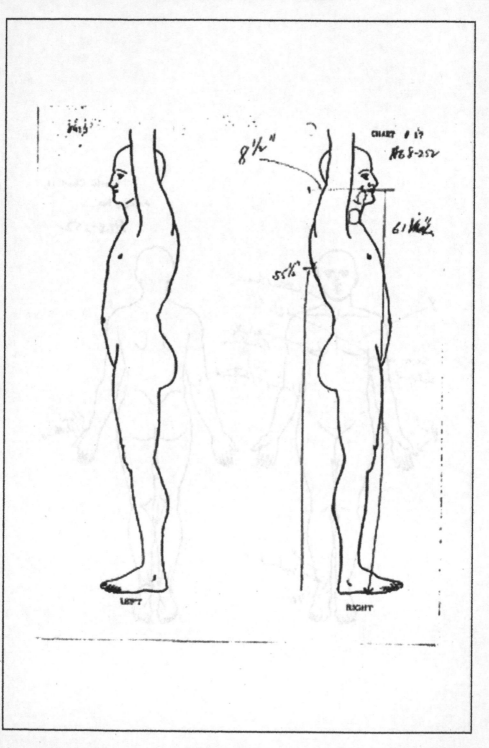

A68-252   MICROSCOPIC SUMMARY

LUNG: Focal areas of intra-alveolar hemorrhage are present
                throughout. Otherwise the alveoli are well preserved
                without hyperdistention or collapse. There is a loss
                of bronchial epithelium free within the lumens of the
                bronchioles. The pulmonary vessels reveal no signifi-
                cant changes.

PANCREAS: The pancreatic parenchyma is well preserved. The islets
                and acini are well preserved. There is minimal conges-
                tion present but no fibrosis or hemorrhage.

KIDNEY: The glomeruli and tubules are well preserved. There is
                no parenchymal fibrosis evident or vascular prolifera-
                tion present. The tubules are filled with eosinophilic
                material. There is no collapse of the tubular lumens.

THYROID: The follicles are uniform and regular. There is a small
                quantity of extravasation of mature erythrocytes into
                peri-follicular locations. Cellular inflammatory reac-
                tion is not present. There is no margination of poly-
                morphonuclear leucocytes within the areas of hemorrhage.

LIVER: There is diffuse cytoplasmic vacuolation throughout the
                hepatic cytoplasm being distributed throughout the lo-
                bules and in both pericentral and periportal locations.
                A small number of mononuclear cells are present in por-
                tal areas. There is some variation in size, shape of
                the hepatic nuclei. The vacuoles that are present are
                irregular in size, being numerous in some cells and
                being single large vacuoles in others with a disruption
                of cytoplasmic borders in some.

ADRENAL: There is congestion of the inner cortical zones of the
                adrenal. The cytoplasm is otherwise well maintained.
                The cortico-medullary ratio is maintained.

SPLEEN: The follicles are present but without secondary reactive
                centers. There is some congestion of the pulp but focal
                hemorrhage is not present.

HEART: The myocardial fibers are well preserved. The nuclei
                are regular. Fibrosis is not present throughout the
                myocardium and cellular inflammatory reaction is not
                present. The atrium reveals no significant changes.

SKIN: There is dermal hemorrhage present but no accumulation
                of polymorphonuclear leucocytes. Blackened debris is
                present throughout the hemorrhagic area of the dermis
                having no identifiable form. There is pronounced eo-
                sinophilia of the collagen bundles. There is hemorrhage
                into the dermal layers with an alteration in the tinc-
                torial properties of the epithelium with focal fragmen-
                tation of the epithelium adjacent to the area of dermal
                hemorrhage.

                                                    Continued..........

AA6-252 Continued.................
MICROSCOPIC SUMMARY   Page 2.

CORONARY: There is moderate intimal proliferation along with an
                  extra cellular deposition of lipid within the sub-
                  intimal areas along with lipid filled macrophages pre-
                  sent in this location. Small foci of perivascular mono-
                  nuclear cells are present in the regions of most pro-
                  nounced intimal proliferation.

PROSTATE: The glandular elements are well preserved without any
                  significant increase in collagenous connective tissue.
                  Inflammatory reaction is not present.

BILL OF COST

4-2-68
DATE

Charges for autopsy performed on the body of

Martin L. King   4-5-68
Name of Decedent   Date of Autopsy

by order of the District Attorney General, Shelby County, Tennessee
under provisions of Tennessee Code Annotated, 38-706.

J. T. Francisco, M. D.
Physician Performing Autopsy

Malcolm X

Given Name: Malcolm Little
Born: May 19, 1925, Omaha, Nebraska
Died: February 21, 1965, New York, New York
Cause of Death: Assassination

Malcolm X was an avid leader in the civil rights movement. He believed in furthering the cause "by any means necessary." He started his career as a member of the Nation of Islam and an advocate for black supremacy. As time went on, he left the Nation of Islam and began advocating for an end to segregation and an increase in equality for all. He received constant death threats, and he emphasized his willingness to defend himself and his family. He was assassinated during a speech in the Audubon Ballroom in New York City. The autopsy report notes his body sustained twenty-one gunshot wounds.

P.D. 5 (Rev. 8-63)

SUPPLEMENTARY COMPLAINT REPORT [DO NOT FOLD THIS REPORT]

U.F. 61 File No.

Complainant's Surname   First Name   Telephone No.

People State of New York

Complainant's Address   Apt. No.

(Malcom Little(X))

Date and Time Reported on U.F. 61: Feb. 21, 1965 3.10 PM   19. Pct. **34**   22. U.F. 61 No. **993**

Day, Date and Time of Occurrence: Sunday Feb. 21, 1965 3.10 PM   27. Pct. **29**   26. C.C.D. No. **26615**

36. F.D. Code **110**

FOLLOWING QUESTIONS PERTAIN TO THIS COMPLAINT REPORT	Answer Yes	No

Crime or Offense as Classified on U.F. 61: **Homicide (Gun)**   Div. Sect. Ser. **1022 -**

Crime or Offense Charged to: **do.**   Status of Case **Active**

Date of This Report: **Feb. 22, 1965**

Subject: AUTOPSY OF MALCOM LITTLE (X) M.N. 39 YRS, HOTEL THERESA, 128 WEST 128 STREET.

1.   Autopsy performed at Bellevue Morgue, by Chief Medical Examiner Dr. Helpern. Cause of death: Multiple shotgun and other calibre bullet wounds of Heart and aorta.

2.   Bullet wound entries:
   left chest one inch above left nipple.
   1½ inches to right of left nipple.
   2½ inches to right of left nipple.
   4 inches to left of right nipple
   1½ inches to left of mid line.
   5 inches up from navel to midline.
   3½ inches down from left nipple.
   right chin.
   5 inches above right knee.
   left ankle inoutside.
   left thigh inside.
   left thigh front 4 inches up from knee.
   Web between thumb and index finger right hand.
   right forearm.
   left bicep.

Investigating Officer's Name (Typed): **Peter McPartland**   Det. Shield No. **875**   Command **12N13**

**THIS IS A NEW YORK CITY GOVERNMENT RECORD
AND SHOULD BE ACCURATELY COMPLETED.**

From PRESBYTERIAN HOSPITAL Hospital,

New York, FEBRUARY, 1965 19

To the MEDICAL EXAMINER OF THE CITY OF NEW YORK:

STATEMENT and particulars of the Death of... Body identified as Malcolm "X"

Residence	Admitted 21 day of Feb. 19 65
Age _____ years _____ months _____ days	at 3 15 o'clock P M
Color N Occupation	By _____
Single, Married or Widowed	Ambulance
Place of Birth	From _____
Father's Name	With police
Father's Birthplace	
Mother's Name	
Mother's Birthplace	
How long in United States	
How long in N. Y. City	Examined by John A. Collins M.D.

SYMPTOMS, SUBJECTIVE AND OBJECTIVE: Clinical, X-ray and Laboratory findings:

Pt arrived without pulse, respiration, any spontaneous
respiration, flaccid, pupils dilated and unresponsive. Closed
chest cardiac massage and started intubation ineffective
Direct opened revealing pleural cavity full of blood
multiple holes in myocardium, aspirated air holes
from lung during positive pressure ventilation. Multiple holes

Details not known other than one police officer's
statement that an automatic gun was used.

@ thoracotomy with cardiac massage

Death took place on the 21 day of Feb 19 65 at 3 30 P M

REMARKS:
Pt did not respond at all to resuscitative measures
No cardiac filling during massage. Pronounced dead
3 30 PM although pt was actually dead on arrival.

John P. Coll M.D.
House Surgeon Physician

Page 2

Bullet wound exits
Right palm
left middle back
upper right thigh
3bullet slaps and 1 crease on right knee upward

Bullets recovered at this time
3 "0" buck pellets left chest
3 "0" buck pellets right side back
1 45 Cal entry thru left ankel
1 9MM Cal entry front left thigh
1 9MM Cal entry left inside thigh

autopsy to be completed 9/:265

Peter McPartland
Det. 875 10MB

Leo Ryan

Given Name: Leo Joseph Ryan, Jr.
Born: May 5, 1925, Lincoln, Nebraska
Died: November 18, 1978, Port Kaituma, Guyana
Cause of Death: Assassination

Leo Ryan was a United States Congressman. In November 1978, he was sent to Jonestown, Guyana to visit the Peoples Temple commune led by American church leader Jim Jones. He traveled with some relatives of Jonestown residents and media crews. While in Jonestown, Ryan met several members of the congregation who wanted to return to America. Ryan took these members with him as he left. At the airport, Ryan's delegation was met with gunfire from the guards of Jonestown. Five members of the congressman's delegation were killed, including Ryan himself. Reportedly worried about the US government's possible retaliation to the shooting, an unnerved Jones encouraged his followers to drink poisoned Flavor Aid. The death count was 909 people. To this day, Ryan is the only United States Congressman to be assassinated while in office.

CENTRAL MEDICAL LABORATORY

P.M. No. 729/78

NAME:...???...???...........AGE:...37.???...SEX:...Male. ???? ??????????...

PLACE OF P.M. EXAMINATION: PHG Mortuary............DATE: 20/11/78 TIME: 9.00.a.m.

DIED: 18/11/78.............TIME: Not known. PLACE: Port.Kaituma. North.West.Dist.
                                                                       -rict.

IDENTIFICATION: James T. Schollaert, c/o U.S. Embassy, Georgtown.....................

WITNESS: Assistant Superintendent, Law, C.I.D. Headquarters.

EXTERNAL EXAMINATION: The body is that of a male of Caucasian descent,
measuring 6ft. 2 ins. It was fully clothed as follows:

(1) Long sleeved shirt (light-green).

(2) Blue striped pants held in position by a buckle.

(3) Brown pair of shoes.

(4) Pair of socks.

The shirt, pants and shoes were blood-stained. There were tears of
varying diameters in the pants (3) in the (R) buttock and (2) in the
(L) buttock; in front of pants 6 cms. tear on (L) groin area. The
pockets (2) in back on the pants were turned inside out.

(1) In the (L) front pocket there was an electioneering pin of
Congressman Leo Ryan.

The body was identified by:-

James T. Schollaert Esq. of the U.S. Embassy in Georgtown, Guyana.

EXTERNAL EXAMINATION:

(1) Perforated wound (L) groin 2½ cms. elliptical in outline and 1½ cms.
wide at its greatest/running downwards in line with the (L) inguinal
ligament and parallel to it.

(2) Above wound (1) was another perforated wound 1c.m. x ½ c.m. above
wound (1).

(3) Linear contusion 2 cms. above wound No.2 running across abdomen for
6 c.ms.

(4) Twelve c.ms. above wound No.3. perforated wound 2c.ms. by 1 c.m. with
contusion parallel to upper and lower ellipse. Wound is on the (L)
lower aspect of the abdomen 10 c.ms. lateral to umbilicus.

(5) There was a raised area under the skin at the (L) subcostal area
15 c.ms. above wound No.4. Incision revealed a metal object
(deformed bullet).

(6) Perforated wound on (L) chest 6 c.ms. above (L) nipple wound 2c.ms.x
1 c.m.

(7) There was a raised area under skin parallel with wound number (6),
3c.ms. from mid sternum metal object removed (deformed bullet).

(8) Perforating wound. (L) upper limb medial aspect 3c.ms. by 1½ c.m.s.
6 c.ms. below axilla. Contusions around wound with 2 parallel cuts
in the skin above and below the perforating wound 1½ c.ms. one above
2 c.ms. the one below.

(9) Two perforating wounds on the (R) aspect of the neck 0.9c.m. diameter
each, the lower one 1½ c.ms. from tip of (R) ear the upper one 11c.ms.
from tip of (R) ear.

(10) Massive lacerated wound (R) side of neck 6c.ms. Muscles of neck
exposed long upper end of wound 2½ c.ms. from tip of ear (R) medial
to wound irregular abrasion extending from neck to angle of jaw.
Under angle of jaw perforating wound 3c.ms. by 1½ c.ms.; bone of angle
of jaw exposed.

(11) (L) lateral aspect of shoulder perforating wound 3c.ms. by 2½c.ms.
bony fragments at orifice - wound is 3c.ms. from root of neck.

(12) On the (L) neck mastoid lateral aspect perforating wound 4c.ms.
by 3c.ms. bony fragment protruding from wound. Wound is 2 c.ms. from

.lp of (R) ear.

(13) Back of (L) ear perforating wound 3c.mm. by 3c.mm. The posterior attachment of the ear was detached.

(14) (L) aspect of parieto-occipital region of skull, compound comminuted fracture excavating scalp with herniation and protrusion of Brain. Brain substance blood-stained oozing out.

(15) Puncture wound mid position of (L) thigh posterior aspect 26 c.mm. from popliteal fossa.

(16) Perforating wound 3c.mm. by 1c.m. on fold of (R) buttocks.

(17) 12 punctured wounds of varying sizes, both buttocks.

(18) (R) loin two areas of contusion.

(19) Contusion of (R) scotal.

(20) Bilateral ecchymosis with bilateral subconjunctival haemorrhages.

(21) Perforating wound (R) posterior lateral aspect of arm in line with shoulder joint wound 1c.m. diameter.

(22) On the (R) thigh 8 c.mm. below the inguinal ligament two parallel linear contusions 3c.mm. and 2c.mm. in length each and 1½c.mm. from each other.

INTERNAL EXAMINATION:

OESOPHAGUS: Some amount of congestion upper ⅓ with large amount of submucous haemorrhage between thyroid cornua and hyoid bone.

TRACHEA & BRONCHI: Congestion in upper aspect with blood-stained froth in Bronchii.

THORACIC CAVITY:

LUNGS: (R) was adherent to the pericardium and there were some pleural reaction at base. Small puncture wound in lower lobe.
(L) lung perforation of the basal lobe bony fragments in substance of (L) lung.

HEART: Some increase of epicardial fat - normal in size. Myocardial normal; Coronary vessels patent and normal. Arch of aorta normal in appearances.

The chest cavity contained 125 ml. of blood on the (R) side and 200 ml. on the (L) side. Fracture of the 2nd and 3rd ribs on the (L) side.

ABDOMEN:

STOMACH: signs of gastritis (patchy) rugae normal - stomach empty except for mucous.

LIVER: Some petechial subcapsular haemorrhage other wise pale in appearances.

GALL BLADDER: No gall stones.

PANCREAS: Normal appearances.

KIDNEYS: Normal appearances except slight increase of hilar fat.

BLADDER: Filled with urine straw coloured.

INTESTINES: Normal appearances.

APPENDIX: Normal.

HEAD AND NECK:

SKULL: Small pieces of the skull on the left side were missing, in the parietal and occipital areas. There was a compound comminuted fracture of the vault extending from the (L) fronto parieto-region and extending upwards and backwards in-to the parietal and occipital region and involving the bones of the (R) aspect of the vault. The bones of the base were also fractured in a comminuted manner - all the bones of the anterior, middle and posterior cranial fossae bilateral - fracture lines extending in all directions.

BRAIN: Only the Cerebellum was in the skull all the cerebrum had fallen out. Cerebellum shows some congestion.

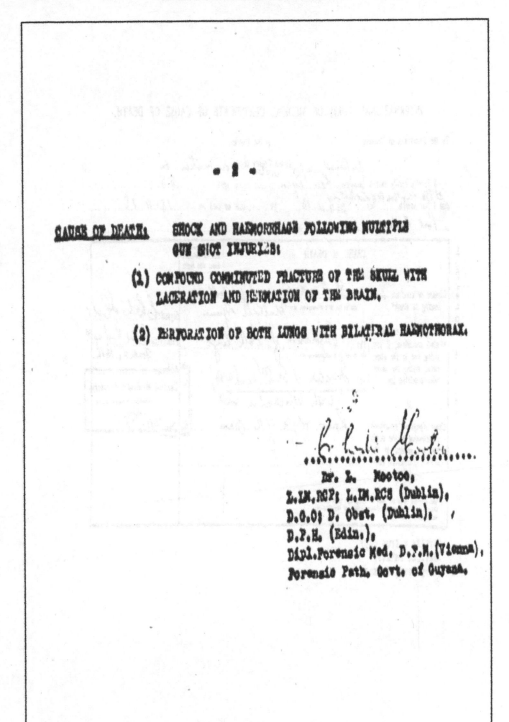

- 2 -

<u>CAUSE OF DEATH:</u> SHOCK AND HAEMORRHAGE FOLLOWING MULTIPLE
GUN SHOT INJURIES:

(1) COMPOUND COMMINUTED FRACTURE OF THE SKULL WITH
LACERATION AND HERNIATION OF THE BRAIN.

(2) PERFORATION OF BOTH LUNGS WITH BILATERAL HAEMOTHORAX.

Dr. L. Mootoo,
L.M.RCP; L.M.RCS (Dublin),
D.O.O; D. Obst. (Dublin),
D.P.H. (Edin.),
Dipl.Forensic Med. D.F.M.(Vienna),
Forensic Path. Govt. of Guyana.

INTERNATIONAL FORM OF MEDICAL CERTIFICATE OF CAUSE OF DEATH.

To the Registrar of Division _____ in the District,

I hereby certify that I _____ Leo Ryan _____ aged _____ 53

that I last saw h _____ on _____ 24.11.78 _____ 19 ___, that he died on _____ 18.11.78

at _____ Port Kaituma _____ and that the cause of h _____ death was _____

CAUSE of DEATH	Approximate interval between onset and death
Disease or condition directly leading to death* (a) Shock and Haemorrhage following — due to (or as a consequence of) Multiple injuries	
Antecedent causes. Morbid conditions, if any, giving rise to the above cause, stating the underlying condition last (b) Perforation of both lungs due to (or as a consequence of)	
(c) Fracture of Skull (multiple) with laceration and haemorrhage of the brain	
II Other significant conditions contributing to the death but not related to the disease or condition causing it	

Signed _____

Prof. Title _____

Address Central Medical Laboratory, Georgetown, Guyana

Date 30.11.78

Certify a true copy
American Embassy
Georgetown, Guyana

Adolf Hitler

Born: April 20, 1889, Braunau am Inn, Austria
Died: April 30, 1945, Berlin, Germany
Cause of Death: Apparent Cyanide Poisoning

Adolf Hitler was the leader of the Nazi party and the cause of the Second World War. The man who once aspired to be an artist in his younger years was ultimately responsible for the death of millions of people both in concentration camps and in battle. During the war, Hitler was a powerful and charismatic leader, and the German Army followed his every order. He spent most of the end of his life in a bunker before committing suicide along with his new wife and long-time partner Eva Braun. After his death, his body was doused with gasoline and burned, making it difficult to identify the body.

Text of Autopsy Report on Hitler Prepared After .

Following is the text, as printed in "The Death of Adolf Hitler" by Lev A. Bezymenski, of the official Soviet autopsy report on the Nazi dictator:

From "The Death of Adolf Hitler" by Lev A. Bezymenski. Copyright © 1968 by Christian Wegner Copyright © 1968 by Christian Wegner English translation copyright © 1968 by Harcourt, Brace & World, Inc.

DOCUMENT NO. 12: CONCERNING THE FORENSIC EXAMINATION OF A MALE CORPSE DISFIGURED BY FIRE (HITLER'S BODY)

Berlin-Buch, 8.V., 1945
Mortuary CAFS¹ No. 496

The Commission consisting of Chief Expert, Forensic Medicine, First Byelorussian Front, Medical Service, Lieutenant Colonel F. I. Shkaravski; Chief Anatomist, Red Army, Medical Service, Lieutenant Colonel N. A. Krayevski; Acting Chief Anatomical Pathologist, First Byelorussian Front, Medical Service, Major A. Y. Marants; Army Expert, Forensic Medicine, Third Shock Army, Medical Service, Major Y. I. Boguslavski; and Army Anatomical Pathologist, Third Shock Army, Medical Service, Major Y. V. Gulkevich, on orders of the member of the Military Council First Byelorussian Front, Lieutenant General Telegin, performed the forensic-medical examination of a male corpse (presumably the corpse of Hitler).

Results of the examination:

A. External Examination

The remains of a male corpse disfigured by fire were delivered in a wooden box (Length 163 cm., Width 55 cm., Height 53 cm.). On the body was found a piece of yellow jersey, 25 x 8 cm., charred around the edges, resembling a knitted undervest.

In view of the fact that the corpse is greatly damaged, it is difficult to gauge the age of the deceased. Presumably it lies between 50 and 60 years. The dead man's height is 165 cm. (the measurements are approximate since the tissue is charred), the right shinbone measures 39 cm. The corpse is severely charred and smells of burned flesh.

Part of the cranium is missing.¹

Parts of the occipital bone, the left temporal bone, the lower cheekbones, the nasal bones, and the upper and lower jaws are preserved. The burns are more pronounced on the right side of the cranium than on the left. In the brain cavity parts of the fire-damaged brain and of the dura mater are visible. On face and body the skin is completely missing; only remnants of charred muscles are preserved. There are many small cracks in the nasal bone and the upper jawbones. The tongue is charred, its tip is firmly locked between the teeth of the upper and lower jaws.

In the upper jaw there are nine teeth connected by a bridge of yellow metal (gold.) The bridge is anchored by pins on the second left and the second right incisor. This bridge consists of 4 upper incisors ([2 [1 1] 2]), 2 canine teeth (3 3), the first left bicuspid ([4], and the first and second right bicuspids (4 5), as indicated in the sketch. The first left incisor (1) consists of a white platelet, with cracks and a black spot on the porcelain (enamel) at the bottom. This platelet is inset into the visible side of the metal (gold) tooth. The second incisor, the canine tooth, and the left bicuspid, as well as the first and second incisors and the first bicuspid on the right, are the usual porcelain (enamel) dental plates, their posterior parts fastened to the bridge. The right canine tooth is fully capped by yellow metal (gold). The maxillary bridge is vertically sawed off behind the second left bicuspid (15). The lower jawbone lies loose in the singed oral cavity. The alveolar processes are broken in the back and have ragged edges. The front surface and the lower edge of the mandibula are scorched. On the front surface the charred prongs of dental roots are recognizable. The lower jaw consists of fifteen teeth, ten of which are artificial. The incisors (2 1 1 2) and the first right bicuspid (4]) are natural, exhibiting considerable wear on the masticating surface and considerably exposed necks. The dental enamel has a bluish shimmer and a dirty yellow coloration around the necks. The teeth to the left (4, 5, 7, and 8) are artificial, of yellow metal (gold), and consist of a bridge of gold crowns. The bridge is fastened to the third, the fifth (in the bridge, the sixth tooth), and the eighth tooth (in the bridge, the ninth tooth). The second bicuspid to the right (5) is topped by a crown of yellow metal (gold) which is linked to the right canine tooth by an arching plate. Part of the masticating surface and the posterior surface of the right canine tooth is capped by a yellow metal (gold) plate as part of the bridge. The first right molar is artificial, white, and secured by a gold clip connected with the bridge of the second bicuspid and the right incisor.

Splinters of glass, parts of the wall and bottom of a thin-walled ampule, were found in the mouth.

The neck muscles are charred, the ribs on the right side are missing, they are burned. The right side of the thorax and the abdomen are completely burned, creating a hole through which the right lung, the liver, and the intestines are open to view. The genital member is scorched. In the scrotum, which is singed but preserved, only the right testicle was found. The left testicle could not be found in the inguinal canal.

The right arm is severely burned, the ends of the bone of the upper arm and the bones of the lower arm are broken and charred. The dry muscles are black and partially brown; they disintegrate into separate fibers when touched. The remnants of the burned part (about two thirds) of the left upper arm are preserved. The exposed end of the bone of the upper arm is charred and protrudes from the dry tissue. Both legs, too, are charred. The soft tissue has in many places disappeared; it is burned and has fallen off. The bones are partially burned and have crumbled. A fracture in the right thighbone and the right shinbone were noted. The left foot is issuing.

B. Internal Examination

The position of the internal organs is normal. The lungs are black on the surface, dark red on the cut surface, and of fairly firm consistence. The mucous membrane of the upper respiratory tracts is dark red. The cardiac ventricles are filled with coagulated reddish-brown blood. The heart muscle is tough and looks like boiled meat. The liver is black on the surface and shows burns; it is of fairly firm consistence and yellowish brown on the cut surface. The kidneys are somewhat shrunken and measure 9 x 5 x 3.5 cm. Their capsule is easily detachable; the surface of the kidneys is smooth, the pattern effaced, they appear as if broiled. The bladder contains 5 cc. yellowish urine, its mucous membrane is gray. Spleen, stomach and intestines show severe burns and are nearly black in parts.

NOTE 1. The following objects taken from the corpse were handed over to the Smersh section of the Third Shock Army on May 8, 1945: (a) a maxillary bridge of yellow metal, consisting of 9 teeth; (b) a singed lower jaw, consisting of 15 teeth.

2. According to the record of the interrogation of Frau Käthe Heusermann it may be presumed that the teeth as well as the bridge described in the document are those of Chancellor Hitler.

3. In her talk with chief expert of forensic medicine, Lieutenant Colonel Shkaravski, which took place on May 11, 1945,¹ in the offices of CAFS No. 496, Frau Käthe Heusermann described the state of Hitler's teeth in every detail. Her description tallies with the anatomical data pertaining to the oral cavity of the unknown man whose burned corpse we dissected.

Appended: A test tube with glass splinters from an ampule which were found in the mouth of the body.

SHKARAVSKI
Chief Expert, Forensic Medicine, First Byelorussian Front, Medical Service, Lieutenant Colonel.

SHKARAVSKI
Chief Anatomical Pathologist, Medical Service, Red Army, Lieutenant Colonel.

—MARANTS
Acting Chief Anatomical Pathologist First Byelorussian Front, Medical Service, Major.

BOGUSLAVSKI
Army Expert, Forensic Medicine, Third Shock Army,

Soviet Inquiry

Medical Service,
Major.
GULKEVICH
Army Anatomical Pathologist,
Third Shock Army,
Medical Service,
Major.

Conclusion

Based on the forensic-medical examination of the partially burned corpse of an unknown man and the examination of other corpses from the same group, the Commission reaches the following conclusions:

1. *Anatomical characteristics of the body:*

Since the body parts are heavily charred, it is impossible to describe the features of the dead man. But the following could be established:

(a) Stature: about 165 cm. (one hundred sixty-five).

(b) Age (based on general development, size of organs, state of lower incisors and of the right bicuspid), somewhere between 50 and 60 years (fifty to sixty).

(c) The left testicle could not be found either in the scrotum or on the spermatic cord inside the inguinal canal, nor in the small pelvis.

(d) The most important anatomical finding for identification of the person are the teeth, with much bridgework, artificial teeth, crowns, and fillings (see documents).

2. *Cause of death:*

On the body, considerably damaged by fire, no visible signs of severe lethal injuries or illness could be detected.

The presence in the oral cavity of the remnants of a crushed glass ampule and of similar ampules in the oral cavity of other bodies, the marked smell of bitter almonds emanating from the bodies and the forensic-chemical test of internal organs which established the presence of cyanide compounds permit the Commission to arrive at the conclusion that death in this instance was caused by poisoning with cyanide compounds.

1. Abbreviation for *Chirurgisches Armeefeldlazarett.*

2. At a somewhat later date occipital parts of a cranium were found, quite probably belonging to Hitler's corpse.

3. I asked M. Krajewski how it was possible for this date to appear in an autopsy report that had been written on May 8. He explained that the report had originally been written by hand; only later was it decided to add the statements of Bezymenski, As mentioned above, the delay between evidence and conclusion is absolutely normal.

Vladimir Lenin

Given Name: Vladimir Illyich Ulyanov
Born: April 22, 1870, Ulyanovsk, Russia
Died: January 21, 1924, Gorki, Russia
Cause of Death: Stroke

Vladimir Lenin was the father of Russian Communism and the first Premier of the Soviet Union—a position he held until his death. Charged with sedition in 1895 he was sentenced without trial to exile in Siberia, after which he traveled Europe. He returned sporadically to assist with ongoing revolutions against the Russian ruling class. He became the leader of the Bolshevik party and the first Premier of the USSR. After dodging two serious assassination attempts, Lenin died at the age of fifty-three from a series of strokes. Some modern scientists disagree as to the cause of Lenin's death and speculate he died of complications from neurosyphilis. His body has been on display in Moscow's Red Square since 1924.

VLADIMIR LENIN'S AUTOPSY REPORT

REPORT

ON THE PATHOLOGICAL-ANATOMICAL EXAMINATION OF THE BODY OF VLADIMIR ILYICH ULYANOV (LENIN), CARRIED OUT ON JANUARY 22, 1924, STARTED AT 11 HOURS 10 MINUTES IN THE MORNING AND COMPLETED AT 3 HOURS 50 MINUTES.

The examination was carried out by Prof. A. 1. Abrikosov in the presence of Prof. 0. Foerster, Prof. V. N. Osipov, Prof. A. A. Deshin, Prof. B. S. Weissbrod, Prof. V. V. Bunak, Dr. F. A. Guetier, Dr. N. I. Elistratov, Dr. V. N. Rozanov, Dr. V. A. Obukh and the Commissar of Health of the R.S.F.S.R., N. A. Semashko.

EXTERNAL EXAMINATION

Body of an elderly man of normal build, adequately nourished. Small pig-mented spots are noted on the interior aspect of the chest (acne). Obvious signs of cadaveric hypostasis are noticeable on the posterior aspect of the trunk and the extremities. A linear cicatrice 2 c.m. in length is noted on the skin in the area of the anterior end of the clavicle. Another cicatrice having an irregular outline and measuring 2 x 1cm. is located on the external surface of the left shoulder area. A round cicatrice about 1cm. in diameter is found on the skin of the spine above the ridge of the scapula.

The outlines of the skeletal muscles are quite prominent.

In the left clavicle at the border of the lower and middle third there is a slight thickening of the bone (bone callus). Above this area in the posterior part of the deltoid muscle, a solid roundish body can be palpated. Upon incision of this area, a deformed bullet is found, enclosed in a capsule of connective tissue at the border between the subcutaneous fatty tissue and the deltoid muscle.

INTERNAL EXAMINATION

The cranial bones are unchanged. Upon removing the skull cover, a solid fusion of the dura mater with the inner surface of the cranium is noted, primarily along the course of the longitudinal sinus. The outer surface of the dura is dun, pale; pigmentation of a yellowish hue is noted in its left temporal and partly frontal area. The anterior part of the left hemisphere seems slightly collapsed in comparison with the corresponding part of the right hemisphere. The longitudinal sinus contains a small quantity of liquid blood. The internal surface of the dura mater is smooth, shiny-moist, easily separating from the underlying arachnoid membrane except in areas bordering the

saggital suture where there are areas of fusion in the region of the Pacchionian granulations. The dura of the base of the brain is normal; the basal sinuses contain liquid blood.

Brain. Weight immediately after removal, freed of the dura mater, is 1,340 Gm. In the left hemisphere: 1. in the anterior central gyrus; 2. in the area of the temporal and occipital pole; 3. in the area of the fissura paracentralis, and 4. in the area of the high gyri, there are noticeable signs of pronounced collapse of the cerebral surface. In the right hemisphere at the border between the temporal and occipital poles there are also two adjacent spots of collapse of the brain surface.

Above the described areas of collapse, the arachnoid membrane is dull, whitish, in places yellowish.

In some areas overlying the fissures, including even some parts where there is no collapse, whitish regions are noted in which the arachnoid is hard and appears thickened upon section.

Vessels of the base of the brain. Both arteriae vertibrales, and also the arteria basilaris are thickened, do not collapse; their walls are hard, irregularly thickened, of a whitish and in places yellowish color. Upon section, their lumen is seen to be extremely narrowed in places down to the dimensions of a tiny slit. Identical changes are also found in branches of the arteries in question (aa. cerebri posteriores). The internal carotid arteries, and also the anterior cerebral arteries are similarly hardened, with an irregularly thickened wall and in spots greatly narrowed lumen. The left internal carotid artery in its intracranial course has a completely obliterated lumen and upon section appears merely as a homogeneous solid whitish band. The left Sylvian (i.e. middle cerebral) artery is very thin, hardened, but upon section still shows a thin small slit.

Incision into the vermiform process of the cerebellar convolutions reveals no change of the brain tissue.

The fourth ventricle is free of any pathological contents.

Resection of the brain according to Flessing shows the brain ventricles, particularly on the left side, to be widened and containing a transparent fluid.

In the above noted areas of collapse of the brain there are areas of softening of the tissue, having a yellowish color and accompanied by formation of cyst-like structures filled with a turbid liquid. The areas of malacia involve the white as well as the gray brain matter. In other parts of the brain the tissue is moist, pale. The vascular plexus overlying the corpora quadrigemina is well irrigated with blood and there are signs of fresh hemorrhage in this area.

Upon removing the skin of the trunk the good development of the subcutaneous and fatty tissue is noted. The muscular system is adequately developed. The muscular tissue is of the usual maroon color.

The positions of the organs of the abdominal cavity are regular with the exception of the cecum which lies somewhat higher than is the norm. The omentum and the mesentery are rich in fat. The diaphragm runs from the level of the fourth rib on the right hand side to the fourth intercostal space on the left. At the region of the pulmonary apex, fibrous synechiae are visible in the right pleura. The left pleura also forms synechiae with the diaphragm in its lower part. No pathological conditions are noted in the region of the heart sac; the mediastinum shows no particular changes.

Heart. Dimensions: transverse 11 cm.; longitudinal 9 cm.; thickness 7 cm. The epicardial surface is smooth and shiny; under the epicardium, mainly in the area of the left ventricle, spotty accumulations of fat are noted. The semilunar valves of the aorta are somewhat thickened at their bases. The mitral valve shows some thickenings at its margins and whitish opaque spots of the anterior cusp. The valves of the right half of the heart are without special changes. The interior of the ascending aorta shows a small number of convex yellowish plaques. The wall thickness of the left ventricle is 13/4 cm. and of the right one % cm. The coronary arteries gape upon section; their walls are very bard and thickened; their lumen definitely constricted.
The inner surface of the descending aorta and also the inner surfaces of the large arteries in general show numerous very prominent yellowish plaques, partly undergoing ulceration and calcification.

Lungs. The right lung is of the normal size and configuration; soft throughout, feels spongy. Resection of pulmonary tissue reveals it full of blood, a foamy liquid appears. The pulmonary apex shows a small retracted scar. The left lung is of the usual size and shape, its consistency being soft throughout. The posterior inferior part of the upper lobe has a scar reaching from the surface to a depth of 1 cm. into the pulmonary tissue. At the apex of the lung there is a small fibrous thickening of the pleura.

The **spleen** is slightly enlarged and moderately filled with blood upon section. The form and size of the **liver** are normal. The border of the left lobe is somewhat sharp. The surface is smooth. Section reveals a moderate degree of so-called grapiness. The gall bladder and the bile ducts reveal no special changes.

The **stomach** is empty. Its walls are collapsed. The mucosa shows clearly visible and normally arranged creases. No special conditions to

be noted regarding the intestines.

The **kidneys** are of normal size. Their tissues are clearly identifiable and the substance of the cortex can be easily distinguished from the medullary part. The capsule comes off easily. The surface of the kidney is smooth with exception of some small areas where small depressions of the surface are present. The lumina of the renal arteries gape upon section.

GLANDS OF INTERNAL SECRETION

The pancreas is of normal size. No special changes are noted following its section.

No special changes are noted in the pituitary gland.

The adrenals are somewhat smaller than the norm, especially the left one; the cortical substance is rich in stipples; the medulla is pigmented and brownish in color.

ANOTOMICAL DIAGNOSIS

Generalized arteriosclerosis with pronounced degree of affection of the cerebral arteries.

Arteriosclerosis of the descending aorta.

Hypertrophy of the right ventricle of the heart.

Multiple foci of yellow cerebromalacia (based on vascular sclerosis) of the left cerebral hemisphere in a stage of resolution and of cystic change.

Fresh hemorrhage into the vascular plexus overlying the corpora quadrigemina.

Bone callus of the left clavicle.

Incapsulated bullet in the soft tissue of the left shoulder.

CONCLUSION

The basic disease of the deceased was disseminated vascular arteriosclerosis based on premature wearing out of the vessels (Abnutzungssklerose). The narrowing of the lumen of the cerebral arteries and the disturbances of the cerebral blood supply brought about focal softening of the brain tissue which can obtain all symptoms of the disease (paralysis, disturbance of speech). The

immediate cause of death was: 1. The aggravation of the circulatory disturbance of the brain, and 2.

Hemorrhage into the arachnoid pia mater in the area of the corpora quadrigemina.

Gorki, 22 January 1924

Prof. A. I. Abrikosov
Prof. Foerster
Prof. V. Osipov
Prof. V. Bunak
Prof. A. Deshin
Prof. B. Weissbrod
Dr. V. Obukh
Dr. Elistratov
Dr. V. Rozanov
N. Semashko

Simón Bolívar

Given Name: Simón José Antonio de la Santísima Trinidad Bolívar y Palacios Ponte y Blanco
Born: July 24, 1783, Caracas, Venezuela
Died: December 17, 1830, Santa Marta, Columbia
Cause of Death: Tuberculosis

Known as *El Libertador*, Simón Bolívar was a general of the Venezuelan army who lead the Venezuelan people to independence from the Spanish. In the course of his career, he also helped to liberate Colombia, Peru, and Ecuador from Spanish rule. Bolívar became president of Venezuela and soon he named himself dictator. After an assassination attempt, he resigned his presidency and committed himself to exile in Europe. He died before he made it across the ocean. Along with countless streets, towns, and monuments across South America, the country of Bolivia is named after him.

1. **Appearance of the body:** Cadaver in state of two thirds of decay; universal discolouration; swelling in the sacral region; musculature very little discoloured–normal consistency.

   - **Head:** The arachnoid vessels in the posterior half [were] slightly injected; the irregularities and convolutions of the cerebrum [were] covered by a brownish material with the consistency and transparency of gelatine; [there was] a little semi-red serous material beneath the dura mater; the rest of the cerebrum and cerebellum did not demonstrate any pathological abnormality.

   - **Chest:** Posteriorly and superiorly on both sides the pleurae were adherent as the result of semi-membranous material; there was hardening of the superior two thirds of each lung. The right, which was almost completely disorganised, looked like a fountain [sic] the colour of wine dregs studded with tubercles of different sizes – not very soft. The left lung although less disorganised showed the same tuberculous affection. Dividing this with a scalpel I found an irregular, angular, calcareous concretion about the size of a hazelnut.1 On opening the rest of the lungs with the instrument, I spilled some brown serous material which as a result of the pressure was rather frothy. The heart did not demonstrate anything particular although it was bathed in a liquid of a light green colour which was contained within the pericardium.

   - **Abdomen:** The stomach [was] dilated by a yellowish fluid with which its walls were heavily impregnated but nonetheless it did not show any lesion nor inflammation. The intestines [were] attenuated and showed slight evidence of tympanites. The bladder [was] completely empty; it was collapsed and lying low in the pelvis; it did not exhibit any pathological signs. The liver [was] of a considerable size and was a little excoriated on its convex surface. The gall bladder [was] much extended. The mesenteric glands [were] obstructed. The spleen and kidneys were healthy. In general the visceral organs did not suffer from any serious lesions.

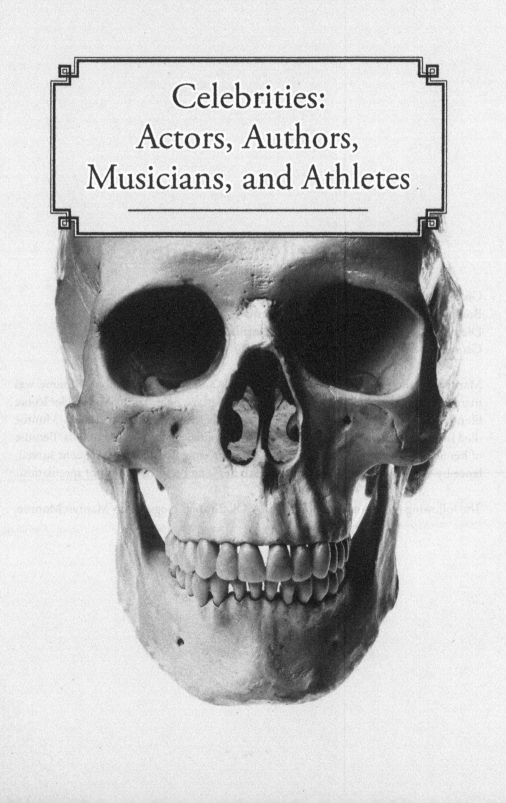

Celebrities:
Actors, Authors,
Musicians, and Athletes

Marilyn Monroe

Given Name: Norma Jeane Mortenson
Born: June 1, 1926, Los Angeles, California
Died: August 5, 1962, Los Angeles, California
Cause of Death: Accidental Drug Overdose

Marilyn Monroe was an actress, singer, model, and major sex symbol. Monroe was married to and divorced from Joe DiMaggio and playwright Arthur Miller. Her iconic blond hair is one of the most recognized symbols in American pop culture. Monroe died in her apartment in Los Angeles after she ingested a large amount of pills. Because of her alleged affairs with both John and Robert Kennedy, and her subsequent surveillance by the FBI, the true cause of her death has long been the subject of speculation.

The following is the autopsy performed by Dr. Thomas Noguchi on Marilyn Monroe.

External examination: The unembalmed body is that of a 36-year-old well-developed, well-nourished Caucasian female weighing 117 pounds and measuring 65-1/2 inches in length. The scalp is covered with bleached blond hair. The eyes are blue. The fixed lividity is noted in the face, neck, chest, upper portions of arms and the right side of the abdomen. The faint lividity which disappears upon pressure is noted in the back and posterior aspect of the arms and legs. A slight ecchymotic area is noted in the left hip and left side of lower back. The breast shows no significant lesion. There is a horizontal 3-inch long surgical scar in the right upper quadrant of the abdomen. A suprapubic surgical scar measuring 5 inches in length is noted. The conjunctivae are markedly congested; however, no ecehymosis or petechiae are noted. The nose shows no evidence of fracture. The external auditory canals are not remarkable:. No evidence of trauma is noted in the scalp, forehead, cheeks, lips or chin. The neck shows no evidence of trauma. Examination of the hands and nails shows no defects. The lower extremities show no evidence of trauma.

Body cavity: The usual Y-shaped incision is made to open the thoracic and abdominal cavities. The pleural and abdominal cavities contain no excess of fluid or blood. The mediastinum shows no shifting or widening. The diaphragm is within normal limits. The lower edge of the liver is within the costal margin. The organs are in normal position and relationship.

Cardiovascular system: The heart weighs 300 grams. The pericardial cavity contains no excess of fluid. The epicardium and pericardium are smooth and glistening. The left ventricular wall measures 1.1 cm. and the right 0.2 cm. The papillary muscles are not hypertrophic. The chordae tendineac are not thickened or shortened. The valves have the usual number of leaflets which are thin and pliable. The tricuspid valve measures 10 cm., the pulmonary valve 6.5 cm., mitral valve 9.5 cm. and aortic valve 7 cm in circumference. There is no septal defect. The foramen ovale is closed. The coronary arteries arise from their usual location and are distributed in normal fashion. Multiple sections of the anterior descending branch of the left coronary artery with a 5 mm. interial demonstrate a patent lumen throughout. The circumflex branch and the right coronary artery also demonstrate a patent lumen. The pulmonary artery contains no thrombus. The aorta has a bright yellow smooth intima.

Respiratory system: The right lung weighs 465 grams and the left 420 grams. Both lungs are moderately congested with some edema. The surface is dark and red with mottling. The posterior portion of the lungs show severe congestion. The tracheobronchial tree contains no aspirated material or blood. Multiple sections

of the lungs show congestion and edematous fluid exuding from the cut surface. No consolidation or suppuration is noted. The mucosa of the larynx is grayish white.

Liver and biliary system: The liver weighs 1890 grams. The surface is dark brown and smooth. There are marked adhesions through the omentum and abdominal wall in the lower portion of the liver as the gallbladder has been removed. The common duct is widely patent. No calculus or obstructive material is found. Multiple sections of the liver show slight accentuation of the lobular pattern; however, no hemorrhage or tumor is found.

Hemic and lymphatic system: The spleen weighs 190 grams. The surface is dark red and smooth. Section shows dark red homogeneous firm cut surface. The Malpighian bodies are not clearly identified. There is no evidence of lymphadenopathy. The bone marrow is dark red in color. Endocrine system: The adrenal glands have the usual architectural cortex and medulla. The thyroid glands are of normal size, color and consistency. Urinary system: The kidneys together weigh 350 grams. Their capsules can be stripped without difficulty. Dissection shows a moderately congested parenchyma. The cortical surface is smooth. The pelves and ureters are not dilated or stenosed. The urinary bladder contains approximately 150 cc. of clear straw-colored fluid. The mucosa is not altered.

Genital system: The external genitalia shows no gross abnormality. Distribution of the pubic hair is of female pattern. The uterus is of the usual size. Multiple sections of the uterus show the usual thickness of the uterine wall without tumor nodules. The endometrium is grayish yellow, measuring up to 0.2 cm in thickness. No polyp or tumor is found. The cervix is clear, showing no nabothian cysts. The tubes are intact. The right ovary demonstrates recent corpus luteum haemorrhagicum. The left ovary shows corpora lutea and albicantia. A vaginal smear is taken.

Digestive system: The esophagus has a longitudinal folding mucosa. The stomach is almost completely empty. The contents is brownish mucoid fluid. The volume is estimated to be no more than 20 cc. No residue of the pills is noted. A smear made from the gastric contents and examined under the polarized microscope shows no refractile crystals. The mucosa shows marked congestion and submucosal petechial hemorrhage diffusely. The duodenum shows no ulcer. The contents of the duodenum is also examined under polarized microscope and shows no refractile crystals. The remainder of the small intestine shows no gross abnormality. The appendix is absent. The colon shows marked congestion and

purplish discoloration. The pancreas has a tan lobular architecture. Multiple sections shows a patent duct.

Skeletomuscular system: The clavicle, ribs, vertebrae and pelvic bones show fracture lines. All bones of the extremities are examined by palpation showing no evidence of fracture.

Head and central nervous system: The brain weighs 1440 grams. Upon reflection of the scalp there is no evidence of contusion or hemorrhage. The temporal muscles are intact. Upon removal of the dura mater the cerebrospinal fluid is clear. The superficial vessels are slightly congested. The convolutions of the brain are not flattened. the contour of the brain is not distorted. No blood is found in the epidural, subdural or subarachnoid spaces. Multiple sections of the brain show the usual symmetrical ventricles and basal ganglia. Examination of the cerebellum and brain stem shows no gross abnormality. Following removal of the dura mater from the base of the skull and calvarium no skull fracture is demonstrated.

Liver temperature taken at 10:30 A.M. registered 89 F

Specimen: Unembalmed blood is taken for alcohol and barbiturate examination. Liver, kidney, stomach and contents, urine and intestine are saved for further toxicological study. A vaginal smear is made.

T NOGUCHI, M.D. DEPUTY MEDICAL EXAMINER 8-13-62

Whitney Houston

Born: August 9, 1963, Newark, New Jersey
Died: February 11, 2012, Beverly Hills, California
Cause of Death: Accidental drowning

Whitney Houston was one of the most celebrated pop singers of all time and holds the Guinness World Record for most awarded female artist. During her career, she won six Grammy awards and twenty-two American Music Awards. At one point in her career, she had seven consecutive number one hits. After her success, Houston publicly battled drugs and alcohol for most of her life. She died in the bathtub of her hotel room in Beverly Hills. Though the main cause of death on the coroner's report is drowning, cocaine use and heart problems are speculated to have been major contributors.

CASE REPORT

COUNTY OF LOS ANGELES

DEPARTMENT OF CORONER

1	APPARENT MODE **ACCIDENT**								CASE NO **2012-01022**
	SPECIAL CIRCUMSTANCES Celebrity, Media Interest								DR/VT **SEC1**

LAST, FIRST, MIDDLE
HOUSTON, WHITNEY ELISEBETH

AKA
HOUSTON, WHITNEY #

ADDRESS
360 HAMILTON AVENUE #100

CITY
WHITE PLAINS

STATE
NY

ZIP
10601

| SEX FEMALE | RACE APPEARS BLACK | DOB 8/9/1963 | AGE 48 | HGT 66 in | WGT 151 lbs | EYES BROWN | HAIR BLACK | TEETH ALL NATURAL TEETH | FACIAL HAIR NONE | ID VIEW Yes | CONDITION FAIR |

| MARK TYPE SCAR | MARK LOCATION LEFT FOREARM | MARK DESCRIPTION INNER, LOWER-OLD HEALED | | | | |

| | ADDRESS | | CITY | STATE | ZIP |

| RELATIONSHIP | PHONE | NOTIFIED BY | | DATE 2/11/2012 | TIME |

| SSN | DL # D9834026 | STATE CA | PENDING SS # |

ID METHOD
CALIFORNIA DRIVER'S LICENSE

| LA # | MAR # | CII # | FBI # | MILITARY # | POB NEW JERSEY |

| IDENTIFIED BY NAME (PRINT) KRISTY MCCRACKEN | RELATIONSHIP NONE | PHONE (323) 343-0714 | DATE 2/12/2012 | TIME 00:30 |

| PLACE OF DEATH/PLACE FOUND HOTEL/MOTEL | ADDRESS OR LOCATION 9876 WILSHIRE BOULEVARD #434 | CITY BEVERLY HILLS | ZIP 90210 |

| PLACE OF INJURY HOTEL/MOTEL | AT WORK No | DATE 2/11/2012 | TIME | LOCATION OR ADDRESS 9876 WILSHIRE BOULEVARD #434, BEVERLY HILLS, CA 90210 | ZIP |

| GOD 2/11/2012 | TIME 15:55 | FOUND OR PRONOUNCED BY PARAMEDICS |

| OTHER AGENCY INV. OFFICER BEVERLY HILLS P.D. - DETECTIVE HYON | PHONE (310) 285-2156 | REPORT NO 12-0806 | NOTIFIED BY | NO |

| TRANSPORTED BY JOHN GREEN | TO LOS ANGELES FSC | DATE 2/11/2012 | TIME 01:10 |

FINGERPRINTED	Yes	CLOTHING	No	PROPERTY	No	MORTUARY	
MED EV	Yes	INVEST PHOTO #	35	SEAL TYPE	NOT SEALED	HOSP ADM	No
PHYS EV	Yes	EVIDENCE LOG	Yes	PROPERTY	Yes	HOSP CHART	No
SUICIDE NOTE	No	GSR NO		RCPT NO	257946	PF NO	

SYNOPSIS
ACCORDING TO THE REPORTED INFORMATION, THE DECEDENT IS A 48 YEAR-OLD BLACK FEMALE WITH A MEDICAL HISTORY OF USING NARCOTIC SUBSTANCES. THE DECEDENT WAS LAST SEEN ALIVE ON SATURDAY 02/11/2012 BETWEEN 1445-1500 HOURS BY HER PERSONAL ASSISTANT. THE DECEDENT COMPLAINED OF HAVING A SORE THROAT, BUT SHE HAD BEEN COMPLAINING OF THAT FOR THE PAST FEW DAYS. THE DECEDENT TOLD THE DECEDENT TO TAKE A BATH, TO START GETTING READY FOR TONIGHT. THE ASSISTANT THEN LEFT THE ROOM TO RUN SOME ERRANDS. AT APPROXIMATELY 1535 HOURS, THE ASSISTANT RETURNED AND USED HER KEY TO ENTER THE LOCKED AND SECURED ROOM. ONCE INSIDE, SHE FOUND THE DECEDENT LYING FACE DOWN IN THE BATHTUB FILLED WITH WATER, UNRESPONSIVE. THE ASSISTANT CALLED FOR HER BODYGUARD, AND TOGETHER THEY PULLED THE DECEDENT OUT OF THE BATHTUB. THE ASSISTANT CALLED DOWNSTAIRS TO CALL 911. 911 WAS CALLED AT 1543 HOURS AND OFFICERS FROM THE BEVERLY HILLS POLICE DEPARTMENT AND PARAMEDICS FROM THE BEVERLY HILLS FIRE DEPARTMENT ARRIVED ON SCENE. ON SATURDAY 02/11/2012 AT 1555 HOURS, PARAMEDICS FROM RESCUE 1 DETERMINED DEATH. THE DECEDENT POSSIBLY OVERDOSED ON A NARCOTIC SUBSTANCE, PRESCRIPTION MEDICATIONS, OVER THE COUNTER MEDICATIONS, AND ALCOHOL. MINOR EXTERNAL TRAUMA WAS NOTED AND THERE ARE NO SIGNS OF FOUL PLAY. DETECTIVE HYON REQUIRES A 2-HOUR NOTIFICATION PRIOR TO THE EXAMINATION. PLEASE SEE CASE NOTES FOR HIS CONTACT INFORMATION.

| KRISTY MCCRACKEN 491917 | INVESTIGATOR | DATE 2/12/2012 | TIME 04:45 | REVIEWED BY | DATE 2/12/12 | TIME |

FORM #3 NARRATIVE TO FOLLOW? ☑

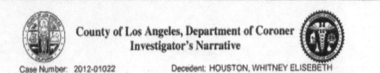

County of Los Angeles, Department of Coroner
Investigator's Narrative

Case Number: 2012-01022   Decedent: HOUSTON, WHITNEY ELISEBETH

Information Sources:

(1)   Beverly Hills Police Department-Report #12-0806   (310)285-2156
       Detective Hyon

Investigation:

On Saturday 02/11/2012 at 2104 hours, Sergeant Publicker from the Beverly Hills Police Department called the Los Angeles County Coroner's Office to report a natural versus accidental death of a 48 year-old black female that possibly drowned in a bathtub. On Saturday 02/11/2012 at 2120 hours, Lieutenant Brian Elias assigned this case to me. I arrived on-scene at 2220 hours and I cleared the scene on Sunday 02/12/2012 at 0135 hours. Prior to my arrival, the decedent was removed from the bathtub by her personal assistant and bodyguard, and then Paramedics placed the decedent onto the living room floor in order to render First-Aid. Also prior to my arrival, Paramedics moved the couch from out of the living room, and placed it on the patio in order to render First-Aid on the decedent. The decedent's purse was on that couch, and the decedent's California driver's license had been removed from the wallet, which was inside the purse, prior to my arrival. Also prior to my arrival, the majority of the decedent's prescription medication bottles had been removed from a brown bag that was on top of the table in the southeast corner of the living room, and then placed on top of that same table. After completing my investigation, I changed this from a natural versus accident to an accident. The decedent possibly overdosed on a narcotic substance, prescription medications, over the counter medications, and alcohol. Minor trauma was noted and there are no signs of foul play.

Location:

The incident occurred and the decedent died in the bathroom inside her room #434 at the Beverly Hilton Hotel located at 9876 Wilshire Boulevard, Beverly Hills CA, 90210.

Informant/Witness Statements:

I spoke with Detective Hyon at the scene, and he told me the following:

The decedent checked into the Beverly Hilton Hotel on Monday 02/06/2012. She was here for the Grammy award ceremony on Sunday 02/12/2012, and there was a pre-Grammy Party at the hotel on Saturday 02/11/2012. The decedent was last seen alive by her personal assistant on Saturday 02/11/2012 between 1445-1500 hours. The decedent complained of having a sore throat that had been lingering for the past few days. Before she left, she told the decedent to go take a bath, to start getting ready for tonight. The personal assistant then left to go pick up items at Neiman Marcus. The personal assistant left Neiman Marcus at 1525 hours, and per the door key, she entered the decedent's locked hotel room at 1536 hours. She went into the bathroom, and she found the decedent lying face down in the bathtub, unresponsive, with the top of her head facing west. The bathtub was filled with water, and there was water on the bathroom floor, however, the water was not running. She called out to the bodyguard, and they pulled the decedent out of the bathtub. The assistant then called downstairs telling them to call 911. They received the 911 call at 1543 hours, and Paramedics from the Beverly Hills Fire Department arrived on-scene. On Saturday 02/11/2012 at 1546 hours, Paramedics from Rescue 1 determined death. On Saturday 02/11/2012 at 2135 hours, the water temperature in the bathtub was 93.5 degrees. There are no signs of foul play.

Scene Description:

The Beverly Hilton Hotel is located at 9876 Wilshire Boulevard in Beverly Hills. Room #434 was located on the 4th floor in the southwest portion of the hotel. The living room was located in the west side of the room. Located in the northwest corner was a chair and then a computer tower with a Fedora on top of it. Located along the north wall, central portion was a dresser with a

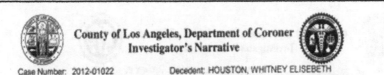

County of Los Angeles, Department of Coroner
Investigator's Narrative

Case Number: 2012-01022   Decedent: HOUSTON, WHITNEY ELISEBETH

mini-bar in it. On top of it was an open bottle of champagne, along with other miscellaneous items. Located in the north wall, northeast portion was the front door to the room. Located in the east wall were doors leading into the bedroom. Located in the southeast corner was a table with multiple bottles of prescription medications, prescribed to the decedent, multiple blister packs, a loose tablet, and other miscellaneous items on top of it. Located in the south wall was a sliding glass door leading onto a balcony. Just south of these sliding glass doors was a couch with a purse on it. Located in the southwest corner was a lamp. Located on the floor in the southwest portion of the room was an empty blister pack. Located along the west wall, central portion were three tables with plates of food, an open can of beer, a single capsule, along with other miscellaneous items on top of it. The decedent was located lying supine on the floor in the central portion of the living room floor.

The bedroom was located in the east side of the room. Located in the north wall, northwest corner was a closet. Just south of the closet were opened suitcases and a lamp. Located in the north wall, central portion was a door leading into the bathroom. Located along the north wall, central portion was a luggage stand. Located in the northeast corner was a table with a bottle of prescription medication, loose tablets, and other miscellaneous items on top of it. Located along the east wall, central portion was a bed. Located along the east wall, southeast portion was a nightstand with a bottle of beer on it. Located in the south wall were sliding glass doors leading onto the same balcony. Located along the south doors, southeast portion was a chaise lounge. Located along the south wall, southwest portion was another luggage stand with an open suitcase on it. Located in the southwest corner was a 3-drawer dresser with a bottle of prescription medication, loose tablets, a bottle of a supplement, and other miscellaneous items on top of it. Located in the west wall were doors leading into the living room. The carpet in the bedroom was soaked with water.

The bathroom was located in the northeast portion of the room. Located along the north wall, central portion was a bathtub. There was approximately 12" of water in the short end and approximately 13" of water in the deep end. In the bathtub was a towel, a bottle of rubbing alcohol, and a pitcher. Located in the north wall, northeast portion was the toilet stall. Located along the east wall was a counter with a sink and drawers below. Located on the counter in front of the sink was an ashtray filled with multiple cigarette butts. Located on the south portion of the counter was a small spoon with a white crystal like substance in it and a rolled up piece of white paper, along with other miscellaneous items. Located on the north portion of the counter was a bottle of prescription medications, and a ripped open small plastic bag, along with other miscellaneous items. Located in the top drawer, in the north side of the counter were remnants of a white powdery substance, and a portable mirror on a base. On the bottom of that base were more remnants of a white powdery substance. Located in the south wall, central portion was the entrance into the bedroom. Located in the southwest portion of the bedroom was a chair with some clothes on it and a blanket on the floor next to it. Located in the west wall, central portion was a door leading into the shower. The bathroom floor was covered with water.

Evidence:

On Saturday 02/11/2012 hours, I collected a plethora of prescription medication bottles, prescribed to the decedent, multiple blister packs, and a loose tablet from off the top of a table in the southeast corner of the living room. I also collected a capsule from off one of the tables in the west central portion of the living room. I also collected an empty blister pack from off the floor in the southwest portion of the living room. I also collected a bottle of prescription medication, prescribed to the decedent from off a table in the northeast corner of the bedroom. I also collected loose tablets from off the same table in the northeast corner of the bedroom. I also collected a bottle of prescription medication, prescribed to the decedent, a bottle of a supplement, and a loose tablet from off a 3-drawer dresser in the southwest corner of the bedroom. I also collected a bottle of prescription medication, prescribed to the decedent, a

County of Los Angeles, Department of Coroner
Investigator's Narrative

Case Number: 2012-01022   Decedent: HOUSTON, WHITNEY ELISEBETH

spoon with a white crystal like substance in it, a rolled up piece of white paper from off the top of a counter along the east wall in the bathroom. I also collected remnants of a white powdery substance from out of a drawer and from the bottom of a mirror in the same drawer in the bathroom counter along the east wall of the bathroom. I later booked all of the bottles of prescription medications, the bottle of the supplement, all of the blister packs, all of the loose tablets and capsules, the spoon, and the white powdery substance at the Forensic Services Center as evidence.

On Saturday 02/11/2012 at 2342 hours, Criminalist Mark Schuchardt used a pubic hair kit on the decedent at the scene. On Saturday 02/11/2012 at 2355 hours, Criminalist Mark Schuchardt collected fingernail clippings from the decedent's hands at the scene. On Sunday 02/12/2012 at 0004 hours, Criminalist Mark Schuchardt collected hair standards from the decedent at the scene. On Sunday 02/12/2012 at 0015 hours, Criminalist Mark Schuchardt used a sexual assault kit on the decedent at the scene. Criminalist Mark Schuchardt later booked the pubic hair kit, the fingernail clippings, the hair standards, and the sexual assault kit at the Forensic Services Center as evidence.

Body Examination:

The decedent is a 48 year-old black female with short black hair, brown eyes, and she has all of her natural teeth. There is an old healed vertical scar approximately 2" in length on her inner lower left forearm. No other scars and no tattoos were noted. The decedent was nude, lying supine on the living room floor. The top of her head was facing south. Her right arm was bent at the elbow with her right hand resting on the floor, against the right central portion of her torso. Her left arm was slightly bent at the elbow with her left hand resting on the floor against her outer upper left thigh. Both of her legs were straight with her right foot pointing north and her left foot was pointing northwest. There was a defibrillator patch on the upper right side of her chest and there was another defibrillator patch on the left central portion of her torso. Both of her eyes were congested and there was a bloody purge coming from her nose. There were 2 superficial abrasions to the left side of her forehead and there was a superficial abrasion to the left side of the bridge of her nose. There was a superficial abrasion to the top of her right shoulder. There was minor skin slippage to the upper central portion of her chest, to the inner left central portion of her chest, and to the lower central portion of her chest. There was minor skin slippage to the upper left side of her abdomen. There was a superficial abrasion to her outer lower left arm. There was a possible old puncture wound to her inner left elbow. There was a superficial abrasion to her inner central left forearm and there were minor abrasions to the top of her left hand, between the middle and ring fingers. There was minor skin slippage to the front of both of her knees and to both of the front central portion of her legs. There was minor skin slippage to her inner upper right calf and to her outer lower left leg. There was skin slippage to the lower central portion of her back. On Sunday 02/12/2012 at 0005 hours, the water temperature in the bathtub was 89.0 degrees. On Sunday 02/12/2012 at 0025 hours, the air temperature inside the living room was 67.0 degrees. On Sunday 02/12/2012 at 0031 hours, the decedent's liver temperature was 96.0 degrees.

Identification:

On Sunday 02/12/2012 at 0030 hours, I positively identified the decedent as Whitney Elisebeth Houston with a DOB of 08/09/1963 by the photograph on her California driver's license at the scene.

Next of Kin Notification:

On Saturday 02/11/2012 at an unknown time, friends notified   , the decedent's daughter, of her mother's death. I have not spoken with   at the time of completion of this report. Please see case notes for further information.

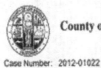 **County of Los Angeles, Department of Coroner**
Investigator's Narrative

Case Number: 2012-01022   Decedent: HOUSTON, WHITNEY ELISEBETH

Tissue Donation:

I did not discuss tissue donation with the decedent's family.

Exam Notification:

Detective Hyon requires a 2-hour notification prior to the examination.   Please see case notes for his contact information.

KRISTY MCCRACKEN #491917   SUPERVISOR

Date of Report

COUNTY OF LOS ANGELES

MEDICAL EVIDENCE

DEPARTMENT OF CORONER

CASE # 2012-01022

DECEDENT'S NAME: HOUSTON, WHITNEY ELISEBETH

DOD: 2/11/2012

INCOMING MODE:

Page 1 of 2

3A

Drug Name	Rx Number	Date of Issue	Number Issued	Number Remaining	Form	Dosage	Rx Directions	Physician	Pharmacy Phone/ Comments
ACIPHEX	0847361-057	1/18/2012	30	1	TABLET	20 MG	TAKE 1 TABLET BY...	DR. K. DOCKERY	WALGREENS (679)566-3284
ALPRAZOLAM	0457299-047	11/1/2011	90	0	TABLET	1 MG	TAKE 1 TABLET BY...	DR. G. CHASE	WALGREENS (313)567-4239
ALPRAZOLAM	0938462-057	12/6/2011	15	0	TABLET	1 MG	TAKE 1 TABLET BY...	DR. R. COLLINS	WALGREENS (679)566-3284 FOR: XANAX
AMOX TR-K CLV	205867	10/22/2011	14	1	TABLET	875-125 MG	TAKE 1 TABLET BY...	DR. S. NASSERI	CVS PHARMACY (313)963-1007 GENERIC FOR: AUGMENTIN
AMOXK CLAV	196205	1/31/2012	20	0	TABLET	875 MG	TAKE 1 TABLET BY...	DR. S. NASSERI	MICKEY FINE PHARMACY (310)271-6123 GENERIC FOR: AUGMENTIN
AMOXK CLAV	197174	2/7/2012	20	15	TABLET	875 MG	TAKE 1 TABLET BY...	DR. S. NASSERI	MICKEY FINE PHARMACY (310)271-6123 GENERIC FOR: AUGMENTIN
DEXAMETHASON	196204	1/31/2012	3	0	TABLET	2 MG	TAKE 1 TABLET BY...	DR. S. NASSER	MICKEY FINE PHARMACY (310)271-6123
DEXAMETHASONE	2130999	9/30/2011	6	0	TABLET	1 MG	TAKE 2 TABLETS BY...	DR. S. NASSERI	RITE AID (310)272-3561

Paraphernalia Description

1-SMALL SPOON WITH A WHITE CRYSTAL LIKE SUBSTANCE IN ONE END. 1-WHITE ROLLED UP PIECE OF PAPER. 2-PIECES FROM SMALL PLASTIC BAGS. REMNANTS OF A WHITE POWDERY SUBSTANCE. 1-OPEN BOTTLE OF CVS PHARMACY IBUPROFEN 200 MG TABLETS ORIGINALLY WITH 30 TABLETS NOW WITH 9 TABLETS. 4-EMPTY BLISTER PACKS ORIGINALLY WITH 8 TABLETS OF MIDOL COMPLETE. 2-EMPTY BLISTER PACKS OF MIDOL EXTENDED TABLETS. 2-BLISTER PACKS CONTAINING 2 MAXIMUM STRENGTH MUCINEX DM TABLET. 3-EMPTY BLISTER PACKS FOR DIPHENHYDRAMINE HCl 25 MG TABLET. 24-BLISTER PACKS CONTAINING 1 DIPHENHYDRAMINE HCl 25 MG

Investigator: KRISTY McCRACKEN (491917)

Date: 2/12/2012

COUNTY OF LOS ANGELES

MEDICAL EVIDENCE

DEPARTMENT OF CORONER

3A

CASE #: 2012-01022
DECEDENT'S NAME: HOUSTON, WHITNEY ELISEBETH
DOD: 2/11/2012
INCOMING MODE:

Page 2 of 2

Drug Name	Rx Number	Date of Issue	Number Issued	Number Remaining	Form	Dosage	Rx Directions	Physician	Pharmacy Phone/ Comments
MINOCYCLINE HCL	2017695	12/10/2010	30	6	TABLET	100 MG	TAKE 1 TABLET BY...	DR. H. LANCER	RITE AID (310)273-3541 GENERIC FOR: DYNACIN
NYSTATIN 100000 SUS MORIT	199206	1/31/2012	150	40	LIQUID		TAKE 2 TEASPOONFULS	DR. S. NASSERI	MICKEY FINE PHARMACY (310)271-6123
PREDNISONE	0947372-057	1/16/2012	21	0	TABLET	5 MG	TAKE 6 TABLETS BY...	DR. K. DOCKERY	WALGREENS (678)566-3284
XANAX	0947847-057	1/20/2012	15/90	0	TABLET	1 MG	TAKE 1 TABLET BY...	DR. R. COLLINS	WALGREENS (678)566-3284

Paraphernalia Description

1-SMALL SPOON WITH A WHITE CRYSTAL LIKE SUBSTANCE IN ONE END. 1-WHITE ROLLED UP PIECE OF PAPER. 2-PIECES FROM SMALL PLASTIC BAGS. REMNANTS OF A WHITE POWDERY SUBSTANCE. 1-OPEN BOTTLE OF CVS PHARMACY IBUPROFEN 200 MG TABLETS ORIGINALLY WITH 30 TABLETS NOW WITH 8 TABLETS. 4-EMPTY BLISTER PACKS ORIGINALLY WITH 8 TABLETS OF MIDOL COMPLETE. 2-EMPTY BLISTER PACKS OF MIDOL EXTENDED TABLETS. 2-BLISTER PACKS CONTAINING 2 MAXIMUM STRENGTH MUCINEX DM TABLET. 3-EMPTY BLISTER PACKS FOR DIPHENHYDRAMINE HCL 25 MG TABLET. 24-BLISTER PACKS CONTAINING 1 DIPHENHYDRAMINE HCL 25 MG

Investigator: KRISTY MCCRACKEN (48197)

Date: 2/12/2012

PRELIMINARY EXAMINATION REPORT - FIELD

COUNTY OF LOS ANGELES   DEPARTMENT OF CORONER

6

WAS ORIGINAL SCENE DISTURBED BY OTHERS? Y(X) N( )
IF YES, NOTE CHANGES IN NARRATIVE FORM #3.

DATE 02/11/12 - 02/12/12

AMBIENT #1 67.0 °F   TIME 0025

AMBIENT #2 ___ °F   TIME ___

WATER 89.0 °F   TIME 0005

LIVER TEMPERATURE #1 96.0 °F   TIME 0031

LIVER TEMPERATURE #2 ___ °F   TIME ___

2012-01022
HOUSTON
WHITNEY
ACC-01?

THERMOMETER # ___

DATE & TIME FOUND 02/11/12 1536   LAST KNOWN ALIVE 02/11/12 1445-1500

APPROX. AGE 48   SEX F   EST. HEIGHT 66   EST. WEIGHT 151   CLOTHED? YES ☐ NO ☒ IF YES, DESCRIBE:

N/A

DESCRIPTION AS TO WHERE REMAINS FOUND AND CONTACT MATERIAL TO BODY.

Lying supine on the living room floor

SCENE TEMPERATURE REGULATED? YES ☐ NO ☒ IF YES, THERMOSTAT SET AT ___ DEGREES F.

LIVOR MORTIS: TIME OBSERVED Unk   RIGOR MORTIS: TIME OBSERVED Unk

NECK FLEXION:

Fixed

ANTERIOR 2+

POSTERIOR 2+

RT. LATERAL 2+

LT LATERAL 2+

JAW 2+	HIP 2+
SHOULDER 2+	KNEE 2+
ELBOW 2+	ANKLE 2+
WRIST 2+	

R   L   L   R

SCALE

0 - ABSENT/NEGATIVE
1 -
2 -
3 -
4 - EXTREME DEGREE

USE SCALE TO DESCRIBE INTENSITY OF RIGOR MORTIS

SHADE DIAGRAMS TO ILLUSTRATE THE LOCATION OF LIVOR MORTIS

DESCRIBE INTENSTIY OF COLORATION AND WHETHER LIVOR MORTIS IS PERMANENT OR BLANCHES UNDER PRESSURE.

K. McCracken #491917
CORONER'S INVESTIGATOR

REVIEWED BY:

76P530 12/93 PS 7-85   NOTE: ALL DATA COLLECTED FOR THIS FORM MUST BE COLLECTED AT SCENE.

COUNTY OF LOS ANGELES

DEPARTMENT OF CORONER

12

AUTOPSY REPORT

No.

2012-01022

HOUSTON, WHITNEY E.

I performed an autopsy on the body of
the DEPARTMENT OF CORONER

at _____

Los Angeles, California _____ on February 12, 2012 @ 1125 Hours
(Date)   (Time)

From the anatomic findings and pertinent history I ascribe the death to:

(A)   DROWNING

DUE TO OR AS A CONSEQUENCE OF

(B)   EFFECTS OF ATHEROSCLEROTIC HEART DISEASE AND COCAINE USE

DUE TO OR AS A CONSEQUENCE OF

(C)

DUE TO OR AS A CONSEQUENCE OF

(D)

OTHER CONDITIONS CONTRIBUTING BUT NOT RELATED TO THE IMMEDIATE CAUSE OF DEATH

Anatomical Summary:

 I. History of substance abuse.

    A) Perforation of posterior nasal septum.

 II. Atherosclerotic heart disease.

    A) 60% narrowing of right coronary artery.

 III. Pulmonary edema.

 IV. Mild emphysema.

 V. Leiomyomas of uterus.

 VI. Adenomyosis (stroma only).

 VII. Congestion, right colon.

 VIII. Perimortem and postmortem scald burns.

 IX. Antemortem injuries:

    A) Contusion and abrasion of left forehead.

    B) Scald burn of sacrum.

    C) Abrasion of left hand.

    D) Abrasion of right lower leg.

    E) Superficial incision of upper lip.

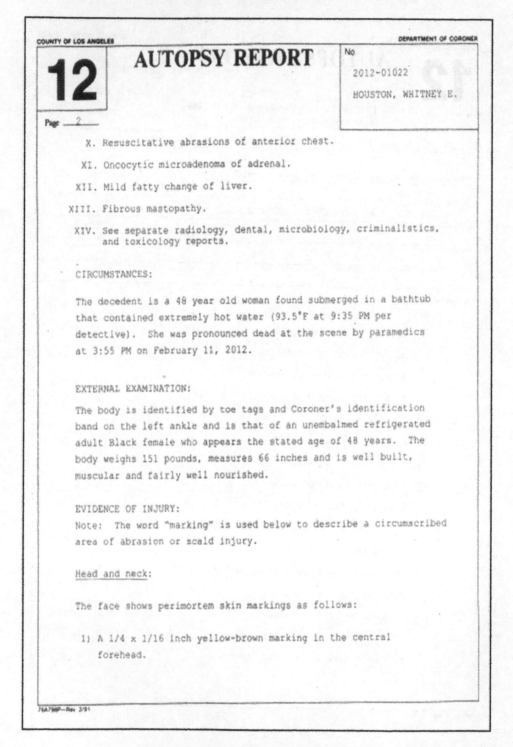

COUNTY OF LOS ANGELES

AUTOPSY REPORT

12

DEPARTMENT OF CORONER

No

2012-01022

HOUSTON, WHITNEY E.

Page ___2___

 X. Resuscitative abrasions of anterior chest.

 XI. Oncocytic microadenoma of adrenal.

 XII. Mild fatty change of liver.

 XIII. Fibrous mastopathy.

 XIV. See separate radiology, dental, microbiology, criminalistics,
and toxicology reports.

CIRCUMSTANCES:

The decedent is a 48 year old woman found submerged in a bathtub
that contained extremely hot water (93.5°F at 9:35 PM per
detective). She was pronounced dead at the scene by paramedics
at 3:55 PM on February 11, 2012.

EXTERNAL EXAMINATION:

The body is identified by toe tags and Coroner's identification
band on the left ankle and is that of an unembalmed refrigerated
adult Black female who appears the stated age of 48 years. The
body weighs 151 pounds, measures 66 inches and is well built,
muscular and fairly well nourished.

EVIDENCE OF INJURY:
Note: The word "marking" is used below to describe a circumscribed
area of abrasion or scald injury.

Head and neck:

The face shows perimortem skin markings as follows:

1) A 1/4 x 1/16 inch yellow-brown marking in the central
forehead.

76A7980—Rev 3/91

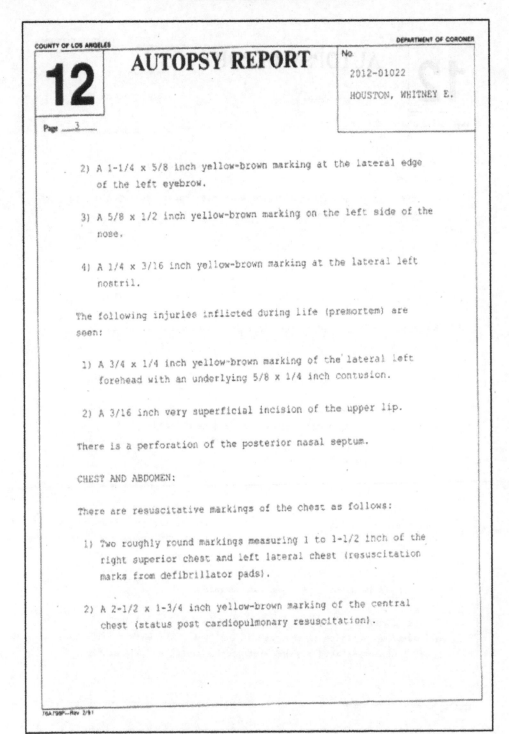

COUNTY OF LOS ANGELES

DEPARTMENT OF CORONER

12

AUTOPSY REPORT

No.

2012-01022

HOUSTON, WHITNEY E.

Page ___3___

2) A 1-1/4 x 5/8 inch yellow-brown marking at the lateral edge
   of the left eyebrow.

3) A 5/8 x 1/2 inch yellow-brown marking on the left side of the
   nose.

4) A 1/4 x 3/16 inch yellow-brown marking at the lateral left
   nostril.

The following injuries inflicted during life (premortem) are
seen:

1) A 3/4 x 1/4 inch yellow-brown marking of the lateral left
   forehead with an underlying 5/8 x 1/4 inch contusion.

2) A 3/16 inch very superficial incision of the upper lip.

There is a perforation of the posterior nasal septum.

CHEST AND ABDOMEN:

There are resuscitative markings of the chest as follows:

1) Two roughly round markings measuring 1 to 1-1/2 inch of the
   right superior chest and left lateral chest (resuscitation
   marks from defibrillator pads).

2) A 2-1/2 x 1-3/4 inch yellow-brown marking of the central
   chest (status post cardiopulmonary resuscitation).

76A/99P--Rev 2/91

COUNTY OF LOS ANGELES   DEPARTMENT OF CORONER

12 AUTOPSY REPORT

No.

2012-01022

HOUSTON, WHITNEY E.

Page ___1___

The following perimortem skin markings are present:

1) .5/8 inch yellow-brown marks of both clavicular regions and
   the left upper chest.

2) A 5/8 inch marking of the left breast.

An antemortem 5 x 3-1/4 inch area of yellow-brown skin slippage
with erythema of the superior margin located over the sacrum.

A postmortem liver temperature incision is present at the right
costal margin.

EXTEMITIES:

In the area of the right elbow are three 3/8 inch yellow-brown
abrasions. On the back of the right hand is a 3/8 inch contusion
and a 1/16 inch yellow-brown abrasion. There is an additional
yellow-brown abrasion of the tip of the right ring finger
measuring 1/8 inch.

On the inner surface of the left upper arm there are four
contusions measuring 1/4 to 3/8 inch. On the posterior surface
of the left arm around the elbow area are two yellow-brown
abrasions measuring 3/8 x 1/4 inch and another measuring 3/8 x
1/3 inch. On the back of the left hand at the knuckle of the
ring finger is a small yellow-brown abrasion.

On the anterior surface of the right leg is a 1/4 x 3/8 inch
yellow-brown abrasion in the area of the knee. There is a 2-1/2
x 1/8 inch hook-shaped red abrasion of the medial surface of the

76A788P—Rev. 2/91

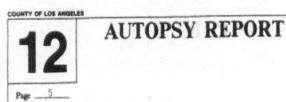

COUNTY OF LOS ANGELES

DEPARTMENT OF CORONER

AUTOPSY REPORT

No.

2012-01022

HOUSTON, WHITNEY E.

Page 5

right lower leg. There is a 2-1/2 inch zone of skin slippage at the right shin. A smaller zone of skin slippage is present at the lateral right ankle.

On the front of the left leg are 3/4 x 1/2 inch yellow-brown abrasions of the knee and shin. Over the dorsum of the left foot is a 3 x 3 inch area of skin slippage.

Tattoos are not present. Rigor mortis is present in the limbs and jaw. Livor mortis is fixed and distributed posteriorly. The head is normocephalic and is covered by black hair. A brown wig is tightly attached to the hair. This is removed and placed in a paper bag to accompany the body. There is no balding and the hair can be described as wavy. The eyebrows are sparse and show irregular hair distribution. Mustache and beard are absent. Examination of the eyes reveals irides that are brown and sclerae that show injection but no jaundice. There are no petechial hemorrhages of the conjunctivae of the lids or the sclerae. The oronasal passages are unobstructed and show bloody purge. The upper teeth have been replaced with a full arch maxillary dental prosthesis supported by dental implants. There are natural lower teeth present (see dental consultant report). There is no removable denture. The neck is unremarkable. There is no chest deformity. There is no increase in the anterior-posterior diameter of the chest. The abdomen is flat. The genitalia are those of an adult female. There is no genital or anal trauma. The extremities show no edema, joint deformity, abnormal mobility or needle tracks. There is evidence of old surgery. The following scars are present:

1) A 3/8 x 1/2 inch scar of the anterior neck near the center.

COUNTY OF LOS ANGELES   DEPARTMENT OF CORONER

12

AUTOPSY REPORT

No.

2012-01022

HOUSTON, WHITNEY E.

Page ___6___

2) Small scars of the inferior margins of the areolae, associated with breast implants.

3) A linear scar of the anterior left forearm.

4) A faint scar at the anterior pelvic brim.

5) A scar at the area of the left hip.

6) Two piercings are present in each ear.

There has not been postmortem intervention for organ procurement.

CLOTHING:

The body was not clothed and we did not see the clothing. The decedent was reportedly found nude in the bathtub.

INITIAL INCISION:

The body cavities are entered through the standard coronal incision and the standard Y-shaped incision. No foreign material is present in the mouth, upper airway or trachea except for bloody purge.

NECK:

The neck organs are removed en bloc with the tongue. No lesions are present nor is trauma of the gingiva or oral mucosa demonstrated. There is no edema of the larynx. Both hyoid bone and larynx are intact and without fractures. No hemorrhage is

76A798P—Rev 2/91

COUNTY OF LOS ANGELES

AUTOPSY REPORT

DEPARTMENT OF CORONER

No
2012-01022
HOUSTON, WHITNEY E.

12

Page ___7___

present in the adjacent throat organs, investing fascia, strap
muscles, thyroid or visceral fascia. There are no prevertebral
fascial hemorrhages. The tongue shows no trauma.

CHEST AND ABDOMINAL CAVITIES:

Both pleural cavities contain a small quantity of straw colored
fluid. No pneumothorax is demonstrated. The parietal pleurae
are intact. The lungs are well expanded. Soft tissues of the
thoracic and abdominal walls are well-preserved. Breast tissue
is sectioned and shows no abnormality. The organs of the
abdominal cavity have a normal arrangement and none are absent.

There is no fluid collection. The peritoneal cavity is without
evidence of peritonitis. There are no adhesions.

SYSTEMIC AND ORGAN REVIEW

The following observations are limited to findings other than
injuries described above.

MUSCULOSKELETAL SYSTEM:

No abnormalities of the bony framework or muscles are present.

CARDIOVASCULAR SYSTEM:

The aorta is elastic and of even caliber throughout with vessels
distributed normally from it. It shows lipid streaking. There is
no tortuosity or widening of the thoracic segment. The abdominal
aorta has minimal atherosclerosis without calcification. There is

76A796P—Rev 2/91

COUNTY OF LOS ANGELES

AUTOPSY REPORT

DEPARTMENT OF CORONER

No.

2012-01022

HOUSTON, WHITNEY E.

Page 8

no dilatation of the lower abdominal segment. No aneurysm is present. The major branches of the aorta show no abnormality. Within the pericardial sac there is a minimal amount of serous fluid. The heart weighs 340 grams. It has a normal configuration. The chambers are normally developed and are without mural thrombosis. The valves are thin, leafy and competent. There is no endocardial discoloration. There are no focal lesions of the myocardium. There is no abnormality of the apices of the papillary muscles. There are no defects of the septum. The great vessels enter and leave in a normal fashion. The ductus arteriosus is obliterated. The coronary ostia are widely patent. There is segmental coronary atherosclerosis resulting in up to 60% occlusion of the right coronary artery at 4 cm from the ostium, and minimal atherosclerosis of the left anterior descending artery. No focal endocardial, valvular or myocardial lesions are seen. The blood within the heart and large blood vessels is liquid.

RESPIRATORY SYSTEM:

A moderate amount of froth is found in the upper respiratory passages. The mucosa is intact. The lungs are subcrepitant and there is dependent congestion. The left lung weighs 610 grams and the right lung weighs 680 grams. The visceral pleurae are smooth and intact. The parenchyma is moderately edematous. The pulmonary vasculature is without thromboembolism.

GASTROINTESTINAL SYSTEM:

The esophagus is intact. The stomach is not distended. It contains 400 grams of watery fluid with portions of food

76A756P—Rev 2/91

COUNTY OF LOS ANGELES

AUTOPSY REPORT

DEPARTMENT OF CORONER

No
2012-01022
HOUSTON, WHITNEY E.

Page ___10___

GENITAL SYSTEM:

The uterus is asymmetrical and the uterine cavity is not enlarged.
There are several intramural and subserosal masses measuring 2.3
to 4 cm in diameter. The masses are well-demarcated and the cut
surface is gray-white with a whorled pattern. The fallopian tubes
are unremarkable. The endometrium is thin and red-brown. The
cervix and vagina have a normal appearance for the age. The
ovaries show hemorrhagic luteal cysts.

HEMOLYMPHATIC SYSTEM:

The spleen weighs 120 grams. The capsule is intact. The
parenchyma is dark red and firm. There is no increase in the
follicular pattern. Lymph nodes throughout the body are small
and inconspicuous. The bone is not remarkable. The bone marrow
of the vertebra is red and moist.

ENDOCRINE SYSTEM:

The thyroid gland weighs 40 grams. The consistency is
unremarkable. Tissue from the parathyroid region is submitted
for microscopic evaluation. The adrenals are unremarkable. The
thymus is not identified. The pituitary gland is of normal size.

HEAD AND CENTRAL NERVOUS SYSTEM:

There is a small amount of subcutaneous hemorrhage in the region
of the left forehead. The hemorrhage does not extend into the
orbits or the temporal muscles. The external periosteum and dura
mater are stripped showing no fractures of the calvarium or base

AUTOPSY REPORT

No.

2012-01022

HOUSTON, WHITNEY E.

Page ___11___

of the skull. There are no tears of the dura mater. There is no epidural, subdural or subarachnoid hemorrhage. The brain weighs 1410 grams. The leptomeninges are thin and transparent. A normal convolutionary pattern is observed. Coronal sectioning demonstrates a uniformity of cortical gray thickness. The cerebral hemispheres are symmetrical. There is no softening, discoloration or hemorrhage of the white matter. The basal ganglia are intact. Anatomic landmarks are preserved. Cerebral contusions are not present. The ventricular system is symmetrical without distortion or dilatation. Pons, medulla and cerebellum are unremarkable. There is no evidence of uncal or cerebellar herniation. Vessels at the base of the brain have a normal pattern of distribution. There are no aneurysms. The cranial nerves are intact, symmetrical and normal in size, location and course. The cerebral arteries are without arteriosclerosis.

SPINAL CORD:

The spinal cord is not dissected.

HISTOLOGIC SECTIONS:

Representative specimens from various organs are preserved in two storage jars in 10% formalin. The sections are submitted for slides.

The slide key is: a) skin of the sacral region, b) right coronary atherosclerotic plaque, c) adrenal gland and aorta, d) cardiac intraventricular septum with left anterior descending artery, e) left ventricle, left atrium and circumflex artery, f) right

AUTOPSY REPORT

No

2012-01022

HOUSTON, WHITNEY E.

Page __12__

atrium, right ventricle and right coronary artery, g) and h) sinoatrial node area, i) atrioventricular node area, j) right lung, k) left lung, l) epiglottis and trachea, m) tissue from parathyroid region and thyroid gland, n) esophagogastric junction and gastric mucosa, o) pancreas and liver, p) spleen and right kidney, q) bladder and left kidney, r) uterus and fibroid, s) ovary and right colon mucosa, t) tonsil, u) left frontal scalp, v) breast and appendix.

The following neuropathology slides are submitted: 1) occipital cortex, 2) cerebellum, 3) thalamus, 4) hippocampus, 5) frontal cortex, 6) hypothalamus with mammilary body, 7) brainstem.

TOXICOLOGY:

Blood from the heart, left femoral vein, right femoral vein, bile, liver, urine, stomach contents, vitreous, tracheal air, serum from heart blood, and centrifuged red cells from heart blood have been submitted to the laboratory. A comprehensive screen, vitreous glucose, electrolytes and urea nitrogen, hemoglobin S screen, and alprazolam are requested.

SPECIAL PROCEDURES:

Viral culture of the nasopharynx and bacterial culture of throat have been submitted to the laboratory.

PHOTOGRAPHY:

The investigator took seventy-five scene photographs on February 11, 2012. Thirty-two photographs have been taken prior to and during the autopsy (one intake, 28 pre-autopsy and 3 during

76A798P—Rev 2/91

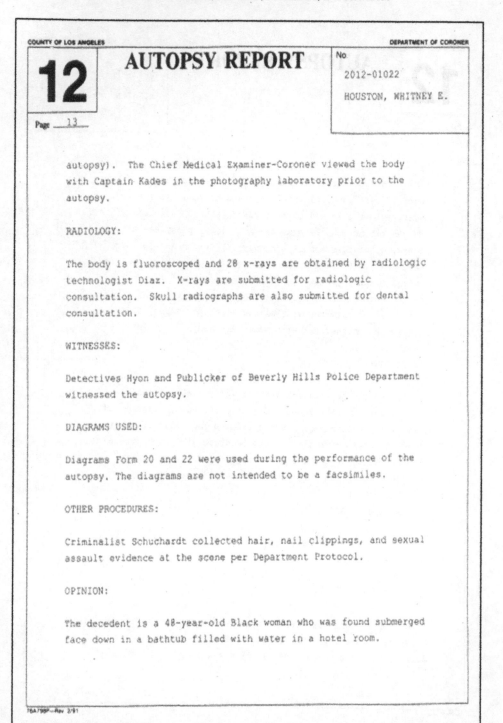

COUNTY OF LOS ANGELES

DEPARTMENT OF CORONER

12

AUTOPSY REPORT

No.
2012-01022
HOUSTON, WHITNEY E.

Page __13__

autopsy). The Chief Medical Examiner-Coroner viewed the body
with Captain Kades in the photography laboratory prior to the
autopsy.

RADIOLOGY:

The body is fluoroscoped and 28 x-rays are obtained by radiologic
technologist Diaz. X-rays are submitted for radiologic
consultation. Skull radiographs are also submitted for dental
consultation.

WITNESSES:

Detectives Hyon and Publicker of Beverly Hills Police Department
witnessed the autopsy.

DIAGRAMS USED:

Diagrams Form 20 and 22 were used during the performance of the
autopsy. The diagrams are not intended to be a facsimiles.

OTHER PROCEDURES:

Criminalist Schuchardt collected hair, nail clippings, and sexual
assault evidence at the scene per Department Protocol.

OPINION:

The decedent is a 48-year-old Black woman who was found submerged
face down in a bathtub filled with water in a hotel room.

76A799P—Rev 3/91

COUNTY OF LOS ANGELES

DEPARTMENT OF CORONER

12

AUTOPSY REPORT

No.

2012-01022

HOUSTON, WHITNEY E.

Page ___14___

Autopsy showed atherosclerotic heart disease. Toxicology testing
showed cocaine, benzoylecgonine, cocaethylene, marijuana,
alprazolam (Xanax), cyclobenzaprine, (Flexeril), and
diphenhydramine (Benadryl).

Microbiology and virology studies were not contributory.

Death was due to drowning due to effects of atherosclerotic heart
disease and cocaine use. No foul play is suspected. The mode of
death is accident.

Christopher Rogers, M.D., MBA
Chief Forensic Medicine Division

3-29-12
DATE

Lakshmanan Sathyavagiswaran, M.D.,FRCP(C),FCAP,FACP
Chief Medical Examiner-Coroner

3-29-2012
DATE

CR:LS:mtm:c
D-02/12/12
T-02/13/12

76A798P—Rev 2/91

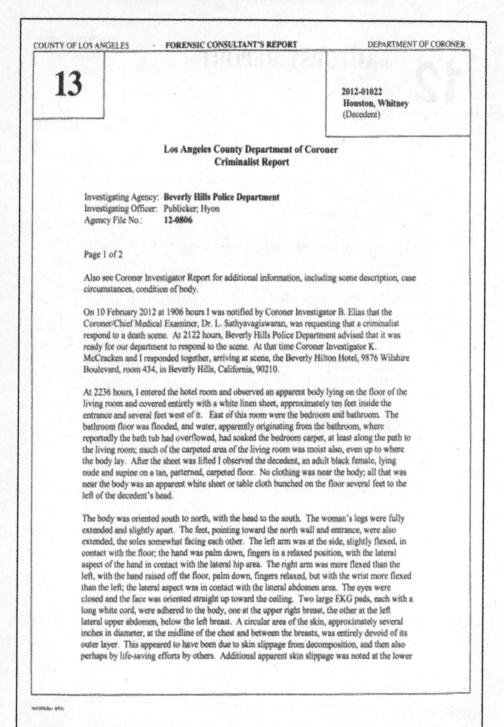

COUNTY OF LOS ANGELES · **FORENSIC CONSULTANT'S REPORT** DEPARTMENT OF CORONER

13

2012-01022
Houston, Whitney
(Decedent)

Los Angeles County Department of Coroner
Criminalist Report

Investigating Agency: **Beverly Hills Police Department**
Investigating Officer: Publicker; Hyon
Agency File No.: **12-0806**

Page 1 of 2

Also see Coroner Investigator Report for additional information, including scene description, case circumstances, condition of body.

On 10 February 2012 at 1906 hours I was notified by Coroner Investigator B. Elias that the Coroner/Chief Medical Examiner, Dr. L. Sathyavagiswaran, was requesting that a criminalist respond to a death scene. At 2122 hours, Beverly Hills Police Department advised that it was ready for our department to respond to the scene. At that time Coroner Investigator K. McCracken and I responded together, arriving at scene, the Beverly Hilton Hotel, 9876 Wilshire Boulevard, room 434, in Beverly Hills, California, 90210.

At 2236 hours, I entered the hotel room and observed an apparent body lying on the floor of the living room and covered entirely with a white linen sheet, approximately ten feet inside the entrance and several feet west of it. East of this room were the bedroom and bathroom. The bathroom floor was flooded, and water, apparently originating from the bathroom, where reportedly the bath tub had overflowed, had soaked the bedroom carpet, at least along the path to the living room; much of the carpeted area of the living room was moist also, even up to where the body lay. After the sheet was lifted I observed the decedent, an adult black female, lying nude and supine on a tan, patterned, carpeted floor. No clothing was near the body; all that was near the body was an apparent white sheet or table cloth bunched on the floor several feet to the left of the decedent's head.

The body was oriented south to north, with the head to the south. The woman's legs were fully extended and slightly apart. The feet, pointing toward the north wall and entrance, were also extended, the soles somewhat facing each other. The left arm was at the side, slightly flexed, in contact with the floor; the hand was palm down, fingers in a relaxed position, with the lateral aspect of the hand in contact with the lateral hip area. The right arm was more flexed than the left, with the hand raised off the floor, palm down, fingers relaxed, but with the wrist more flexed than the left; the lateral aspect was in contact with the lateral abdomen area. The eyes were closed and the face was oriented straight up toward the ceiling. Two large EKG pads, each with a long white cord, were adhered to the body, one at the upper right breast, the other at the left lateral upper abdomen, below the left breast. A circular area of the skin, approximately several inches in diameter, at the midline of the chest and between the breasts, was entirely devoid of its outer layer. This appeared to have been due to skin slippage from decomposition, and then also perhaps by life-saving efforts by others. Additional apparent skin slippage was noted at the lower

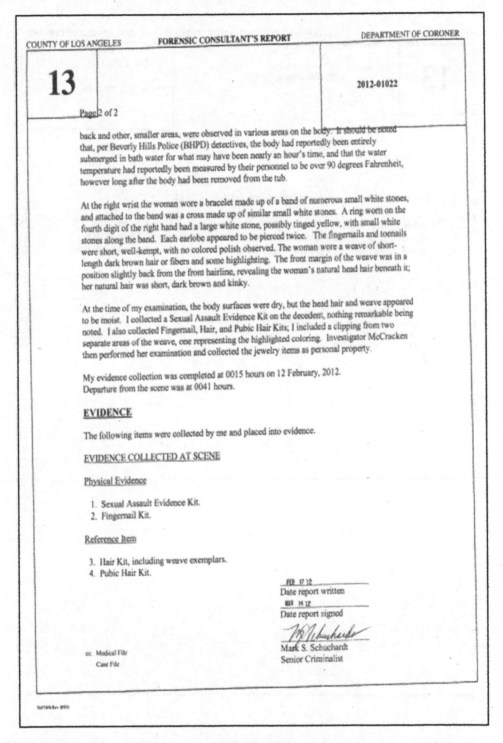

COUNTY OF LOS ANGELES   **FORENSIC CONSULTANT'S REPORT**   DEPARTMENT OF CORONER

13

2012-01022

Page 2 of 2

back and other, smaller areas, were observed in various areas on the body. It should be noted that, per Beverly Hills Police (BHPD) detectives, the body had reportedly been entirely submerged in bath water for what may have been nearly an hour's time, and that the water temperature had reportedly been measured by their personnel to be over 90 degrees Fahrenheit, however long after the body had been removed from the tub.

At the right wrist the woman wore a bracelet made up of a band of numerous small white stones, and attached to the band was a cross made up of similar small white stones. A ring worn on the fourth digit of the right hand had a large white stone, possibly tinged yellow, with small white stones along the band. Each earlobe appeared to be pierced twice. The fingernails and toenails were short, well-kempt, with no colored polish observed. The woman wore a weave of short-length dark brown hair or fibers and some highlighting. The front margin of the weave was in a position slightly back from the front hairline, revealing the woman's natural head hair beneath it; her natural hair was short, dark brown and kinky.

At the time of my examination, the body surfaces were dry, but the head hair and weave appeared to be moist. I collected a Sexual Assault Evidence Kit on the decedent, nothing remarkable being noted. I also collected Fingernail, Hair, and Pubic Hair Kits; I included a clipping from two separate areas of the weave, one representing the highlighted coloring. Investigator McCracken then performed her examination and collected the jewelry items as personal property.

My evidence collection was completed at 0015 hours on 12 February, 2012.
Departure from the scene was at 0041 hours.

EVIDENCE

The following items were collected by me and placed into evidence.

EVIDENCE COLLECTED AT SCENE

Physical Evidence

    1. Sexual Assault Evidence Kit.
    2. Fingernail Kit.

Reference Item

    3. Hair Kit, including weave exemplars.
    4. Pubic Hair Kit.

FEB 17 12
Date report written
FEB 14 12
Date report signed

Mark S. Schuchardt
Senior Criminalist

cc: Medical File
    Case File

COUNTY OF LOS ANGELES   **FORENSIC CONSULTANT'S REPORT**   DEPARTMENT OF CORONER

13

DENTAL CONSULTATION

2012-01022

Houston, Whitney

March 15, 2012

Reviewed one frontal and one lateral skull radiograph dated 2-12-12.

Decedent has an extensive maxillary dental prosthesis supported by 11 endosseous dental implants. Decedent has one dental implant with a restoration in the lower right molar area. There does not appear to be any active dental disease at the time these radiographs were taken.

_____   3-28-12
Cathy Law, DDS, DABFO   Date
Forensic Dental Consultant

CL/mtm:f
T-3/19/12

County of Los Angeles   **FORENSIC CONSULTANT'S REPORT**   Department of Coroner

13

RADIOLOGY CONSULT

2012-01022
Houston, Whitney E.

REQUEST:

48 year old black female who died unexpectedly. Evaluate x-ray for abnormal findings.

RADIOGRAPHIC IMAGES:

Whole Body Radiographic Survey-adult.

FINDINGS:

Radiopaque linear densities are present, adjacent to the apical calvarium and the posterior occipital. These are identified as "hair clips" by the attending pathologists. There has been extensive dental prosthetic replacement. There are no visible calvarial or facial bone defects. Mild osteoarthritic changes are present in both a/c joints. The outlines of bilateral breast prostheses are visible. The remainder of the radiographic examination is normal.

IMPRESSIONS:

1. No acute or post traumatic changes are visible.
2. Extensive prosthetic dental replacement.
3. Mild osteoarthritic changes are present in the acromioclavicular joints.
4. Bilateral breast prosthesis.
5. Otherwise negative radiographic examination.

Donald C. Boger   2/13/12
Donald C. Boger, M.D.   Date
Radiology Consultant

DCB/ic
hw 2/13/12

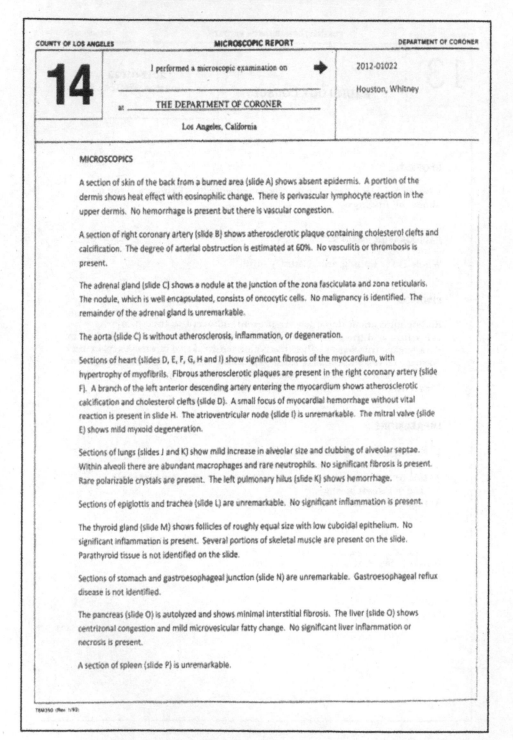

COUNTY OF LOS ANGELES   **MICROSCOPIC REPORT**   DEPARTMENT OF CORONER

14

I performed a microscopic examination on ➡ 2012-01022

Houston, Whitney

at _____ THE DEPARTMENT OF CORONER _____

Los Angeles, California

MICROSCOPICS

A section of skin of the back from a burned area (slide A) shows absent epidermis. A portion of the dermis shows heat effect with eosinophilic change. There is perivascular lymphocyte reaction in the upper dermis. No hemorrhage is present but there is vascular congestion.

A section of right coronary artery (slide B) shows atherosclerotic plaque containing cholesterol clefts and calcification. The degree of arterial obstruction is estimated at 60%. No vasculitis or thrombosis is present.

The adrenal gland (slide C) shows a nodule at the junction of the zona fasciculata and zona reticularis. The nodule, which is well encapsulated, consists of oncocytic cells. No malignancy is identified. The remainder of the adrenal gland is unremarkable.

The aorta (slide C) is without atherosclerosis, inflammation, or degeneration.

Sections of heart (slides D, E, F, G, H and I) show significant fibrosis of the myocardium, with hypertrophy of myofibrils. Fibrous atherosclerotic plaques are present in the right coronary artery (slide F). A branch of the left anterior descending artery entering the myocardium shows atherosclerotic calcification and cholesterol clefts (slide D). A small focus of myocardial hemorrhage without vital reaction is present in slide H. The atrioventricular node (slide I) is unremarkable. The mitral valve (slide E) shows mild myxoid degeneration.

Sections of lungs (slides J and K) show mild increase in alveolar size and clubbing of alveolar septae. Within alveoli there are abundant macrophages and rare neutrophils. No significant fibrosis is present. Rare polarizable crystals are present. The left pulmonary hilus (slide K) shows hemorrhage.

Sections of epiglottis and trachea (slide L) are unremarkable. No significant inflammation is present.

The thyroid gland (slide M) shows follicles of roughly equal size with low cuboidal epithelium. No significant inflammation is present. Several portions of skeletal muscle are present on the slide. Parathyroid tissue is not identified on the slide.

Sections of stomach and gastroesophageal junction (slide N) are unremarkable. Gastroesophageal reflux disease is not identified.

The pancreas (slide O) is autolyzed and shows minimal interstitial fibrosis. The liver (slide O) shows centrizonal congestion and mild microvesicular fatty change. No significant liver inflammation or necrosis is present.

A section of spleen (slide P) is unremarkable.

T8A350 (Rev. 1/93)

COUNTY OF LOS ANGELES   MICROSCOPIC REPORT   DEPARTMENT OF CORONER

2012-01022

Houston, Whitney

14

Page 2

Sections of right kidney (slide P) and left kidney (slide Q) show mild arteriolar sclerosis. Glomeruli, tubules and interstitium are unremarkable. There is no significant inflammation or infarction.

The bladder (slide Q) is denuded of mucosa. The muscularis is unremarkable.

The uterus (slide R) shows a mass of interlacing bundles of spindle cells. No mitotic figures, calcification, or hyalinization are identified. The myometrium contains scattered portions of endometrial stroma without endometrial glands. A short segment of proliferative endometrium is present.

A section of ovary (slide S) shows a hemorrhagic corpus luteum as well as several corpora albicantia.

The right colon (slide S) shows mucosal autolysis. Blood vessels in the muscularis are congested, but there is no hemorrhage.

A section of tonsil (slide T) shows no acute inflammation.

A section of subcutaneous tissue from the left forehead (slide U) shows no hemorrhage or inflammation.

Sections of breasts (slide V) show scattered normal glands in extensive fibrous stroma. No malignancy or significant inflammation is present.

The appendix (slide W) shows fibrous obliteration of the tip.

NEUROPATHOLOGY MICROSCOPICS

Sections of cerebral cortex (slide 1), cerebellum (slide 2), thalamus (slide 3), frontal cortex (slide 5), and brain stem (slide 7) are unremarkable. Slide 4, taken as hippocampus, shows basal ganglia region. Slide 6, taken as hypothalamus with mammillary body, shows globus pallidus, internal capsule, thalamus and hypothalamus. All are unremarkable.

Note: Slides A through W were reviewed by Drs. Chandrasoma, Lakshmanan and Rogers on 3-5-12. Slides B, D, E, F, G, H and I were reviewed by Drs. Fishbein and Rogers on 2-23-12. Slides 1 through 7 are reviewed by Drs. Itabashi and Rogers on 2-23-12.

DIAGNOSIS

1. Atherosclerotic heart disease

    a. Atherosclerosis of right and left coronary arteries

    b. Myocardial fibrosis and fiber hypertrophy

COUNTY OF LOS ANGELES   MICROSCOPIC REPORT   DEPARTMENT OF CORONER

14

2012-01022

Houston, Whitney

Page 3

2. Antemortem scald burn of back

3. Oncocytic microadenoma of adrenal

4. Mild emphysema

5. Mild fatty change of liver

6. Uterine leiomyoma

7. Adenomyosis (stroma only)

8. Fibrous mastopathy

9. Evidence of therapy

    a. Hemorrhages of myocardium and left pulmonary hilus

_____   3.29-12
CHRISTOPHER ROGERS, M.D., MBA   DATE
CHIEF FORENSIC MEDICINE DIVISION

_____   3.29.2012
LAKSHMANAN SATHYAVAGISWARAN, M.D., FRCP(C), FCAP, FACP   DATE
CHIEF MEDICAL EXAMINER-CORONER

CR:LS:mtm/f
T-3/7/12

Rev 2 97i

COUNTY OF LOS ANGELES — **MEDICAL REPORT** — **DEPARTMENT OF CORONER**

15

AUTOPSY CLASS: ☒A ☐B ☐C ☐ Examination Only D

☐ FAMILY OBJECTION TO AUTOPSY

Date: 2-17-12 Time: 1125 Dr. Rogers/Lakshmanan
(Print)

FINAL ON: 3-21-2012 By: Lakshmanan
(Print)

APPROXIMATE INTERVAL BETWEEN ONSET AND DEATH

DEATH WAS CAUSED BY: (Enter only one cause per line for A, B, C, and D)

IMMEDIATE CAUSE:

(A) DROWNING ◄ Unknown

DUE TO, OR AS A CONSEQUENCE OF:

(B) EFFECTS OF ATHEROSCLEROTIC HEART DISEASE ◄ Unknown

DUE TO, OR AS A CONSEQUENCE OF: AND COCAINE USE

(C) ◄

DUE TO, OR AS A CONSEQUENCE OF:

(D) ◄

OTHER CONDITIONS CONTRIBUTING BUT NOT RELATED TO THE IMMEDIATE CAUSE OF DEATH:

☐ NATURAL   ☐ SUICIDE   ☐ HOMICIDE

☒ ACCIDENT   ☐ COULD NOT BE DETERMINED

If other than natural causes, HOW DID INJURY OCCUR? 1) FOUND SUBMERGED IN BATHTUB FILLED WITH WATER 2) COCAINE INTAKE

WAS OPERATION PERFORMED FOR ANY CONDITION STATED ABOVE: ☐ YES ☒ NO

TYPE OF SURGERY: _____ DATE: _____

☐ ORGAN PROCUREMENT   ☐ TECHNICIAN: McDowell

PREGNANCY IN LAST YEAR   ☐ YES ☐ NO ☐ UNK ☐ NOT APPLICABLE

☒ WITNESS TO AUTOPSY   ☐ EVIDENCE RECOVERED AT AUTOPSY
Item Description:

Hyon
Publicker, BHPD

3) Autopsy photos 3 in autopsy room, 28 in photo lab] Reviewed 2-14-12

1 intake photos

✓ Viral culture nasophar
✓ Throat culture

RESIDENT _____   DME _____

WHITE - File Copy   CANARY - Forensic Lab   PINK - Certification   GOLDENROD - DME   (Rev 04-08)

Age: 48   Gender: Male / Female

PRIOR EXAMINATION REVIEW BY DME

☒ BODY TAG   ☐ CLOTHING
☒ X-RAY (No. ___)   ☐ FLUORO
☐ SPECIAL PROCESSING TAG   ☐ MED. RECORDS
☒ AT SCENE PHOTOS (No. 15)

CASE CIRCUMSTANCES

☐ EMBALMED
☐ DECOMPOSED
☐ >24 HRS IN HOSPITAL
☐ OTHER

TYPING SPECIMEN

TYPING SPECIMEN TAKEN BY: OR
SOURCE: Heart

TOXICOLOGY SPECIMEN

COLLECTED BY: OR
☒ HEART BLOOD   ☒ STOMACH CONTENTS
☒ FEMORAL BLOOD (L)   ☒ VITREOUS (2)
   TECHNIQUE: External   ☒ Tracheal air
☒ Femoral R BLOOD   ☐ SPLEEN
   BLOOD   ☐ KIDNEY
☒ BILE   ☒ Serum (heart)
☒ LIVER   ☒ Red cell (heart)
☒ URINE   ☐ heart (2)
URINE GLUCOSE DIPSTICK RESULT: 4+ 3+ 2+ 1+ 0
TOX SPECIMEN RECONCILIATION BY: ___

HISTOLOGY

☒ Regular (No. 2)   ☐ Oversize (No. ___)
Histopath Cut: ☒ Autopsy ☐ Lab

TOXICOLOGY REQUESTS

FORM 3A: ☒ YES ☐ NO
☐ NO TOXICOLOGY REQUESTED
SCREEN ☒ C ☐ H ☐ T ☐ S ☐ O
☐ ALCOHOL ONLY
☐ CARBON MONOXIDE
☐ OTHER (Specify drug and tissue)
   ✓ Vitreous glucose electrolytes, urea
   Hemoglobin 5 screen
   Alprazolam

REQUESTED MATERIAL ON PENDING CASES

☐ POLICE REPORT   ☒ MED HISTORY
☐ TOX FOR COD   ☒ HISTOLOGY
☐ TOX FOR R/O   ☐ INVESTIGATIONS
☒ MICROBIOLOGY   ☐ EYE PATH. CONS.
☒ RADIOLOGY CONS.
☐ CONSULT ON: _____
☐ BRAIN SUBMITTED
☐ NEURO CONSULT   ☐ DME TO CUT
☐ CRIMINALISTICS
☐ GSR ☐ SEXUAL ASSAULT ☐ OTHER

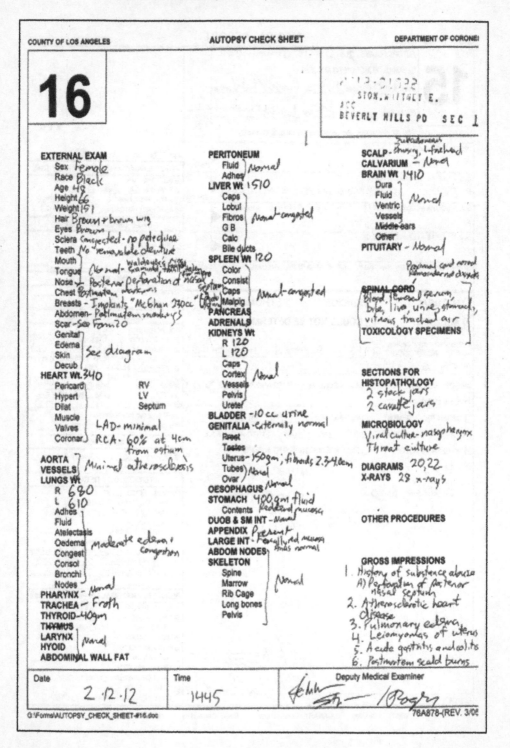

COUNTY OF LOS ANGELES   AUTOPSY CHECK SHEET   DEPARTMENT OF CORONER

16

```
          -13-01722
          STON.WHITNEY E.
          ACC
          BEVERLY HILLS PD    SEC 1
```

EXTERNAL EXAM
Sex Female
Race Black
Age 48
Height 66
Weight 151
Hair Brown + brown wig
Eyes Brown
Sclera Congested - no petechiae
Teeth No remarkable denture
Mouth
Tongue Abnormal - examined Waldeyer's ring
Nose Posterior perforation of nasal Septum
Chest Postmortem markings
Breasts - Implants "McGhan 270cc"
Abdomen- Postmortem markings
Scar - See Form 20
Genital
Edema
Skin   See diagram
Decub

HEART Wt. 340
Pericard   RV
Hypert   LV
Dilat   Septum
Muscle
Valves   LAD - minimal
Coronar   RCA- 60% at 4cm from ostium

AORTA
VESSELS   Minimal atherosclerosis
LUNGS Wt
R 680
L 610
Adhes
Fluid
Atelectasis
Oedema   Moderate edema + congestion
Congest
Consol
Bronchi
Nodes
PHARYNX - Normal
TRACHEA - Froth
THYROID - 40gm
THYMUS
LARYNX   Normal
HYOID
ABDOMINAL WALL FAT

PERITONEUM
Fluid   Normal
Adhes
LIVER Wt 1510
Caps
Lobul
Fibros   Normal - congested
G B
Calc
Bile ducts
SPLEEN Wt 120
Color
Consist
Caps   Normal - congested
Malpig
PANCREAS
ADRENALS
KIDNEYS Wt
R 120
L 120
Caps
Cortex   Normal
Vessels
Pelvis
Ureter
BLADDER - 10 cc urine
GENITALIA - externally normal
Rest
Testes
Uterus - 150gm; fibroids 2.3-4.0cm
Tubes   Normal
Ovar
OESOPHAGUS Normal
STOMACH 400 gm fluid
Contents Reddened mucosa
DUOB & SM INT - Normal
APPENDIX Present
LARGE INT - Focally red mucosa
ABDOM NODES Anus normal
SKELETON
Spine
Marrow   Normal
Rib Cage
Long bones
Pelvis

SCALP - Subcutaneous bruising, L forehead
CALVARIUM - Normal
BRAIN Wt 1410
Dura
Fluid   Normal
Ventric
Vessels
Middle-ears
Other
PITUITARY - Normal

Proximal cord normal
Remainder no damage

SPINAL CORD
Blood, Femoral serum, bile, liver, urine, stomach, vitreous, tracheal air
TOXICOLOGY SPECIMENS

SECTIONS FOR HISTOPATHOLOGY
2 stock jars
2 cassette jars

MICROBIOLOGY
Viral culture - nasopharynx
Throat culture

DIAGRAMS 20,22
X-RAYS 28 x-rays

OTHER PROCEDURES

GROSS IMPRESSIONS
1. History of substance abuse
   A) Perforation of posterior nasal septum
2. Atherosclerotic heart disease
3. Pulmonary edema
4. Leiomyomas of uterus
5. Acute gastritis and colitis
6. Postmortem scald burns

Date   2·12·12   Time   1445   Deputy Medical Examiner

G:\Forms\AUTOPSY_CHECK_SHEET-#16.doc   76A878-(REV. 3/05)

Coroner Case Number: 2012-01022 **Decedent:** HOUSTON, WHITNEY ELIZABETH

SPECIMEN	SERVICE	DRUG	RESULT	ANALYST
	Phenytoin	Phenytoin	ND	E. Fu
Urine				
	Alcohol	Ethanol	Negative	M. Schuchardt
Vitreous				
	Outside Test	Electrolytes	* Done	NMS Labs, Inc.
	Outside Test	Glucose	* Done	NMS Labs, Inc.

NOTE: Blood*=Blood drawn from right Femoral Vein. Blood, Femoral=Blood drawn from left Femoral Vein. *Vitreous sample was submitted to NMS Labs, Inc. at a dilution due to the viscosity of the specimen.

Legend:

		mg\dL	Milligram per Deciliter	QNS	Quantity Not Sufficient	
g	Grams	mg/L	Milligram per Liter	TNP	Test Not Performed	
g%	Gram Percent	ND	Not Detected	ug	Micrograms	
Inc.	Inconclusive	ng/g	Nanograms per Gram	ug/g	Micrograms per Gram	
mg	Milligrams	ng/mL	Nanograms per Milliliter	ug/mL	Micrograms per Milliliter	

In accordance with the Department's Evidence Retention Policy, the blood specimen(s) will be retained for one year and all other specimen for six-months from Autopsy.

Administratively reviewed by: _[signature]_

Daniel T. Anderson, M.A, FTS-ABFT, D-ABC
Supervising Criminalist II
TOXICOLOGY

ER 39.12

Joseph M. Quashnock, PhD   **PerkinElmer Genetics, Inc.**   <u>Date of Report</u>
Laboratory Director   **PO Box 219**   02/18/2012

Bridgeville, PA 15017

(412) 220-2300 Phone
(412) 220-0784 Fax   Page 1 of 1

Initial Release: 02/18/2012 14:58

Date Collected: 02/12/2012	Date Recvd: 02/17/2012	Birth Date: 08/09/1963
Submittor: Los Angeles Coroner		Cond. of Spec: S
Filter Paper: 3996042	Patient's Name: DOE, JANE	Sex: F
PS ID: 4951371	AKA Name:	
Accession No: 2012045767	Med. Rec. No: 2012-01022	
Mother's Name:		Physician: ROGERS

Autopsy Specimen Report

Screening Test	Outcome
Acylcarnitine Profile	Negative
CAH 17-OHP	Negative
Congenital Hypothyroidism-TSH	Negative
Galactose- (Gal and Gal-1-P)	Negative
Hemoglobinopathies	Negative

OUTCOME DEFINITIONS

NEGATIVE - The analyte detected does not exceed the concentration usually found in such analyses. Interpretation should be in conjunction with other findings.

SELECTED REFERENCE RANGE

17 OH P
Cutoff values for 17 hydroxyprogesterone are age dependent. For infants less than 91 days of age, abnormal is defined as a value > 19.0 ng/mL; for infants 91 days to 1 year of age, abnormal is > 5.0 ng/mL; for age > 1 year, abnormal is > 4.0 ng/mL. Note new reference range for 17-hydroxyprogesterone effective November 1, 2010.

TSH
Cutoff values for TSH are age dependent. For infants < 7 days of age, abnormal is defined as a TSH value >50 uIU/mL; for infants 7 days or older, abnormal is > 30 uIU/mL.

GAL
Abnormal is defined for all infant ages as a total galactose > 20 mg/dL.

Comments:

The results of PerkinElmer Genetics post-mortem testing are analytically accurate within the limits of the test technology used. Factors including specimen source, quality of specimen and patient variables will affect results. Limited information on reference ranges is available. Interpretation of results should be in conjunction with additional clinical or laboratory evidence to help support or disprove the presence of a specific disorder.

Laboratory Report

NMS
LABS

NMS Labs

CONFIDENTIAL

3701 Welsh Road, PO Box 433A, Willow Grove, PA 19090-0437
Phone: (215) 657-4900 Fax: (215) 657-2972
e-mail: nms@nmslabs.com
Robert A. Middleberg, PhD, DABFT, DABCC-TC, Laboratory Director

Toxicology Report

Report Issued   03/07/2012 09:02

To: 10139
Los Angeles County Coroner Medical Examiner
Attn: Joseph Muto
1104 N. Mission Road
Los Angeles, CA 90033

Patient Name	DOE, JANE
Patient ID	2012-01022
Chain	11392960
Age	Not Given
Gender	Not Given
Workorder	12058575

Page 1 of 2

Positive Findings:

Compound	Result	Units	Matrix Source
Potassium (Vitreous Fluid)	8.5	mEq/L	Vitreous Fluid
Chloride (Vitreous Fluid)	53	mEq/L	Vitreous Fluid
Creatinine (Vitreous Fluid)	0.6	mg/dL	Vitreous Fluid
Urea Nitrogen (Vitreous Fluid)	13	mg/dL	Vitreous Fluid
Glucose (Vitreous Fluid)	< 20	mg/dL	Vitreous Fluid

See Detailed Findings section for additional information

** vitreous sample submitted at a
½ dilution due to viscosity*

Testing Requested:

Analysis Code	Description
01919FL	Electrolytes Panel, Fluid

Tests Not Performed:

Part or all of the requested testing was unable to be performed. Refer to the **Analysis Summary and Reporting Limits** section for details.

Specimens Received:

ID	Tube/Container	Volume/ Mass	Collection Date/Time	Matrix Source	Miscellaneous Information
001	Red Top Tube	1.2 mL	02/21/2012 13:00	Vitreous Fluid	

All sample volumes/weights are approximations.
Specimens received on 02/22/2012.

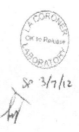

Sp 3/7/12

v.8

▲ NMS
LABS

CONFIDENTIAL

Workorder 12058575
Chain 11392960
Patient ID 2012-01022

Page 2 of 2

＋ all samples at a
½ dilution (see pg 1)

Detailed Findings:

Analysis and Comments	Result	Units	Rpt. Limit	Specimen Source	Analysis By
Potassium (Vitreous Fluid)	8.5	mEq/L		001 - Vitreous Fluid	[Not provided]
Chloride (Vitreous Fluid)	53	mEq/L		001 - Vitreous Fluid	[Not provided]
Creatinine (Vitreous Fluid)	0.6	mg/dL		001 - Vitreous Fluid	[Not provided]
Urea Nitrogen (Vitreous Fluid)	13	mg/dL		001 - Vitreous Fluid	[Not provided]
Glucose (Vitreous Fluid)	< 20	mg/dL		001 - Vitreous Fluid	[Not provided]

Other than the above findings, examination of the specimen(s) submitted did not reveal any positive findings of toxicological significance by procedures outlined in the accompanying Analysis Summary.

Reference Comments:

1. Glucose (Vitreous Fluid) - Vitreous Fluid:

    Analysis for Electrolytes Panel, including Sodium, Potassium, Chloride, Creatinine, Urea Nitrogen and Glucose was performed by:
    Health Network Laboratories
    2024 Lehigh Street
    Allentown, PA 18103

Chain of custody documentation has been maintained for the analyses performed by NMS Labs.

Unless alternate arrangements are made by you, the remainder of the submitted specimens will be discarded six (6) weeks from the date of this report; and generated data will be discarded five (5) years from the date the analyses were performed.

Analysis Summary and Reporting Limits:

Acode 01919FL - Electrolytes Panel, Fluid - Vitreous Fluid

-Analysis by [Not provided] for:

Compound	Rpt. Limit	Compound	Rpt. Limit
Chloride (Vitreous Fluid)	N/A	Potassium (Vitreous Fluid)	N/A
Creatinine (Vitreous Fluid)	N/A	Sodium (Vitreous Fluid)	N/A
Glucose (Vitreous Fluid)	N/A	Urea Nitrogen (Vitreous Fluid)	N/A

SP 3/9/12

02329-12 v.8

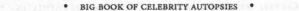

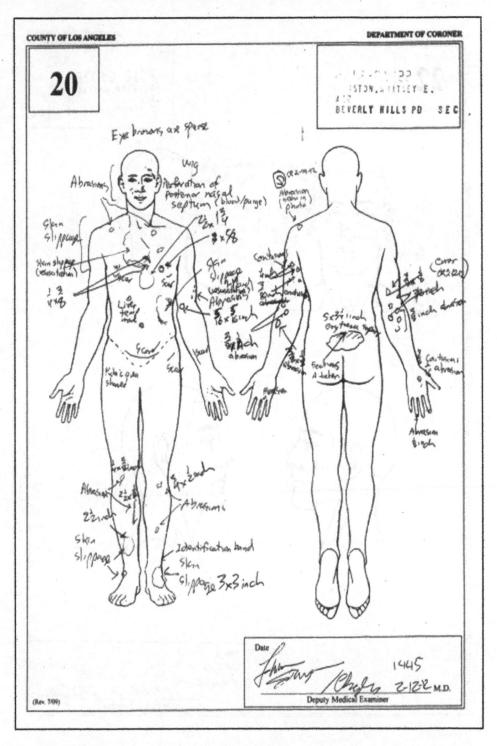

Deputy Medical Examiner

(Rev. 7/09)

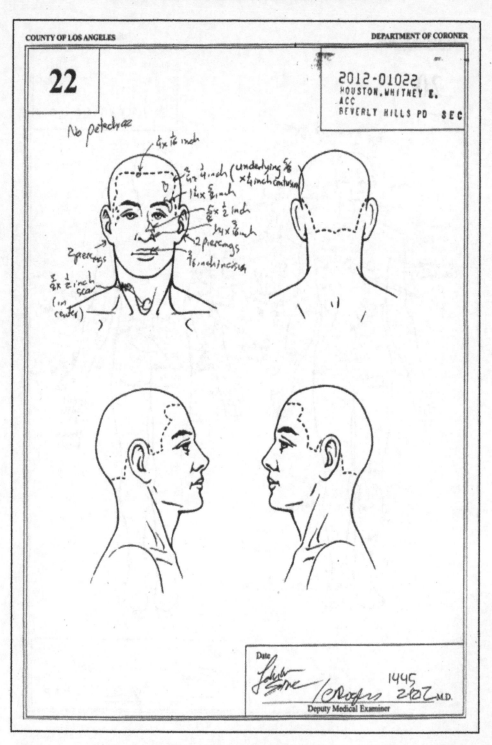

COUNTY OF LOS ANGELES   **SEXUAL ASSAULT EVIDENCE DATA SHEET**   DEPT OF CORONER

81

Case Reported to Coroner (Date/Time): _02/11/12_ _3104h_

Criminalist: _SCHUELDART_ _L_

Forensic Science Laboratories
Phone #: 323-343-0530   Fax #: 323-222-5171

CC#: _2012-01022_

Decedent: _HOUSTON, WHITNEY_

Male   (Female)

SEXUAL ASSAULT EVIDENCE COLLECTION STARTED: Location: _scene_   Date: _02/11/12_ Time: _2330_

SEXUAL ASSAULT EVIDENCE COLLECTION COMPLETED: Location: _scene_   Date: _02/12/12_ Time: _0015_

	Collected Scene	FSC	INITIALS	Not Collected
1. ORAL CAVITY: Swab set & slide set	☒	☐		☐
2. NECK: Wet swab set	☐	☐		☒
3. LEFT BREAST: Wet swab set	☒	☐		☐
4. RIGHT BREAST: Wet swab set	☒	☐		☐
5. EXTERNAL GENITAL: Wet swab set & slide set	☒	☐		☐
6. VAGINAL CAVITY: Swab set & slide set	☒	☐		☐
7. CERVICAL: Swab set & slide set	☐	☐		☒
8. PENILE SHAFT: Wet swab set & slide set	☐	☐		☐
9. ANAL OPENING: Wet swab set & slide set	☒	☐		☐
10. RECTAL: Swab set & slide set	☒	☐		☐
11. VAGINAL ASPIRATE	☐	☐		☒
12. PUBIC HAIR COMBING	☒	☐		☐

13. OTHER EVIDENCE packaged with the sexual assault evidence:

-
-
-
-

14. ALTERNATE LIGHT SOURCE utilized ....YES ☐   NO ☒

Wavelength	Color of Goggles	Findings

COMMENTS: _BODY NUDE - REMATELY SUBMERGED ENTIRELY IN 98" BATH WATER FOR AT/AS ONE HOUR; M4 CLOTHING COLLECTED._

Reviewed by DME: _CRoss_ , M.D.   Date: _2-14-12_   Time: _1145_

Revised 94-61-001

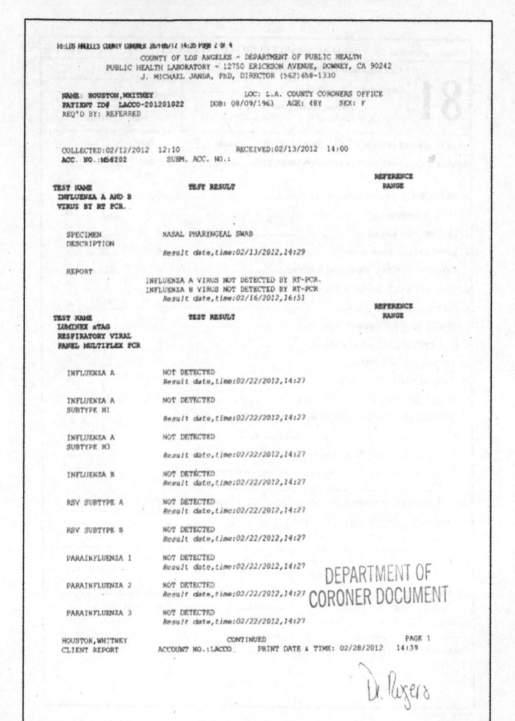

COUNTY OF LOS ANGELES - DEPARTMENT OF PUBLIC HEALTH
PUBLIC HEALTH LABORATORY - 12750 ERICKSON AVENUE, DOWNEY, CA 90242
J. MICHAEL JANDA, PhD, DIRECTOR (562)658-1330

NAME: HOUSTON,WHITNEY   LOC: L.A. COUNTY CORONERS OFFICE
PATIENT ID# LACCO-201201022   DOB: 08/09/1963   AGE: 48Y   SEX: F
REQ'D BY: REFERRED

COLLECTED:02/12/2012 12:10   RECEIVED:02/13/2012 14:00
ACC. NO.:M56202   SUBM. ACC. NO.:

TEST NAME	TEST RESULT	REFERENCE RANGE
INFLUENZA A AND B VIRUS BY RT PCR.		

SPECIMEN DESCRIPTION   NASAL PHARYNGEAL SWAB
Result date,time:02/13/2012,14:29

REPORT
INFLUENZA A VIRUS NOT DETECTED BY RT-PCR.
INFLUENZA B VIRUS NOT DETECTED BY RT-PCR
Result date,time:02/16/2012,16:51

TEST NAME	TEST RESULT	REFERENCE RANGE
LUMINEX xTAG RESPIRATORY VIRAL PANEL MULTIFLEX PCR		
INFLUENZA A	NOT DETECTED Result date,time:02/22/2012,14:27	
INFLUENZA A SUBTYPE H1	NOT DETECTED Result date,time:02/22/2012,14:27	
INFLUENZA A SUBTYPE H3	NOT DETECTED Result date,time:02/22/2012,14:27	
INFLUENZA B	NOT DETECTED Result date,time:02/22/2012,14:27	
RSV SUBTYPE A	NOT DETECTED Result date,time:02/22/2012,14:27	
RSV SUBTYPE B	NOT DETECTED Result date,time:02/22/2012,14:27	
PARAINFLUENZA 1	NOT DETECTED Result date,time:02/22/2012,14:27	
PARAINFLUENZA 2	NOT DETECTED Result date,time:02/22/2012,14:27	
PARAINFLUENZA 3	NOT DETECTED Result date,time:02/22/2012,14:27	

DEPARTMENT OF CORONER DOCUMENT

HOUSTON,WHITNEY   CONTINUED   PAGE 1
CLIENT REPORT   ACCOUNT NO.:LACCO   PRINT DATE & TIME: 02/28/2012 14:39

Dr. Rogers

COUNTY OF LOS ANGELES - DEPARTMENT OF PUBLIC HEALTH
PUBLIC HEALTH LABORATORY - 12750 ERICKSON AVENUE, DOWNEY, CA 90242
J. MICHAEL JANDA, PhD, DIRECTOR (562)658-1330

NAME: HOUSTON,WHITNEY   LOC: L.A. COUNTY CORONERS OFFICE
PATIENT ID# LACCO-201201022   DOB: 08/09/1963 AGE: 48Y   SEX: F
REQ'D BY: REFERRED

COLLECTED:02/12/2012 12:10   RECEIVED:02/13/2012 14:00
ACC. NO.:M56202   SUBM. ACC. NO.:

                                                          REFERENCE
                                                          RANGE
TEST NAME   TEST RESULT
LUMINEX xTAG   (CONTINUED)
RESPIRATORY VIRAL
PANEL MULTIPLEX PCR
                          Result date,time: 02/22/2012,14:27

  HUMAN   NOT DETECTED
  METAPNEUMOVIRUS
                          Result date,time:02/22/2012,14:27

  RHINOVIRUS   NOT DETECTED
                          Result date,time:02/22/2012,14:27

  ADENOVIRUS   NOT DETECTED
                          Result date,time:02/22/2012,14:27

                    VIROLOGY

     COLLECTED: 02/12/2012 /12:10   RECEIVED: 02/13/2012 /14:00

     ACC. NO.: M56203 BATTERY ORDERED: VIRAL CULTURE, COMPREHENSIVE

     SPECIMEN DESCRIPTION: NASAL PHARYNGEAL SWAB

     REPORT STATUS: FINAL 02/27/2012

     DIRECT EXAM: 1.   NOT DONE

     CULTURE: 1.   NO VIRUS ISOLATED IN TISSUE CULTURE

                    DEPARTMENT OF
                  CORONER DOCUMENT

HOUSTON,WHITNEY   END OF REPORT   PAGE 2
CLIENT REPORT   ACCOUNT NO.:LACCO   PRINT DATE & TIME: 02/28/2012 14:39

02/14/2012 07:59 FAX 3234415108   MICROBIOLOGY LAB   → CORONER'S   ☒003/004

LAC + USC Medical Center
1200 N. State St., Los Angeles, CA 90033
Ira A. Shulman, M.D., Director, Laboratories & Pathology
02/14/2012 07:00

Page: 1

X186954 COLL: 02/12/2012 1215   REC: 02/12/2012 1402 PHYS: ILLEGIBLE, PHYSICIAN
THROAT/NASOPHARYNGEA   FINAL 02/13/2012
MICRO LAB SETUP: UNKNOWN UNKNOWN
          SPECIMEN DESCRIPTION: AUTOPSY THROAT
          SPECIAL REQUESTS: NONE

     CULTURE: NORMAL ORAL FLORA ISOLATED IN NORMAL NUMBERS.

END OF REPORT

                                        HOUSTON, WHITNEY
                                        CC-201201022
ACCOUNT #: 9068   CC CORONERS CASE
                                        F 08/09/1963
C O N F I D E N T I A L
SUMMARY REPORT

CR 21412

Buddy Holly

Given Name: Charles Hardin Holly
Born: September 7, 1936, Lubbock, Texas
Died: February 3, 1959, Clear Lake, Iowa
Cause of Death: Plane Crash

In his short career, Buddy Holly was considered one of the most influential artists in rock. He died in a plane crash while on tour across the Midwest. Ritchie Valens and J. P. "The Big Bopper" Richardson were also on the plane. Since his death, there have been many songs in tribute of Holly, most notably Don Maclean's "American Pie," which coined the term "the day the music died" in reference to the tragedy.

From the Coroner's Report dated Feb. 4, 1959

The body of Charles H. Holley was clothed in an outer jacket of yellow leather-like material in which 4 seams in the back were split almost full length. The skull was split medially in the forehead and this extended into the vertex region. Approximately half the brain tissue was absent. There was bleeding from both ears, and the face showed multiple lacerations. The consistency of the chest was soft due to extensive crushing injury to the bony structure. The left forearm was factured [sic] 1/3 the way up from the wrist and the right elbow was fractured. Both thighs and legs showed multiple factures [sic]. There was a small laceration of the scrotum.

Personal effects found with the body are listed on a separate sheet in this report.

Fingerprints were taken of the deceased for purposes of identification.

Ralph E. Smiley, MD
Acting coroner
Personal effects, Charles Holley
Cash $193.00 less $11.65 coroner's fees - $181.35. 2 cuff links, silver 1/2 in.
balls having jeweled band. Top portion of ball point pen.

Ritchie Valens

Given Name: Richard Steven Valenzuela
Born: May 13, 1941, Los Angeles, California
Died: February 3, 1959, Clear Lake, Iowa
Cause of Death: Plane Crash

Ritchie Valens was one of the first musicians to combine Spanish language with rock music. Known as a Chicano rock star, Valens's first hit was "La Bamba," one of the first completely Spanish songs to reach the top of the charts. Valens died in the same plane crash that claimed Buddy Holly in Clear Lake, Iowa.

The coroner took his fee out of the money Valens had on him at the time.

CORONER'S REPORT OF INVESTIGATION Form 205-L, Austin, Mason City, Iowa

Cerro Gordo _____ County, Iowa

In Account With

For Investigation of the Death of

Richard Valentuela

Ralph R. Smiley, M. D. Acting _____ Coroner. Address Racoina, Calif.

BE IT REMEMBERED, That on the _____ day of _____ Feb. _____, 19 59, information was given the undersigned, Ralph R. Smiley M. D. Acting _____, Coroner of _____ Cerro Gordo _____ County, Iowa, that the body of Richard Valenzuela _____ had been found at _____ near Mt Lincoln _____ in said County, supposed to have come to ____ his ____ death by violence, unknown enemy, or has died without attendance of a physician. In the latter case the Coroner, under Chapter 141, Code of Iowa, must be called to sign the death certificate. An investigation conducted ____ Feb. 3 and ____ 19 ____ reveals facts of a financial nature, as follows:

Deceased is resident of _____ Racoina, Calif. _____

Relatives or others financially responsible _____ I do not know _____

Estate left ____ I do not know. _____

Personal effects found on body silver crucifix and religious medal, brown leather pocket case, numerous receipts

Disposition of personal effects on ____ Hollywood office, with keys, watch $ 42.00 $ 11.55 coroner's fees, check $30

Disposition of body ____ Sioux Funeral Home, Fees _____ bracelet with "Donna" attached

Coroner's Transcript of Fees—To County Auditor

CORONER'S FEES (Sec. 340.19, Code of Iowa, and Chap. 12 and 47, 44th G. A.)	Amount	REPORTER'S FEES 50c an hour. (Sec. 339.10)	Amount
Inquest or Investigation, including return, $10	$ 10.00		$
To Comply with Chap. 141, Code of Iowa, $5			
Jury Order, 25 cents		**Total Reporter's Fee** $	
Warrants, 25 cents		**WITNESS FEES—Give Name and Address if Out of Town** Fee $2.00 per day and 10c per mile. (Sec. 339.23)	
Subpoena, 25 cents each			$
Mileage, 7c per mile, not automobile exp.	.65		
Docket Case, $1	1.00		
	$		
Total Coroner's Fees $	11.65		
CONSTABLE'S FEES (Sec. 601.129)		**Total Witness Fees** $	
Name	$	**MISCELLANEOUS COSTS** (Unusual Items)	
Summoning Jury, $1.00 (no mileage)			$
Subpoena, 15 cents each			
Mileage, 7c per mile			
Total Constable's Fees $		**Total Miscellaneous Costs** $	
JURY FEES—Give Names Fee $2.00 per day; Mileage 10c one way. (Sec. 339.23)		**RECAPITULATION**	
1:		Coroner's Fees	$ 11.65
2:		Constable's Fees	
3:		Juror's Fees	
Total Jury Fees $		Physician's Fees	
PHYSICIAN'S AND SURGEON'S FEES (Give Names and Addresses)		Reporter's Fees	
	$	Witness Fees	
		Miscellaneous Costs	
Total Physician's and Surgeon's Fees $		**Total Amount of Claims** $ 11.65

I swear that the above account is just and true, is under authority of law and has not been paid, or any part thereof. I make this statement for the purpose of obtaining payment of said claim.

Subscribed and sworn to before me this ____ 11th ____ day of ____ Feb. ____, 19 59.

The body of Richard Valenzuela was clothed in a black wool cloth overcoat containing a label "Harris & Drank, Los Angeles, Cal.", a black wool cloth suit containing inside, the coat label "Sobel's, San Fernando, Cal.", a white shirt and underclothing. On the volar surface of the right forearm was a dark tattoo of initials "R.V." The head was badly crushed and deformed, the calvarium region wide open and the brain tissue almost completely eviscerated; the right side of the face was crushed and flattened and the right eye-socket eviscerated. The facial features were not identifiable. There was marked deformity of the left forearm due to fracture, a 1-inch laceration on the dorsum of the left hand at its junction with the little finger. The left upper femur had marked deformity with fracture while the right tibia showed a compound fracture. There were two shallow lacerations in the medial mid-left shin region. Internal injuries were not appraised because autopsy was not done. Personal effects are listed on a separate sheet in this report.

Fingerprints were taken of the deceased for purposes of identification.

(See attached report of investigation)

A copy of the transcript of fees has been sent to the County Auditor. A copy of this report is filed with the Clerk of the District Court. A copy of each is filed or recorded in the Coroner's Docket.

I, _____ Ralph E. Smiley, M.D. Acting Coroner of _____ Cerro Gordo _____ County, Iowa, on

the __3rd__ day of ____Feb.____, 19_59_, hereby certify that the above facts are made of record after diligent investigation and I believe them to be correct.

_____ Coroner

Michael Jackson

Born: August 9, 1959, Gary, Indiana
Died: June 25, 2009, Los Angeles, California
Cause of Death: Drug overdose

The King of Pop started his career as a member of the Jackson Five before moving onto a solo career. He is one of the most influential and popular singers throughout the world, and his record *Thriller* is the best-selling album of all time. His death came as a shock to many of his fans, and his doctor, Conrad Murray, was convicted of involuntary manslaughter following the singer's death.

CASE REPORT

COUNTY OF LOS ANGELES

1

APPARENT MODE
ACCIDENT/ NATURAL

SPECIAL CIRCUMSTANCES
Celebrity, Media Interest

IN PRESENCE OF CORONER
CASE NO
2009-04415

UNIT
S.C.

LAST, FIRST, MIDDLE
JACKSON, MICHAEL JOSEPH

ADDRESS
100 NORTH CAROLWOOD DRIVE

CITY
LOS ANGELES

STATE
CA

ZIP
90077

SEX	RACE	DOB	AGE	HGT	WGT	EYES	HAIR	TEETH	FACIAL HAIR	EMPLOYED	DVM	CLOTHING
MALE	BLACK	8/29/1958	50	69 in	136 lbs	BROWN	BROWN	ALL NATURAL TEETH			Yes	FAIR

NOTIFIED BY

DATE
6/25/2009

TIME

SSN
XXX-XX-5798

STATE
CA

PERSON BY

ONE TYPE
CALIFORNIA DRIVERS LICENSE

LIC #	SRN #	DOB	FBI #	MILITARY #	POB
					INDIANA

IDENTIFIED BY NAME (PRINT)
CDL

RELEASED #

PHONE

DATE
6/25/2009

TIME

PLACE OF DEATH/PLACE FOUND
HOSPITAL
RONALD REAGAN/UCLA MEDICAL CENTER

ADDRESS OR LOCATION
757 WESTWOOD PLAZA DRIVE

CITY
LOS ANGELES

ZIP
90095

PLACE OF INJURY
RESIDENCE

AT WORK
No

DATE

TIME

LOCATION OR ADDRESS
100 NORTH CAROLWOOD DRIVE, LOS ANGELES, CA

ZIP
90077

DOD	TIME	FOUND OR PRONOUNCED BY
6/25/2009	14:26	DR COOPER

OTHER AGENCY / INV OFFICER
LAPD ROBBERY HOMICIDE DIVISION - DET SKY (213) 485-2167

REPORT NO

NOTIFIED BY

NO

TRANSPORTED BY
ALEXANDER P PEREZ

TO
LOS ANGELES FSC

DATE
6/25/2009

TIME
18:50

PRESUMED/POV	Yes	CLOTHING	No	AS EVT	No	MORTUARY	
MED EV	Yes	INVEST PHOTOS	30	SEAL TYPE	NOT SEALED	HOSP EVT	Yes
PHYS EV	No	EVIDENCE LOG	Yes	PROPERTY	Yes	HOSP CHART	Yes
SUICIDE NOTE	No	CSR NO		RCPT NO	231940	DR NO	397-5944

SYNOPSIS
THE DECEDENT IS A 50-YEAR-OLD BLACK MALE WHO SUFFERED RESPIRATORY ARREST WHILE AT HOME UNDER THE CARE OF HIS PRIMARY PHYSICIAN. ON THE DAY OF HIS DEATH, THE DECEDENT COMPLAINED OF DEHYDRATION AND NOT BEING ABLE TO SLEEP. SEVERAL HOURS LATER, THE DECEDENT STOPPED BREATHING AND COULD NOT BE RESUSITATED. PARAMEDICS TRANSPORTED HIM TO UCLA MEDICAL CENTER, WHERE HE WAS PRONOUNCED DEAD. THE DECEDENT WAS TAKING SEVERAL PRESCRIPTION MEDICATIONS INCLUDING LORAZEPAM, TRAZODONE, DIAZEPAM, TEMAZEPAM AND FLOMAX. IT IS UNKNOWN IF HE WAS COMPLIANT WITH HIS MEDICATION. THE DECEDENT NEVER DIED FROM VERTIGO AND HAD NO HISTORY OF HEART PROBLEMS.

DONNA FIREAK
#7063

DATE
6/26/2009

TIME
04:33

REVIEWED BY

TIME
0700

FORM #3 NARRATIVE TO FOLLOW? ✓

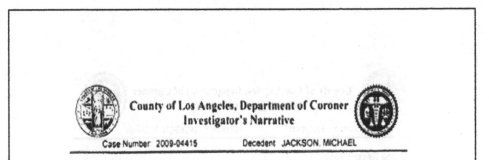

County of Los Angeles, Department of Coroner
Investigator's Narrative

Case Number: 2009-04415   Decedent JACKSON, MICHAEL

Information Sources:

1 Detective W. Porche, LAPD- West Los Angeles Division

2 Detective S. Smith, LAPD- Robbery Homicide Division

3. UCLA Medical Center, medical record #397-5944

Investigation:

On 6/25/09 at 1538 hours, Detective W. Porche from the Los Angeles Police Department (LAPD) reported this case as an accidental vs. natural death to the Los Angeles County Department of Coroner. Lieutenant F. Corral assigned this death investigation to me at 1615 hours. I arrived at UCLA Medical Center at 1720 hours, along with Assistant Chief E. Winter and Forensic Attendant A. Perez. Upon my completion of the body examination at the hospital, the decedent was transported by the Los Angeles Sheriffs Department-Air Bureau to the Coroner's Forensic Science Center (FSC). Forensic Attendant Perez escorted the decedent's body during transport.

Assistant Chief E. Winter and I left the hospital and went to the decedent's residence. We arrived at the residence at 1910 hours and I performed a scene investigation. We departed the scene 2020 hours and returned to the FSC.

Location:

Place of death: UCLA Medical Center, 757 Westwood Plaza Drive, Los Angeles, CA 90095

Informant/Witness Statements:

The following information is preliminary and subject to change pending further investigation by the appropriate law enforcement agency. I spoke with Detective S. Smith from the LAPD and he reported that on the early morning of 6/25/09 at approximately 0100 hours, the decedent placed a call to his primary physician, cardiologist, Dr. Conrad Murray. The decedent complained of being dehydrated and not being able to sleep. Dr. Murray went to the decedent's residence and administered medical care. The details and extent of this medical care are currently unknown; though the decedent slept for several hours and Dr. Murray was at the bedside. Around 1200 hours, Dr. Murray found that the decedent was not breathing and he pulled the decedent onto the bedroom floor and began CPR. 911 was called and paramedics responded to the house.

According to the medical record (listed above), the paramedics arrived at the home at 1225 hours and found the decedent asystolic. Paramedics continued CPR and ACLS protocol including two rounds of epinephrine and atropine. The decedent was then intubated and CPR efforts continued. The decedent remained unresponsive; his pupils were fixed and dilated. Under advisement of Dr. Murray, the decedent was placed in the ambulance and transported to UCLA Medical Center. Throughout the transport, all medical orders were given by Dr. Murray.

The decedent presented asystolic to the hospital. Central lines and an intra-aortic balloon pump were placed but the decedent remained without vital signs. Dr. Cooper pronounced death at 1426 hours on 6/25/09.

According to Detective S. Smith, the decedent had been undergoing daily strenuous exercise in preparation for an upcoming planned music tour, in which it would have been necessary for the decedent to be in strong physical condition. The decedent did not have a history of heart problems. He was taking several prescription medications including clonazepam, trazodone, diazepam, lorazepam and Flomax but it is unknown if he was compliant.

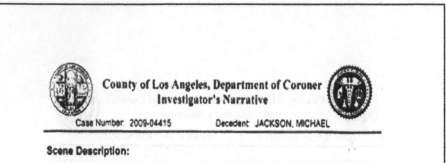

County of Los Angeles, Department of Coroner
Investigator's Narrative

Case Number: 2009-04415   Decedent: JACKSON, MICHAEL

Scene Description:

The decedent's residence is a two-story mansion located in Bel-Air on a quiet residential street. The home is clean and well-groomed. I observed the bedroom on the second floor of the home, to the right of the top of the staircase. Reportedly, this is the bedroom where the decedent had been resting and entered cardiac arrest. His usual bedroom was down the hall.

The bedroom to the right of the staircase contained a queen size bed, numerous tables and chairs, a dresser and a television. There was also a large attached walk-in closet. The bedding was disheveled and appeared as though someone had been lying on the left side of the bed. There was a blue plastic pad lined with cotton on the left side of the fitted sheet near the center of the bed. Near the left foot of the bed, there was a string of wooden beads and a tube of toothpaste. Miscellaneous items remained on the right side of the bed including a book, laptop computer and eyeglasses. Also near the foot of the bed, there was a closed bottle of urine atop a chair.

Next to the left side of the bed, there were two tables and a tan colored sofa chair. Reportedly, the decedent's doctor sat here. A green oxygen tank was also on this side of the bed. The decedent's prescription medication bottles were seen on the tables with various medical supplies including a box of catheters, disposable needles and alcohol pads. Several empty orange juice bottles, a telephone and lamp were on the tables as well. An ambu-bag and latex gloves lay on the floor next to the bed.

Evidence:

I collected medical evidence from the decedent's residence on 6/25/09; see form 3A for details.

Body Examination:

I performed an external body examination at the hospital on 6/25/09. The decedent was wearing a hospital gown. The body is that of an adult Black male who appears to be approximately 50-years-old. He has brown colored eyes, natural teeth and brown hair. The decedent's head hair is sparse and is connected to a wig. The decedent's overall skin has patches of light and dark pigmented areas.

The ambient temperature in the hospital room was 68 degrees F at 1815 hours. At 1811 hours, rigor mortis was not present throughout the body and lividity blanched with light pressure. Lividity was consistent with a supine position.

There was a dark black discoloration on the decedent's upper forehead near his hair line. Dark coloration was present on the decedent's eyebrows, eyelashes and lips. A small piece of gauze was found on the tip of his nose and an ETT, held in place with medical tape, was seen in his mouth. A red discoloration is prominent on the center of his chest.

Gauze covering a puncture wound was taped to his right neck and IV catheters were present in his left neck and bilaterally in the inguinal area. There was also an external urine catheter present. Additional puncture wounds were seen on his right shoulder, both arms and both ankles. There is a bruise on his left inner leg, below his knee and 4 discolored indentations were found on his lower backside.

Identification:

The body was positively identified as Michael Joseph Jackson by visual comparison to his California Drivers License on 6/25/09.

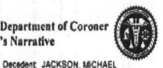

**County of Los Angeles, Department of Coroner
Investigator's Narrative**

Case Number. 2009-04415   Decedent: JACKSON, MICHAEL

Next of Kin Notification:

The decedent was not married and his children are under 18 years of age   His mother,
is the legal next-of-kin and was notified of the death on 6/25/09.

Tissue Donation:

The hospital record does not indicate if the decedent's family was approached regarding
donation

Autopsy Notification:

Detective S. Smith from the LAPD-Robbery Homicide Division requests notification of autopsy.
See file for contact information.

E. Fleak
ELISSA FLEAK, Investigator

John Fleak
Supervisor

6/26/9

6/26/2009

3A

COUNTY OF LOS ANGELES   MEDICAL EVIDENCE   DEPARTMENT OF CORONER

CASE # 2009-04415
DECEDENT'S NAME: JACKSON, MICHAEL JOSEPH
DOD: 6/25/2009
INCOMING MODE

Page 1 of 2

Drug Name	Rx Number	Date of Issue	Number Issued	Number Remaining	Form	Dosage	Rx Directions	Physician	Pharmacy Phone/ Comments
BENOQUIN					LIQUID	20%	LOTION IN TUBE		APPLIED PHARMACY SERVICES, NO SCRIPT INFO
CLORAZEPAM	1753217	4/18/2009	30	8	TABLET	7MG	1 AT BEDTIME	METZGER	RITE AID 310-273-3561
DIAZEPAM	C0222085	6/20/2009	60	57	TABLET	10MG	1/2 TO 1 EVERY 6 HRS	MURRAY	CVS 310-273-3782
FLOMAX	982153	6/2/2009	30	24	CAPSULE	0.4MG	ONCE DAILY	MURRAY	CVS 310-474-2152
HYDROQUINONE					LIQUID	8%	LOTION IN TUBE	MURRAY	
LIDOCAINE	6826273	3/14/2009	60		LIQUID	4%FLO	LOTION IN TUBE	MURRAY	APPLIED PHARMACY SERVICES, NO SCRIPT INFO
LORAZEPAM	C367154	4/28/2009	30	8	TABLET	2MG	ONCE AT BEDTIME	MURRAY	APPLIED PHARMACY SERVICES, NO 304-03779 PRESCRIBED TO DR. MURRAY CVS 310-474-2152
TEMAZEPAM	C541756	12/22/2008	30	3	CAPSULE	30MG	ONCE AT BEDTIME AS N	MURRAY	CVS 310-474-2152

Paraphernalia Description

ONE GREEN OXYGEN TANK; A BROKEN SYRINGE, AN OPEN BOX OF HYPODERMIC DISPOSABLE NEEDLES; AN OPEN BOX OF IV-CATHETERS; UNA ANTHELIOS XL LOTION; OPEN BOTTLE OF BAYER ASPIRIN; EMPTY GLASS VIAL OF PROPOFOL INJECTABLE EMULSION 1%; AND EMPTY GLASS VIAL OF FLUMAZENIL INJECTION 0.5MG/5ML.

Investigator: ELISSA J. FLEAK (#270811)

Date: 6/26/2009

COUNTY OF LOS ANGELES **MEDICAL EVIDENCE** **DEPARTMENT OF CORONER**

3A

CASE #: 2009-04415
DECEDENT'S NAME: JACKSON, MICHAEL JOSEPH
DOD: 6/25/2009
INCOMING MODE:

Page 2 of 2

Drug Name	Rx Number	Date of Issue	Number Issued	Number Remaining	Form	Dosage	Rx Directions	Physician	Pharmacy Phone/ Comments
TEST									
TIZANIDINE	1812059	6/7/2009	10	8	TABLET	4MG	HALF TABLET AT BEDTI...	KLEIN	RITE AID 310-273-3561 PRESCRIBED TO OMAR ARNOLD
TRAZADONE	1700218	4/18/2009	60	36	TABLET	50MG	2 AT BEDTIME AS NEED...	METZGER	RITE AID 310-273-3561

Paraphernalia Description

ONE GREEN OXYGEN TANK; A BROKEN SYRINGE; AN OPEN BOX OF HYPODERMIC DISPOSABLE NEEDLES; AN OPEN BOX OF IV-CATHETERS; UVA ANTHELIOS XL LOTION; OPEN BOTTLE OF BAYER ASPIRIN; EMPTY GLASS VIAL OF PROPOFOL, INJECTABLE EMULSION 1%; AND EMPTY GLASS VIAL OF FLUMAZENIL INJECTION 0.5KGML.

Investigator: ELISSA J. FLEAK (46701...)
Date: 6/26/2009

COUNTY OF LOS ANGELES

DEPARTMENT OF CORONER

MEDICAL EVIDENCE

*** 2ᴺᴰ FORM 3A ***

Initiated on 6/29/2009 for evidence collected from second scene visit

3A

CASE #: 2009-04415
DECEDENT'S NAME: JACKSON, MICHAEL JOSEPH
DOD: 6/25/2009
BECOMING MODE: Accident vs. Natural

Page 1 of 3

Drug Name	Rx Number	Date of Issue	Number Issued	Number Remaining	Form	Dosage	Rx Directions	Physician	Pharmacy Phone/ Comments
Propofol 1% injectable emulsion					liquid		no prescription directions and no patient or doctor names		3 – 100 mL vials
Propofol 1% injectable emulsion					liquid		no prescription directions and no patient or doctor names		8 – 20 mL vials
Lidocaine HCl injectable					liquid		no prescription directions and no patient or doctor names		6 – 30 mL vials
Midazolam injectable					liquid		no prescription directions and no patient or doctor names		5 – 10 mL vials

Paraphernalia Description

2 blue plastic/canvas bags, 1 square black bag, 5 business cards for Dr. Conrad Murray, 1 IV side clamp, 1 blue rubber strip, 1 Sterline steroid sphygmomanometer (blood pressure cuff), 1 red stained piece of gauze, 1 pulse finger monitor (Nonin- Onyx), and 1 bag of medical supplies including crumpled packaging

Investigator: ELISSA FLEAK 427565

Date: 6/29/2009

*** 2ND FORM 3A ***
Initiated on 6/29/2009 for evidence collected from second scene visit

COUNTY OF LOS ANGELES

DEPARTMENT OF CORONER

MEDICAL EVIDENCE

CASE #	2009-04415
DECEDENTS NAME	JACKSON, MICHAEL JOSEPH
DOD	6/25/2009
INCOMING MODE	Accident vs. Natural

3A

Page 2 of 3

Drug Name	Rx Number	Date of Issue	Number Issued	Number Remaining	Form	Dosage	Rx Directions	Physician	Pharmacy Phone/ Comments
Flumazenil injectable			liquid				no prescription directions and no patient or doctor names		4 – 5 mL vials
Lorazepam injectable			liquid				no prescription directions and no patient or doctor names		2 – 4 mL vials
Lorazepam injectable			liquid				no prescription directions and no patient or doctor names		1 – 10 mL vial
Ephedrine, Caffeine, Aspirin				14	black and red capsules				red plastic pill bottle with no prescription directions and no patient or doctor names

Paraphernalia Description	
	Investigator: ELISSA J FLEAK 49575.1
	Date: 6/29/2009

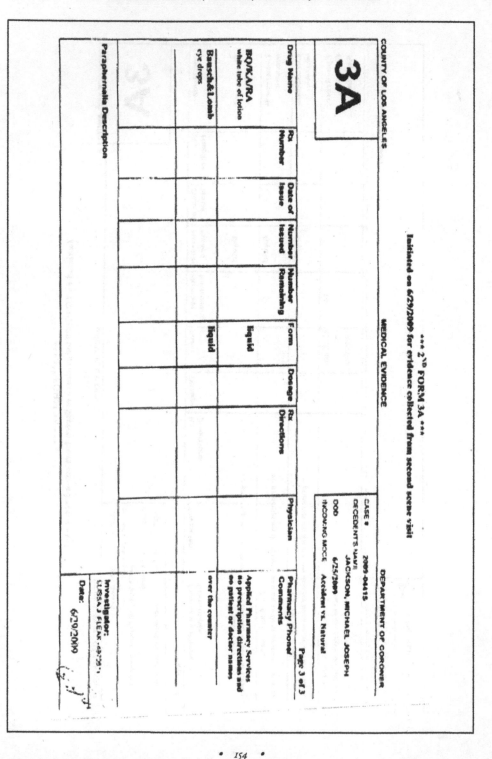

COUNTY OF LOS ANGELES

3A

*** 2ND FORM 3A ***
Initiated on 6/29/2009 for evidence collected from second scene visit

MEDICAL EVIDENCE

DEPARTMENT OF CORONER

CASE # : 2009-04415
DECEDENT'S NAME : JACKSON, MICHAEL JOSEPH
DOD : 6/25/2009
INCOMING MODE : Accident vs. Natural

Page 3 of 3

Drug Name	Rx Number	Date of Issue	Number Issued	Number Remaining	Form	Dosage Rx Directions	Physician	Pharmacy Phoned Comments
BQ/KA/RA white tube of lotion					liquid			Applied Pharmacy Services so prescription directions and so patient or doctor names
Bausch & Lomb eye drops				liquid			I over the counter	

Paraphernalia Description

Investigator: LISSA J FLEAK - 83729 "

Date: 6/29/2009

COUNTY OF LOS ANGELES

3A

*** 3rd FORM 3A ***
Initiated on 7/9/2009 for evidence brought to FSC by family

MEDICAL EVIDENCE

DEPARTMENT OF CORONER

CASE #: 2009-04415
DECEDENT'S NAME: JACKSON, MICHAEL JOSEPH
DOB: 6.25/2009
INCIDENT MODE: Accident vs. Natural

Page 1 of 1

Drug Name	Rx Number	Date of Issue	Number Issued	Number Remaining	Form	Dosage	Rx Directions	Physician	Pharmacy Phone/ Comments
Zanaflex	701E879	11/6/08	4	0	tablet	4mg	½ to 1 tab at bedtime	Klein, Arnold	Mickey Fine Pharm 310-271-6128
Prednisone	1795027	4/25/09	10	0	tablet	10mg	6 tab now, 4 tomorrow	Klein, Arnold	Rite Aid 310-273-3561
Amoxicillin	533380	2/2/09	28	21	caps	500mg	4 times daily	Dwight James/ Cherilyn Lee	Patient name blacked out on label
Azithromycin	54729	3/9/2009	6	2	tablet	250mg	2 tabs first day then 1 for 4 days	Dwight James/ Cherilyn Lee	patient name: Kathlyn Hursey

Paraphernalia Description

OTC - Bausch and Lomb eye drops, small tube of "Ultravate" ointment

Investigator: LUSSA J FLEAK (397.761)

Date: 7/9/2009

COUNTY OF LOS ANGELES   DEPARTMENT OF CORONE

12   AUTOPSY REPORT

I performed an autopsy on the body of ➡

No.
2009-04415

JACKSON, MICHAEL

at _____ the DEPARTMENT OF CORONER

Los Angeles, California _____ on JUNE 26, 2009 @ 1000 HOURS
                              (Date)   (Time)

From the anatomic findings and pertinent history I ascribe the death to:

(A)   **ACUTE PROPOFOL INTOXICATION**
DUE TO OR AS A CONSEQUENCE OF

(B)
DUE TO OR AS A CONSEQUENCE OF

(C)
DUE TO OR AS A CONSEQUENCE OF

(D)
OTHER CONDITIONS CONTRIBUTING BUT NOT RELATED TO THE IMMEDIATE CAUSE OF DEATH:
  BENZODIAZEPINE EFFECT

Anatomical Summary:

1. Toxicology findings (see separate report).

   A) Propofol, lorazepam, midazolam, lidocaine, diazepam and nordiazepam, identified in blood samples (see toxicology report for details).

   B) Propofol, midazolam, lidocaine and ephedrine identified in urine.

   C) Propofol and lidocaine identified in liver tissue.

   D) Propofol identified in vitreous humor.

   E) Lidocaine and propofol identified in stomach contents.

2. Nodular prostatic hyperplasia.

   A) Prominent intravesical median lobe enlargement.

   B) Urinary retention.

3. Vitiligo.

4. Tubular adenoma of colon.

5. Evidence of therapy.

   A) Endotracheal tube.

   B) Intravascular catheters of left neck, and both femoral regions.

UNTY OF LOS ANGELES DEPARTMENT OF CORONER

12

AUTOPSY REPORT

No.
2009-04415

JACKSON, MICHAEL

Page 2

C) Intra-aortic balloon pump, inserted through left femoral artery.

D) Punctures and contusions of right neck, both arms, left calf, and right ankle.

E) Condom catheter.

F) Resuscitative abrasion-contusion of central chest.

G) Resuscitative fractures of sternum, right 4th and 5th ribs, and left 3rd through 5th ribs.

H) Resuscitative alveolar hemorrhage of lungs.

I) Resuscitative transmural hemorrhage of stomach.

6. See separate consultation reports:

A) Neuropathology.
   1. Mild cerebral vascular congestion.
   2. Mild diffuse brain swelling without herniation syndrome.
   3. Mild basal ganglia calcification.

B) Pulmonary pathology.
   1. Marked diffuse congestion and patchy hemorrhage of right and left lungs.
   2. Marked respiratory bronchiolitis, histiocytic desquamation, and multifocal chronic interstitial pneumonitis.
   3. Multifocal fibrocollagenous scars.
   4. Organizing and recanalizing thromboemboli of two small arteries.
   5. Intravascular eosinophilia with occasional interstitial eosinophilic infiltrate.
   6. Suggestive focal desquamation of respiratory lining cells with squamous metaplasia.

C) Radiology.
   1. Minimal degenerative spondylosis of the lower thoracic spine.
   2. Right C7 cervical rib.
   3. Degenerative osteoarthritis of lower lumbar spine facet joints, distal interphalangeal joints of the right index and long fingers, and distal interphalangeal joint of left little finger.

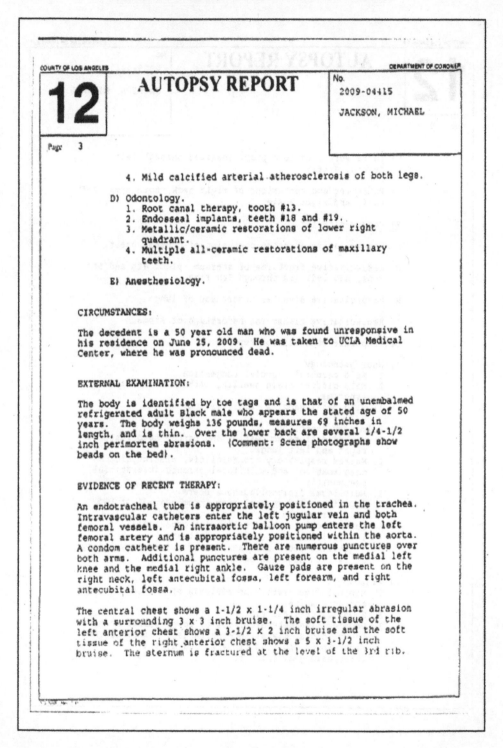

12

AUTOPSY REPORT

No.
2009-04415

JACKSON, MICHAEL

Page 3

        4. Mild calcified arterial atherosclerosis of both legs.

   D) Odontology.
      1. Root canal therapy, tooth #13.
      2. Endosseal implants, teeth #18 and #19.
      3. Metallic/ceramic restorations of lower right
         quadrant.
      4. Multiple all-ceramic restorations of maxillary
         teeth.

   E) Anesthesiology.

CIRCUMSTANCES:

The decedent is a 50 year old man who was found unresponsive in
his residence on June 25, 2009. He was taken to UCLA Medical
Center, where he was pronounced dead.

EXTERNAL EXAMINATION:

The body is identified by toe tags and is that of an unembalmed
refrigerated adult Black male who appears the stated age of 50
years. The body weighs 136 pounds, measures 69 inches in
length, and is thin. Over the lower back are several 1/4-1/2
inch perimortem abrasions. (Comment: Scene photographs show
beads on the bed).

EVIDENCE OF RECENT THERAPY:

An endotracheal tube is appropriately positioned in the trachea.
Intravascular catheters enter the left jugular vein and both
femoral vessels. An intraaortic balloon pump enters the left
femoral artery and is appropriately positioned within the aorta.
A condom catheter is present. There are numerous punctures over
both arms. Additional punctures are present on the medial left
knee and the medial right ankle. Gauze pads are present on the
right neck, left antecubital fossa, left forearm, and right
antecubital fossa.

The central chest shows a 1-1/2 x 1-1/4 inch irregular abrasion
with a surrounding 3 x 3 inch bruise. The soft tissue of the
left anterior chest shows a 3-1/2 x 2 inch bruise and the soft
tissue of the right anterior chest shows a 5 x 3-1/2 inch
bruise. The sternum is fractured at the level of the 3rd rib.

12

AUTOPSY REPORT

No.
2009-04415

JACKSON, MICHAEL

Page 4

The right 4th and 5th ribs are fractured at the chondrocostal junction. The left 3rd, 4th and 5th ribs are fractured at the chondrosternal junction.

The following scars are present:

1. There is a 3/4 inch scar behind the left ear and a scar-like area behind the right ear.
2. There are scars at the lateral border of the alae nasi, 3/5 inch in length on the right and 5/8 inch in length on the left.
3. On the top of the right shoulder is an irregular scar-like area approximately 4 inches in diameter.
4. At the posterior base of the neck are two downsloping scar-like areas measuring 3-1/4 inch on the left and 3 inches on the right. (See microscopic examination, slide U).
5. The left arm shows a 1/4 inch scar on its anterior surface just proximal to the antecubital region. The left wrist shows a 1/8 inch scar.
6. There is a 7/8 inch scar on the right thenar eminence, and a 1/8 inch scar of the right wrist.
7. There is a 2 inch surgical scar in the right lower quadrant of the abdomen.
8. There is a 5/8 inch scar around the area of the umbilicus.
9. There is a 2 x 1/8 inch semicircular scar of the right knee, with several smaller scars distal to it measuring 1/2 to 1/4 inch in length.
10. On the anterior right shin is a 5 x 2-1/2 inch area of hyperpigmentation.

The following tattoos are present:

There is a dark skin discoloration resembling a tattoo on the anterior half of the scalp. There are dark tattoos in the areas of both eyebrows and at the superior and inferior borders of the palpebral fissures. There is a pink tattoo in the region of the lips.

There is focal depigmentation of the skin, particularly over the anterior chest and abdomen, face and arms.

Rigor mortis is present in the limbs and jaw. Livor mortis is fixed and distributed posteriorly.

The head is normocephalic and is partly covered by black hair. There is frontal balding and the hair can be described as short and tightly curled. A mustache and beard are absent.

COUNTY OF LOS ANGELES   DEPARTMENT OF CORONER

12   AUTOPSY REPORT

No.
2009-04415

JACKSON, MICHAEL

Page   5

Examination of the eyes reveals irides that are brown and
sclerae that show no injection or jaundice. There are no
petechial hemorrhages of the conjunctivae of the lids or the
sclerae. The oronasal passages are unobstructed. A bandage is
present on the tip of the nose. Upper and lower teeth are
present and in good repair (see odontology consultation). The
neck is unremarkable. There is no chest deformity. There is no
increase in the anterior-posterior diameter of the chest. The
abdomen is flat. The genitalia are those of an adult male. The
penis appears uncircumcised. The extremities show no edema,
joint deformity, or abnormal mobility.

CLOTHING:

The body was not clothed and no clothing is available for
review.

INITIAL INCISION:

The head and body cavities are entered through the standard
coronal incision and the standard Y-shaped incision,
respectively. No foreign material is present in the mouth,
upper airway and trachea.

NECK:

The neck organs are removed en bloc with the tongue. There are
small contusions inside the lips as well as in the central area
of the tongue. On the mucosa of the left pyriform recess are
three slightly raised nodules measuring 0.2 cm in diameter each.
There is no edema of the larynx. Both hyoid bone and larynx are
intact without fractures. No hemorrhage is present in the
adjacent throat organs, investing fascia, strap muscles, thyroid
or visceral fascia. There are no prevertebral fascial
hemorrhages.

CHEST AND ABDOMINAL CAVITIES:

The pleural cavities contain minimal fluid and no adhesions. No
pneumothorax is demonstrated. The parietal pleurae are intact.
The lungs are well expanded. Soft tissues of the thoracic and
abdominal walls are well-preserved. The organs of the abdominal

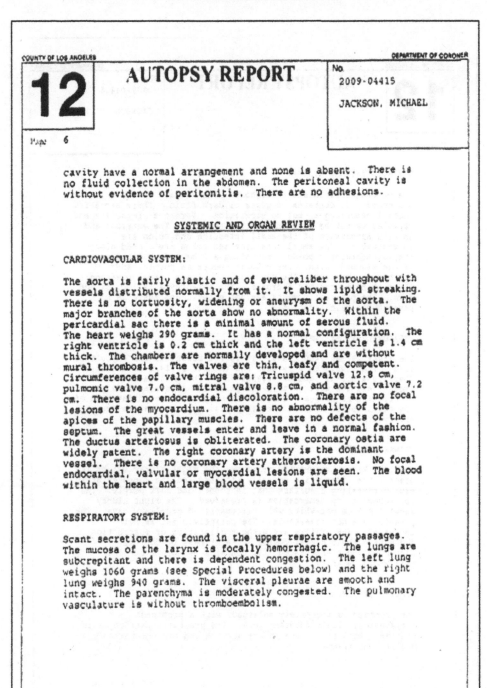

AUTOPSY REPORT

12

No.
2009-04415

JACKSON, MICHAEL

Page   6

cavity have a normal arrangement and none is absent. There is
no fluid collection in the abdomen. The peritoneal cavity is
without evidence of peritonitis. There are no adhesions.

SYSTEMIC AND ORGAN REVIEW

CARDIOVASCULAR SYSTEM:

The aorta is fairly elastic and of even caliber throughout with
vessels distributed normally from it. It shows lipid streaking.
There is no tortuosity, widening or aneurysm of the aorta. The
major branches of the aorta show no abnormality. Within the
pericardial sac there is a minimal amount of serous fluid.
The heart weighs 290 grams. It has a normal configuration. The
right ventricle is 0.2 cm thick and the left ventricle is 1.4 cm
thick. The chambers are normally developed and are without
mural thrombosis. The valves are thin, leafy and competent.
Circumferences of valve rings are: Tricuspid valve 12.8 cm,
pulmonic valve 7.0 cm, mitral valve 8.8 cm, and aortic valve 7.2
cm. There is no endocardial discoloration. There are no focal
lesions of the myocardium. There is no abnormality of the
apices of the papillary muscles. There are no defects of the
septum. The great vessels enter and leave in a normal fashion.
The ductus arteriosus is obliterated. The coronary ostia are
widely patent. The right coronary artery is the dominant
vessel. There is no coronary artery atherosclerosis. No focal
endocardial, valvular or myocardial lesions are seen. The blood
within the heart and large blood vessels is liquid.

RESPIRATORY SYSTEM:

Scant secretions are found in the upper respiratory passages.
The mucosa of the larynx is focally hemorrhagic. The lungs are
subcrepitant and there is dependent congestion. The left lung
weighs 1060 grams (see Special Procedures below) and the right
lung weighs 940 grams. The visceral pleurae are smooth and
intact. The parenchyma is moderately congested. The pulmonary
vasculature is without thromboembolism.

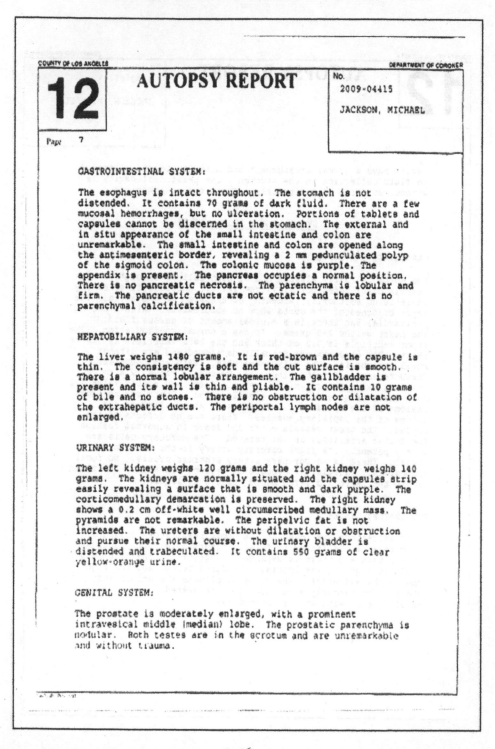

COUNTY OF LOS ANGELES

DEPARTMENT OF CORONER

AUTOPSY REPORT

12

No.
2009-04415

JACKSON, MICHAEL

Page   7

GASTROINTESTINAL SYSTEM:

The esophagus is intact throughout. The stomach is not
distended. It contains 70 grams of dark fluid. There are a few
mucosal hemorrhages, but no ulceration. Portions of tablets and
capsules cannot be discerned in the stomach. The external and
in situ appearance of the small intestine and colon are
unremarkable. The small intestine and colon are opened along
the antimesenteric border, revealing a 2 mm pedunculated polyp
of the sigmoid colon. The colonic mucosa is purple. The
appendix is present. The pancreas occupies a normal position.
There is no pancreatic necrosis. The parenchyma is lobular and
firm. The pancreatic ducts are not ectatic and there is no
parenchymal calcification.

HEPATOBILIARY SYSTEM:

The liver weighs 1480 grams. It is red-brown and the capsule is
thin. The consistency is soft and the cut surface is smooth.
There is a normal lobular arrangement. The gallbladder is
present and its wall is thin and pliable. It contains 10 grams
of bile and no stones. There is no obstruction or dilatation of
the extrahepatic ducts. The periportal lymph nodes are not
enlarged.

URINARY SYSTEM:

The left kidney weighs 120 grams and the right kidney weighs 140
grams. The kidneys are normally situated and the capsules strip
easily revealing a surface that is smooth and dark purple. The
corticomedullary demarcation is preserved. The right kidney
shows a 0.2 cm off-white well circumscribed medullary mass. The
pyramids are not remarkable. The peripelvic fat is not
increased. The ureters are without dilatation or obstruction
and pursue their normal course. The urinary bladder is
distended and trabeculated. It contains 550 grams of clear
yellow-orange urine.

GENITAL SYSTEM:

The prostate is moderately enlarged, with a prominent
intravesical middle (median) lobe. The prostatic parenchyma is
nodular. Both testes are in the scrotum and are unremarkable
and without trauma.

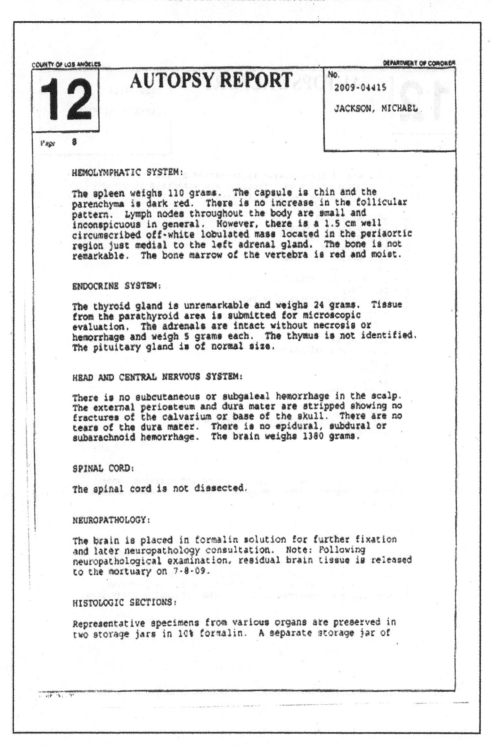

COUNTY OF LOS ANGELES   DEPARTMENT OF CORONER

12

AUTOPSY REPORT

No.
2009-04415
JACKSON, MICHAEL

Page   8

HEMOLYMPHATIC SYSTEM:

The spleen weighs 110 grams. The capsule is thin and the parenchyma is dark red. There is no increase in the follicular pattern. Lymph nodes throughout the body are small and inconspicuous in general. However, there is a 1.5 cm well circumscribed off-white lobulated mass located in the periaortic region just medial to the left adrenal gland. The bone is not remarkable. The bone marrow of the vertebra is red and moist.

ENDOCRINE SYSTEM:

The thyroid gland is unremarkable and weighs 24 grams. Tissue from the parathyroid area is submitted for microscopic evaluation. The adrenals are intact without necrosis or hemorrhage and weigh 5 grams each. The thymus is not identified. The pituitary gland is of normal size.

HEAD AND CENTRAL NERVOUS SYSTEM:

There is no subcutaneous or subgaleal hemorrhage in the scalp. The external periosteum and dura mater are stripped showing no fractures of the calvarium or base of the skull. There are no tears of the dura mater. There is no epidural, subdural or subarachnoid hemorrhage. The brain weighs 1380 grams.

SPINAL CORD:

The spinal cord is not dissected.

NEUROPATHOLOGY:

The brain is placed in formalin solution for further fixation and later neuropathology consultation. Note: Following neuropathological examination, residual brain tissue is released to the mortuary on 7-8-09.

HISTOLOGIC SECTIONS:

Representative specimens from various organs are preserved in two storage jars in 10% formalin. A separate storage jar of

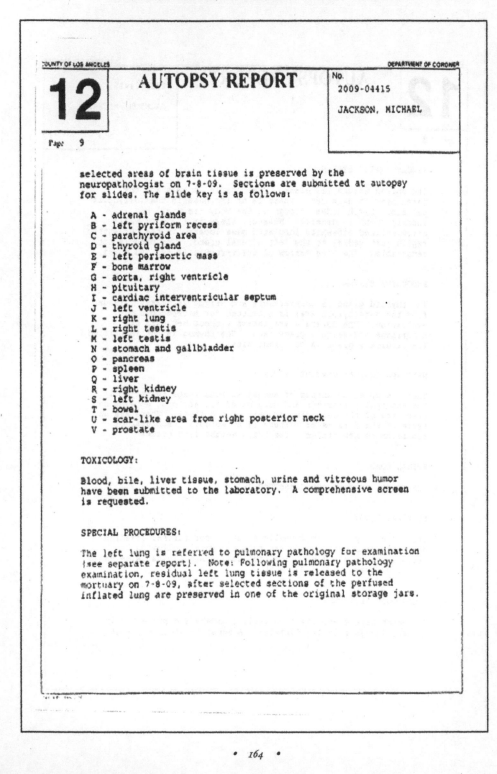

12   AUTOPSY REPORT

No.
2009-04415

JACKSON, MICHAEL

Page 9

selected areas of brain tissue is preserved by the
neuropathologist on 7-8-09. Sections are submitted at autopsy
for slides. The slide key is as follows:

        A - adrenal glands
        B - left pyriform recess
        C - parathyroid area
        D - thyroid gland
        E - left periaortic mass
        F - bone marrow
        G - aorta, right ventricle
        H - pituitary
        I - cardiac interventricular septum
        J - left ventricle
        K - right lung
        L - right testis
        M - left testis
        N - stomach and gallbladder
        O - pancreas
        P - spleen
        Q - liver
        R - right kidney
        S - left kidney
        T - bowel
        U - scar-like area from right posterior neck
        V - prostate

TOXICOLOGY:

Blood, bile, liver tissue, stomach, urine and vitreous humor
have been submitted to the laboratory. A comprehensive screen
is requested.

SPECIAL PROCEDURES:

The left lung is referred to pulmonary pathology for examination
(see separate report). Note: Following pulmonary pathology
examination, residual left lung tissue is released to the
mortuary on 7-8-09, after selected sections of the perfused
inflated lung are preserved in one of the original storage jars.

COUNTY OF LOS ANGELES   DEPARTMENT OF CORONER

12   AUTOPSY REPORT

No.
2009-04415

JACKSON, MICHAEL

Page 10

PHOTOGRAPHY:

Photographs have been taken prior to and during the course of the autopsy. The following photographs taken by the coroner are reviewed prior to signing the autopsy report:

1. 17 photographs taken at the hospital on 6-25-09.
2. 13 photographs taken at the scene on 6-25-09 showing the bedroom where paramedics treated the decedent.
3. One intake photograph taken at the Forensic Science Center on 6-25-09.
4. 61 photographs taken on 6-26-09 before and during autopsy (documenting resuscitative injury and intravesical prostatic enlargement).
5. 3 photographs of a silver BMW 645 Ci taken on 6-29-09.
6. 13 photographs taken at the scene on 6-29-09 showing the dressing room with closets where additional medical evidence was collected.
7. Three contact sheets showing 108 photographs (items 1 to 6 above).
8. Four photographs taken on 7-23-09 of the Stokes litter from Sheriff's Air 5 helicopter used in transporting decedent.
9. Five enlarged scene photographs taken by the police are reviewed with Dr. Calmes, in addition to some of the other police photographs pertaining to medical evidence.

RADIOLOGY:

Sixteen x-rays are obtained.

WITNESS:

Detective Scott Smith of LAPD witnessed the autopsy.

DIAGRAMS USED:

Diagram Forms 20 and 22 were used during the performance of the autopsy. The diagrams are not intended to be a facsimile.

12

AUTOPSY REPORT

No.
2009-04415

JACKSON, MICHAEL

Page   11

OPINION:

Toxicology studies show a high blood concentration of propofol, as well as the presence of benzodiazepines as listed in the toxicology report. The autopsy did not show any trauma or natural disease which would cause death.

The cause of death is acute propofol intoxication. A contributory factor in the death is benzodiazepine effect.

The manner of death is homicide, based on the following:

1. Circumstances indicate that propofol and the benzodiazepines were administered by another.

2. The propofol was administered in a non-hospital setting without any appropriate medical indication.

3. The standard of care for administering propofol was not met (see anesthesiology consultation). Recommended equipment for patient monitoring, precision dosing, and resuscitation was not present.

4. The circumstances do not support self-administration of propofol.

CHRISTOPHER ROGERS, MD, MBA   DATE   8-19-09
CHIEF FORENSIC MEDICINE DIVISION

LAKSHMANAN SATHYAVAGISWARAN, MD   DATE   8-19-09
FRCP(C), FCAP, FACP
CHIEF MEDICAL EXAMINER-CORONER

CR:mtm:c
D-06/26/09
T-06/30/09

COUNTY OF LOS ANGELES   FORENSIC CONSULTANT'S REPORT   DEPARTMENT OF CORONER

13

2009-04415
Jackson, Michael

July 31, 2009

This consultation is provided at the request of the Chief Medical Examiner-Coroner, Dr. Lakshmanan Sathyavagiswaran.

Gross Description:

The weights of the left and right lung are provided in the Autopsy Protocol.

On 6/26/09, the bronchus of the left lung was cannulated with a plastic tube that was slightly smaller in diameter than that of the bronchus. The tube was attached to a perfusion-inflation apparatus containing ~40 gallons of 10% buffered (monobasic and dibasic phosphate) formalin. Perfusion was maintained for ~72 hrs at 30cm water pressure, following which the formalin was replaced with tap water and perfusion continued for ~24 hours.

The formalin-fixed and washed lung was then placed in an electrical rotary slicer and five sagittal slices of whole lung tissue were obtained beginning at the hilum. The inflated left lung measured 25.0 cm in sagittal height, 12.0 cm in coronal width, and 12.0 cm in sagittal depth. The visceral pleural surfaces were generally thin and transparent with the exception that the lateral surface of a large portion of the lower lobe was slightly thickened and had a milky appearance. There was also a patchy anthracotic pigment deposition that involved primarily the superior and lateral portions of the upper and lower lung lobes, with band-like distributions along the rib cage. There were no pleural adhesions or areas of consolidation other than several poorly defined small nodules in the apical portion of the upper lobe in association with a few whitish streaks having an apparent lymphatic distribution. The anterior margin of the upper lobe showed a patchy film-like opacification. The main stem bronchus of the left lung measured 2.5 cm in length and was grossly unremarkable. A few hilar lymph nodes were noted that were grossly unremarkable except for slight anthracotic pigmentation.

Gross examination of the sliced section at the base of the Left Lower Lobe showed three relatively firm and nodular masses of tissue immediately below the pleura surface. On cut section, the largest of the nodular masses was irregular and measured 0.6 cm x 0.8 cm x 0.5 cm. Two other masses, each measuring 0.5 cm x 0.5cm and 0.7 cm, were moderately firm in consistency and, in large part, associated with congestion and hemorrhage. An area of brownish discoloration of the apical pleura overlying the Left Upper Lobe measured 0.5cm x 0.6cm, with superficial involvement (~1.0mm) of the subpleural tissue. Additional small areas of subpleural brownish discolorations were nearby. At the base of the Left Upper Lobe, a reddish-brown and hemorrhagic mass was found that measured 0.6 cm x 0.6cm x 0.4 cm. Five sections of the formalin-perfused lung tissue were excised for microscopic study.

Sections taken for paraffin embedding and processing:

Cassette B - apex, Left Lower Lobe; Cassette D - base, Left Lower Lobe
Cassette A - base, Left Upper Lobe; Cassette E - base, Left Lower Lobe
Cassette C - Main stem bronchus, transverse section

Histopathologic Findings

On examination of the base of the Left Lower Lobe, four roughly rectangular scar areas were found that measured approximately 3.5mm x 1.4mm, 7.6mm x 4.2mm, 4.8mm x 0.9mm, and 1.4mm x 0.6mm. All shared in common acellular fibrocollagenous tissue, derangement of bronchioloalveolar structures, hemorrhage, proteinaceous-fibrinous deposits, and aggregates of heavily pigmented macrophages. In some scar areas there was a fibrous thickening of bronchioloalveolar walls with round cell infiltrates and aggregates of pigmented histiocytes. There is slight to moderate thickening of the pleura that overlies fibro-inflammatory lesions. Several foci of round cells aggregates are noted, including periarteriolar and pericapillary sites.

COUNTY OF LOS ANGELES   **FORENSIC CONSULTANT'S REPORT**   DEPARTMENT OF CORONER

13

July 31, 2009

2009-04415
Jackson, Michael

Page 2

Histopathologic Findings (Cont.)

There is widespread bronchioloalveolar histiocytic infiltration and patchy histiocytic desquamation. Centriacinar derangement is noted with and without chronic inflammation. Two small arteries are observed that contain organizing/recanalizing thromboemboli. One of the vessels with a thromboembolus (base of upper lobe) is associated with a localized, subpleural area of hemorrhage. Eosinophils are often noted within capillaries and other vascular channels, and are also seen occasionally within interstitial tissues of the lung. In two instances, an air space was observed that contained cells consistent with respiratory lining cells that have undergone squamous metaplasia. Histiocytes often contained birefringent particulates in association with anthracotic pigment. Birefringent particles were absent elsewhere in the lung. Slight chronic inflammation was seen in the bronchial section. The foregoing findings were in part observed in the "K" section of the uninflated lung (H&E stained section). PAS and iron stains of Slides D and K were reviewed.

DIAGNOSIS:

Marked diffuse congestion and patchy hemorrhage of right and left lungs.
Marked respiratory bronchiolitis, histiocytic desquamation, and multifocal chronic interstitial pneumonitis.
Multifocal fibrocollagenous scars with and without congestion and hemorrhage.
Organizing and recanalizing thromboemboli of two small arteries.
Intravascular eosinophilia with occasional interstitial eosinophilic infiltrate.
Suggestive focal desquamation of respiratory lining cells with squamous metaplasia.

OPINION

The above findings reflect a depletion of structural and functional reserves of the lung. Reserve depletion is the result of widespread respiratory bronchiolitis and chronic lung inflammation in association with fibrocollagenous scars and organizing/recanalizing thromboemboli of small arteries.

It should be noted that the above lung injury with reserve loss is not considered to be a direct or contributing cause of death. However, such an individual would be especially susceptible to adverse health effects.

Respectfully submitted,

Russell P. Sherwin, M.D.
Deputized Consultant in Pulmonary Pathology
Professor of Pathology
Keck School of Medicine
University of Southern California

RPS/vr

County of Los Angeles   FORENSIC CONSULTANT'S REPORT   Department of Coroner

13

ODONTOLOGY CONSULT

CC #2009-04415
JACKSON, Michael Joseph

REQUEST:

The decedent is a 50 year old black man who died unexpectedly. Please examine for dental contribution to cause of death.

FILMS:

Post Mortem AP and lateral skull

FINDINGS:

Review of the two films reveal history of routine restorative dentistry. There were incomplete dental records from two Las Vegas dentists who performed restorative and surgical treatment for this decedent. There is root canal therapy completed on tooth #13. There are endosseal dental implants in the positions of teeth #18 and #19. There are also metallic/ceramic restorations present in the lower right quadrant. There are multiple all ceramic restorations present in the maxillary teeth. There is no gross pathology seen on these two radiographic views, even though these are not the standard views for a dental exam.

Cathy Law

Cathy Law, D.D.S.
DENTAL CONSULTANT

7-10-09

Date

cl:ECL
hw 7/10/09

COUNTY OF LOS ANGELES   FORENSIC CONSULTANT'S REPORT   DEPARTMENT OF CORONER

13

NEUROPATHOLOGY

2009-04415

JACKSON, MICHAEL J.

July 8, 2009

AGE: 50 years

DATE OF DEATH: June 25, 2009

REFERRING DME: Christopher Rogers, M.D.

CIRCUMSTANCES:

The following information is taken from the Investigator
Report, preliminary autopsy notes, and records from UCLA
Ronald Reagan Medical Center currently in the file.

This 50-year-old man was reportedly found unresponsive in his
residence at approximately 1200 hours on 6/25/09, and arriving
paramedics found him to be in cardiopulmonary arrest. He was
transported to UCLA Ronald Reagan Medical Center, but did not
respond to resuscitative efforts and was pronounced at 1426
hours on 6/25/09. Available records reveal no remarkable
prior neurological symptoms or findings, and no history of
trauma of seizures preceding the cardiopulmonary arrest.

At the time of postmortem examination on 6/26/09 the findings
included evidence of therapy, and no scalp, skull or
intracranial abnormalities were described. Brain weight at
removal was 1380 grams.

GROSS DESCRIPTION:

Specimens available for examination are cranial dura mater and
brain. The specimens are identified as to source by the
identification tag indicating specimen number and decedent
name on the specimen container, and separately on a plastic
card within the specimen container, within the green surgical
cap surrounding the brain.

The cranial dura mater submitted includes dorsal convexities
with falx cerebri, posterior fossa with tentorium cerebelli,
and the bulk of the middle and anterior fossae bilaterally.
External and internal surfaces of the dura mater are smooth
and shiny, without evidence of discoloration, hemorrhage,
subdural neomembranes, mass lesions, or other significant

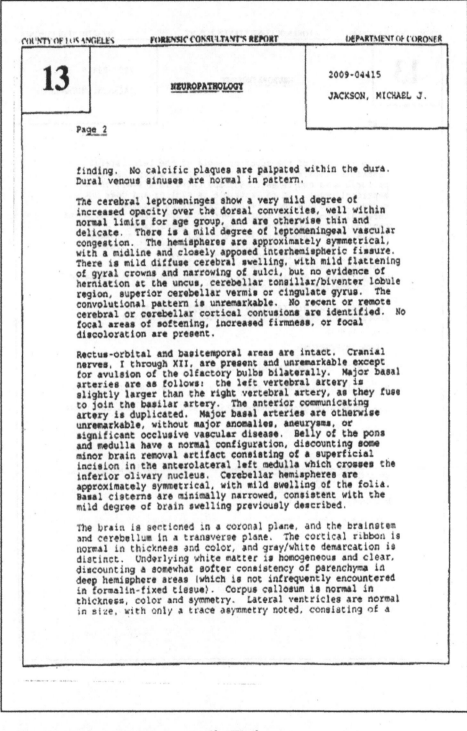

13

NEUROPATHOLOGY

2009-04415

JACKSON, MICHAEL J.

Page 2

finding. No calcific plaques are palpated within the dura. Dural venous sinuses are normal in pattern.

The cerebral leptomeninges show a very mild degree of increased opacity over the dorsal convexities, well within normal limits for age group, and are otherwise thin and delicate. There is a mild degree of leptomeningeal vascular congestion. The hemispheres are approximately symmetrical, with a midline and closely apposed interhemispheric fissure. There is mild diffuse cerebral swelling, with mild flattening of gyral crowns and narrowing of sulci, but no evidence of herniation at the uncus, cerebellar tonsillar/biventer lobule region, superior cerebellar vermis or cingulate gyrus. The convolutional pattern is unremarkable. No recent or remote cerebral or cerebellar cortical contusions are identified. No focal areas of softening, increased firmness, or focal discoloration are present.

Rectus-orbital and basitemporal areas are intact. Cranial nerves, I through XII, are present and unremarkable except for avulsion of the olfactory bulbs bilaterally. Major basal arteries are as follows: the left vertebral artery is slightly larger than the right vertebral artery, as they fuse to join the basilar artery. The anterior communicating artery is duplicated. Major basal arteries are otherwise unremarkable, without major anomalies, aneurysms, or significant occlusive vascular disease. Belly of the pons and medulla have a normal configuration, discounting some minor brain removal artifact consisting of a superficial incision in the anterolateral left medulla which crosses the inferior olivary nucleus. Cerebellar hemispheres are approximately symmetrical, with mild swelling of the folia. Basal cisterns are minimally narrowed, consistent with the mild degree of brain swelling previously described.

The brain is sectioned in a coronal plane, and the brainstem and cerebellum in a transverse plane. The cortical ribbon is normal in thickness and color, and gray/white demarcation is distinct. Underlying white matter is homogeneous and clear, discounting a somewhat softer consistency of parenchyma in deep hemisphere areas (which is not infrequently encountered in formalin-fixed tissue). Corpus callosum is normal in thickness, color and symmetry. Lateral ventricles are normal in size, with only a trace asymmetry noted, consisting of a

COUNTY OF LOS ANGELES   FORENSIC CONSULTANT'S REPORT   DEPARTMENT OF CORONER

13

NEUROPATHOLOGY

2009-04415

JACKSON, MICHAEL J.

Page 3

trace rounding of the superior angle of the left lateral
ventricle compared to the right, which is sharp. Septum
pellucidum is non-fenestrated, and there is a small cavum
septi pellucidi. Third ventricle is midline and does not
exceed 0.3 to 0.4 cm in maximum transverse diameter.
Cerebral aqueduct and fourth ventricle are normal in size and
configuration, and choroid plexus is unremarkable
bilaterally. Basal ganglia are normal in size, symmetry,
contour and color. Substantia nigra is normally pigmented.
Hippocampal formation, amygdaloid complex of nuclei,
mamillary bodies and pineal body are all grossly
unremarkable. Multiple transverse sections of the brainstem
and cerebellum reveal no abnormality.

Selected areas are retained in storage. Representative
sections are submitted for microscopic examination.

GROSS IMPRESSIONS:

A.   Mild cerebral vascular congestion.

B.   Mild diffuse brain swelling without herniation syndrome.

C.   Otherwise grossly unremarkable adult brain and coverings.

JOHN M. ANDREWS, M.D.   DATE
DEPUTY MEDICAL EXAMINER
NEUROPATHOLOGY CONSULTANT

JMA:mtm:c
T-07/08/09

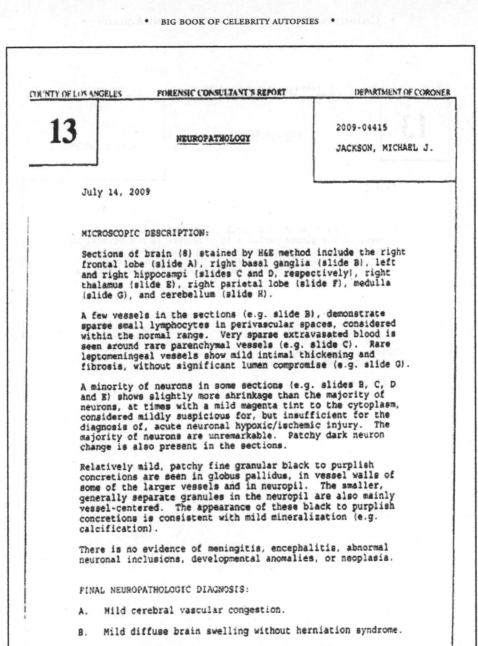

COUNTY OF LOS ANGELES   FORENSIC CONSULTANT'S REPORT   DEPARTMENT OF CORONER

13

NEUROPATHOLOGY

2009-04415

JACKSON, MICHAEL J.

July 14, 2009

MICROSCOPIC DESCRIPTION:

Sections of brain (8) stained by H&E method include the right frontal lobe (slide A), right basal ganglia (slide B), left and right hippocampi (slides C and D, respectively), right thalamus (slide E), right parietal lobe (slide F), medulla (slide G), and cerebellum (slide H).

A few vessels in the sections (e.g. slide B), demonstrate sparse small lymphocytes in perivascular spaces, considered within the normal range. Very sparse extravasated blood is seen around rare parenchymal vessels (e.g. slide C). Rare leptomeningeal vessels show mild intimal thickening and fibrosis, without significant lumen compromise (e.g. slide G).

A minority of neurons in some sections (e.g. slides B, C, D and E) shows slightly more shrinkage than the majority of neurons, at times with a mild magenta tint to the cytoplasm, considered mildly suspicious for, but insufficient for the diagnosis of, acute neuronal hypoxic/ischemic injury. The majority of neurons are unremarkable. Patchy dark neuron change is also present in the sections.

Relatively mild, patchy fine granular black to purplish concretions are seen in globus pallidus, in vessel walls of some of the larger vessels and in neuropil. The smaller, generally separate granules in the neuropil are also mainly vessel-centered. The appearance of these black to purplish concretions is consistent with mild mineralization (e.g. calcification).

There is no evidence of meningitis, encephalitis, abnormal neuronal inclusions, developmental anomalies, or neoplasia.

FINAL NEUROPATHOLOGIC DIAGNOSIS:

A. Mild cerebral vascular congestion.

B. Mild diffuse brain swelling without herniation syndrome.

C. Mild basal ganglia calcification (see comment).

COUNTY OF LOS ANGELES   FORENSIC CONSULTANT'S REPORT   DEPARTMENT OF CORONER

13

NEUROPATHOLOGY

2009-04415

JACKSON, MICHAEL J.

Page 2

Comment: The type of mild basal ganglia mineralization present in the globus pallidus in this case is not unusual in this age group. In the absence of any clinical evidence of endocrine or metabolic disorder, it is interpreted as an incidental finding unrelated to the cause or manner of death.

_____   7/34/c9
JOHN M. ANDREWS, M.D.   DATE
DEPUTY MEDICAL EXAMINER
NEUROPATHOLOGY CONSULTANT

JMA:mtm:c
T-07/16/09

13

ANESTHESIOLOGY CONSULTATION

JACKSON, Michael Joseph
2009-04415

This special consult is at the request of the Los Angeles County Chief Medical Examiner Coroner, Dr. Lakshmanan, for a 50 year old decedent who was found with physical evidence of the anesthetic drug propofol in his home.

RELEVANT INFORMATION ON PROPOFOL AND ITS ADMINISTRATION:

Propofol is an intravenous anesthetic with highly favorable properties: rapid onset of sedation and/or unconsciousness, predictable dose response (usually) and duration of action, rapid return of consciousness, little post-anesthesia "hang-over" and little postoperative nausea and vomiting. Unfavorable properties include respiratory and cardiovascular depression, especially on induction or if the IV bolus is rapid. Respiratory and cardiovascular depression is usually dose dependent and is accentuated if other sedatives, such as benzodiazepines, are present. There is also a narrow margin between mere sedation and full general anesthesia, with possible loss of the patient's ability to breathe and maintain their airway. (These properties are the most relevant to this case; other properties of propofol are not listed.)

Since its introduction into clinical practice in 1989, propofol has been widely used for induction and maintenance of anesthesia for surgery and to supplement regional and local anesthesia. It is widely used for sedation during uncomfortable diagnostic procedures and is also used in ICUs for sedating critically ill patients. It is reported to be used to relieve the pain of acute migraine headaches, in pain clinic settings. There are NO reports of its use for insomnia relief, to my knowledge. The only reports of its use in homes are cases of fatal abuse (first reported in 1992), suicide, murder and accident.

Propofol must be given intravenously. Administration techniques include single IV bolus (for induction of general anesthesia, going on to additional anesthesia drugs), repeat IV boluses (when there is a short-term need for sedation in a quick painful procedure) and IV bolus followed by continuous infusion (used for both general anesthesia with the addition of other drugs or for lengthy diagnostic procedures). The infusion technique requires precision control of the dose by way of a controllable infusion pump, because of the narrow margin between mere sedation and full general anesthesia and build-up of the drug as it is administered long-term. Because propofol is painful on injection, lidocaine (1 cc of 1%) is usually given, either immediately before injection or mixed into the amount to be infused. Propofol solutions easily support bacterial growth, and attention to antisepsis is required as well as discarding vials and syringes within 6 hours of use.

Full patient monitoring is required any time propofol is given. The most essential monitor is a person trained in anesthesia and in resuscitation who is continuously present and not involved in the on-going surgical/diagnostic procedure. Other monitors expected would be a continuous pulse oximeter, EKG and blood pressure cuff, preferably one that automatically inflates. An end-tidal CO_2 monitor would be used for fully anesthetized patients and is also highly desirable in sedated patients. Although the measurement of CO_2 would not be accurate in sedated patients, who have a loose mask or nasal cannula for supplemental oxygen, the presence of CO_2 documents that the patient is breathing and that the airway is open. If CO_2 stops being present, for whatever reason, the monitor will alarm (audible and visual signals), which calls attention to the possible apnea and/or airway obstruction, so action can be taken promptly. Of course, airway devices and drugs for resuscitation must always be present. Supplemental O_2 should always be delivered to patients receiving propofol, and they should always have a recovery period with monitoring and observation by trained recovery nurses.

13

ANESTHESIOLOGY CONSULTATION

Pg. 2 of 2

Because of the risk of sudden onset of full general anesthesia, propofol should be given only by anesthesiologists or other supervised anesthesia providers, who are fully trained to recognize and treat the possible respiratory and cardiac depression. In the ICU setting, propofol should be given by ACLS certified critical care level nurses, following physician orders. (These patients are intubated and ventilated, decreasing the need to deal with respiratory depression or airway problems from propofol.) In procedure rooms such as endoscopy suites, propofol is sometimes given by nurses (hopefully ACLS certified) under the supervision of the physician doing the procedure. This is not ideal and is the subject of conflict between gastroenterologists and anesthesiologists at the national level.

THIS PARTICULAR CASE:

Questions to be answered include was the standard of care for administering propofol met, could the decedent have administered the propofol to himself and what is an anesthesiologist's point of view on the toxicology screen results.

Was the standard of care for giving propofol met? It is not known whether trained medical personnel were continuously observing the decedent while propofol given. There was no evidence of an infusion pump for control of an IV infusion. No monitors were found at the scene; a blood pressure cuff and portable pulse oximeter were recovered from a closet in the next room. A tank of oxygen with some kind of non-rebreathing bag with a clear plastic mask (for positive pressure ventilation) was near where the patient was found by the paramedics. This tank was empty when examined on 7/13/09. A non-rebreathing bag was not attached when the tank was examined. Multiple opened bottles of propofol were found, with small amounts of remaining drug. A used bottle should be discarded 6 hours after opening, to avoid possible bacterial growth. The standard of care for administering propofol was not met.

Could the decedent have given propofol to himself? It is unknown where the propofol physically came from. It would have been difficult for the patient to administer the drugs (others besides propofol were administered) to himself, given the configuration of the IV set-up. The IV catheter was in the left leg. The injection port of the IV tubing was 13.5 cm from the tip in the catheter. He would have had to bend his knee sharply or sit up to reach the injection port and push the syringe barrel, an awkward situation, especially if sleep was the goal. If only bolus injections via a syringe were used, sleep would not have been maintained, due to the short action of propofol. Someone with medical knowledge or experience would have started the IV. Anyone could have drawn up and administered the medications after the IV was started.

What is an anesthesiologist's view point on the toxicology screen results? The levels of propofol found on toxicology exam are similar to those found during general anesthesia for major surgery (intra-abdominal) with propofol infusions, after a bolus induction. During major surgery, a patient with these blood levels of propofol would be intubated and ventilated by an anesthesiologist, and any cardiovascular depression would be noted and treated.

Anesthesiologists would also comment on the presence of other sedative drugs in the toxicology screen. Lorazepam, a long-acting benzodiazepine, is present at a pharmacologically significant level and would have accentuated the respiratory and cardiovascular depression from propofol.

Selma Calmes MD
Anesthesiology Consultant

Date 11/03/2009

County of Los Angeles   **FORENSIC CONSULTANT'S REPORT**   Department of Coroner

13

RADIOLOGY CONSULT

CC #2009-04415
JACKSON, Michael Joseph

REQUEST:

The decedent is a 50 year old black man who died unexpectedly. Please examine for trauma or natural disease.

FILMS:

Whole body radiographic survey—Adult

FINDINGS:

The two views of the skull demonstrate metallic dental "caps" of several right mandibular teeth(pre-molar/molar) with appropriate post operative dental changes, and at least 2 implanted left mandibular dental prostheses (pre-molar/molar). The nasal bones are obscured by overlying cranial and facial structures. The remainder of the craniofacial skeletal structures are unremarkable. An endotracheal tube is in place.

There are no visible significant thoracic skeletal abnormalities other than minimal degenerative spondylosis at T11/12. A small right C7 cervical rib is present. An iatrogenic device with a linear metallic marker is present overlying the left thoracic parasagittal region consistent with a known aortic balloon pump, with the tip located at T6. The superficial soft tissues are unremarkable.

The abdomen and pelvis are unremarkable except for the presence of iatrogenic catheters consistent with femoral vascular catheters as well as the abdominopelvic portion of the aortic balloon pump and what appears to be mild degenerative osteoarthritis of the lumbar spine facet joints at L4/5 and L5-S1.

The right upper extremity is unremarkable, except for probable mild degenerative osteoarthritis of the DIP joints of the index and long fingers. A small portion of the mid right upper extremity (including the proximal third of the forearm) is not included on the films.

The left upper extremity is unremarkable except for moderate degenerative osteoarthritis of the DIP joint of the little finger.

The skeletal and articular structures of the right lower extremity are unremarkable. Incidently noted is a thin 5 cm. long calcific collection in the posterior mid to distal leg consistent with atherosclerotic arterial calcification.

13

RADIOLOGY CONSULT

CC #2009-04415
JACKSON, Michael Joseph

Page 2 of 2

The skeletal structures of the left lower extremity are unremarkable. Incidently noted is a thin 2 cm. long calcific density in the posterior distal leg consistent with calcified arterial atherosclerosis (found at the same level as the ID marker band placed about the lower left leg). There is additional minimal calcified arterial atherosclerotic calcification approximately 1.5 cm distal to the larger calcification.

IMPRESSION:

1. Right mandibular pre-molar/molar metallic "caps" with appropriate post-operative changes.
2. Two (2) mandibular pre-molar/molar implanted dental prostheses.
3. Minimal degenerative spondylosis of the lower thoracic spine.
4. Right C7 cervical rib
5. Vascular iatrogenic devices are in place.
6. Mild degenerative osteoarthritis of the lower lumbar spine facet joints.
7. Probable mild degenerative osteoarthritis of the DIP joints of the right index and long fingers.
8. Moderate degenerative osteoarthritis of the DIP joint of the left little finger.
9. Mild calcified arterial atherosclerosis of both legs.

Donald C. Boger, M.D.   7/2/09

DONALD C. BOGER, M.D.   Date
RADIOLOGY CONSULTANT

DCB/ecl
7/2/09

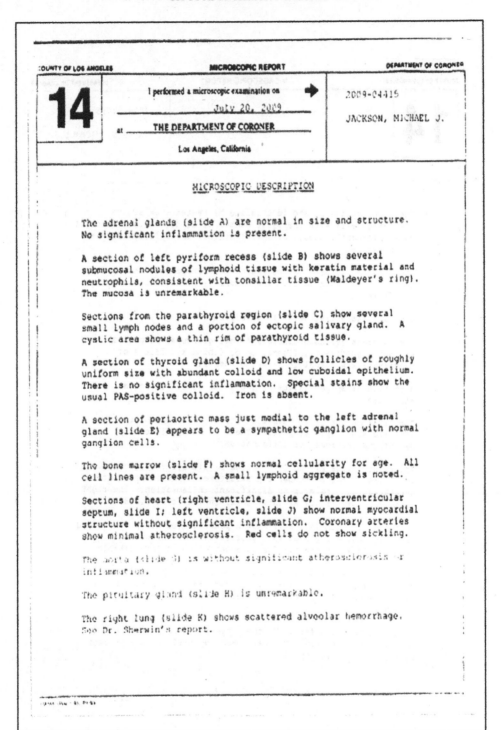

14

I performed a microscopic examination on

July 20, 2009

at **THE DEPARTMENT OF CORONER**

Los Angeles, California

2009-04415

JACKSON, MICHAEL J.

MICROSCOPIC DESCRIPTION

The adrenal glands (slide A) are normal in size and structure. No significant inflammation is present.

A section of left pyriform recess (slide B) shows several submucosal nodules of lymphoid tissue with keratin material and neutrophils, consistent with tonsillar tissue (Waldeyer's ring). The mucosa is unremarkable.

Sections from the parathyroid region (slide C) show several small lymph nodes and a portion of ectopic salivary gland. A cystic area shows a thin rim of parathyroid tissue.

A section of thyroid gland (slide D) shows follicles of roughly uniform size with abundant colloid and low cuboidal epithelium. There is no significant inflammation. Special stains show the usual PAS-positive colloid. Iron is absent.

A section of periaortic mass just medial to the left adrenal gland (slide E) appears to be a sympathetic ganglion with normal ganglion cells.

The bone marrow (slide F) shows normal cellularity for age. All cell lines are present. A small lymphoid aggregate is noted.

Sections of heart (right ventricle, slide G; interventricular septum, slide I; left ventricle, slide J) show normal myocardial structure without significant inflammation. Coronary arteries show minimal atherosclerosis. Red cells do not show sickling.

The aorta (slide G) is without significant atherosclerosis or inflammation.

The pituitary gland (slide H) is unremarkable.

The right lung (slide K) shows scattered alveolar hemorrhage. See Dr. Sherwin's report.

14

2009-04415

JACKSON, MICHAEL J.

Page 2

The right (slide L) and left (slide M) testes show active
spermatogenesis with the usual number of Leydig cells. There is
no significant fibrosis or inflammation. The epididymides are
unremarkable.

The stomach (slide N) shows recent hemorrhage into the mucosa,
submucosa and muscularis. The mucosa is without ulceration or
inflammation.

The gallbladder (slide N) is autolyzed.

The pancreas (slide O) shows a normal glandular structure
without significant inflammation or fibrosis. Islets of
Langerhans are normal in size and number.

A section of spleen (slide P) shows the usual follicular
structure.

The liver (slide Q) is normal in structure. Hepatocytes show no
inclusions or lipid droplets. There is no significant
parenchymal necrosis or inflammation.

The right (slide R) and left (slide S) kidneys show glomeruli
which are normal in number and structure. Tubular cells are
unremarkable. There is no significant inflammation. The right
pyramidal apex (slide R) shows focal interstitial fibrosis.

Sections of colon (slide T) show a pedunculated polyp consisting
of benign colonic glands in a fibrous stroma. Abundant
eosinophils are present. The adjacent colon is unremarkable.

Sections of skin (slide U) show no melanocytic pigment.
Melanocytes, although present, are reduced in number. The skin
is otherwise unremarkable. No scar or suture material is
present.

The prostate gland (slide V) shows hyperplastic glands in a
nodular configuration. Minimal lymphoid infiltrate is present.
There is no malignancy.

14

2009-04415

JACKSON, MICHAEL J.

Page 3

Consultation is obtained with Dr. Chandrasoma, Professor of
Pathology at USC Keck School of Medicine.

Diagnosis: 1. Colon, tubular adenoma
             2. Vitiligo
             3. Nodular prostatic hyperplasia
             4. Evidence of resuscitation
                A) Lung, alveolar hemorrhage
                B) Stomach, transmural hemorrhage

_____   8-19-09
CHRISTOPHER ROGERS, MD, MBA   DATE
CHIEF FORENSIC MEDICINE DIVISION

_____   8-19-09
LAKSHMANAN SATHYAVAGISWARAN, MD   DATE
FRCP(C), FCAP, FACP
CHIEF MEDICAL EXAMINER-CORONER

CR:LS:mtm:f
T-7/29/09

COUNTY OF LOS ANGELES   **MEDICAL REPORT**   DEPARTMENT OF CORONER

15

AUTOPSY CLASS: ☑A ☐B ☐C ☐ Examination Only D

☐ FAMILY OBJECTION TO AUTOPSY

Date 6-36-01 Time: 1000 Dr _Rogers/Lakshmanan_

FINAL ON: 6-7-01 By: _Rogers/Lakshmanan_

DEATH WAS CAUSED BY: (Enter only one cause per line for A, B, C, and D)

IMMEDIATE CAUSE:

(A) _Acute propofol intoxication_   Unk

DUE TO, OR AS A CONSEQUENCE OF:

(B)

DUE TO, OR AS A CONSEQUENCE OF:

(C)

DUE TO, OR AS A CONSEQUENCE OF:

(D)

OTHER CONDITIONS CONTRIBUTING BUT NOT RELATED TO THE IMMEDIATE CAUSE OF DEATH:

Benzodiazepine effect

☐ **NATURAL**   ☐ **SUICIDE**   ☑ **HOMICIDE**

☐ **ACCIDENT**   ☐ **COULD NOT BE DETERMINED**

If other than natural causes,
HOW DID INJURY OCCUR? _Intravenous injection by another_

WAS OPERATION PERFORMED FOR ANY CONDITION STATED ABOVE: ☐ YES ☑ NO

TYPE OF SURGERY: _____ DATE: _____

☐ ORGAN PROCUREMENT ☐ TECHNICIAN: _Sanchez / DelaCruz_

PREGNANCY IN LAST YEAR ☐ YES ☐ NO ☐ UNK ☐ NOT APPLICABLE

☐ WITNESS TO AUTOPSY ☐ EVIDENCE RECOVERED AT AUTOPSY
Item Description:

_'ott Smith, LAPD
Photo memory
card given to
Capt backs_

Age: 50   Gender: ☑ Male / Female

PRIOR EXAMINATION REVIEW BY DME

☑ BODY TAG☑   ☐ CLOTHING
☐ X-RAY (No.   )   ☐ FLUORO
☐ SPECIAL PROCESSING TAG   ☐ MED RECORDS
☐ AT SCENE PHOTOS (No.   )

CASE CIRCUMSTANCES

☐ EMBALMED
☐ DECOMPOSED
☐ >24 HRS IN HOSPITAL
☐ OTHER

TYPING SPECIMEN

TYPING SPECIMEN TAKEN BY: _R_
SOURCE: _Femoral_

TOXICOLOGY SPECIMEN

COLLECTED BY: _R_
☑ HEART BLOOD ☐   ☑ STOMACH CONTENTS
☑ FEMORAL BLOOD ☑   ☑ VITREOUS
TECHNIQUE _____
☐ _____ BLOOD ☐ SPLEEN
☐ _____ BLOOD ☐ KIDNEY
☑ BILE ☐ _____
☑ LIVER ☐ _____
☑ URINE (3) ☐ _____

URINE GLUCOSE DIPSTICK RESULT: 4: 3 2: 1: 0
TOX SPECIMEN RECONCILIATION BY: _VB_

HISTOLOGY

☐ Regular (No. _2_) ☐ Oversize (No. _1_)
Histopath Cut: ☑ Autopsy ☐ Lab

TOXICOLOGY REQUESTS

FORM 3A: ☑ YES ☐ NO
☐ NO TOXICOLOGY REQUESTED
SCREEN ☑C ☐H ☐T ☐S ☐O
☐ ALCOHOL ONLY
☐ CARBON MONOXIDE
☐ OTHER (Specify drug and tissue)

REQUESTED MATERIAL ON PENDING CASES

☐ POLICE REPORT   ☐ MED HISTORY
☑ TOX FOR COD   ☑ HISTOLOGY
☐ TOX FOR R/O   ☐ INVESTIGATIONS
☐ MICROBIOLOGY   ☐ EYE PATH CONS.
☐ RADIOLOGY CONS
☐ CONSULT ON
☑ BRAIN SUBMITTED
☐ NEURO CONSULT ☐ DME TO DDT
☐ CRIMINALISTICS
☐ GSR ☐ SEXUAL ASSAULT ☐ OTHER

RESIDENT _____

DME _____

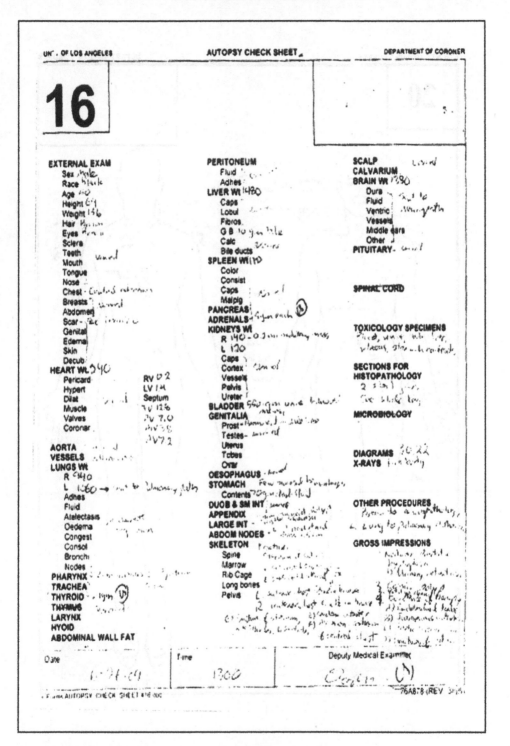

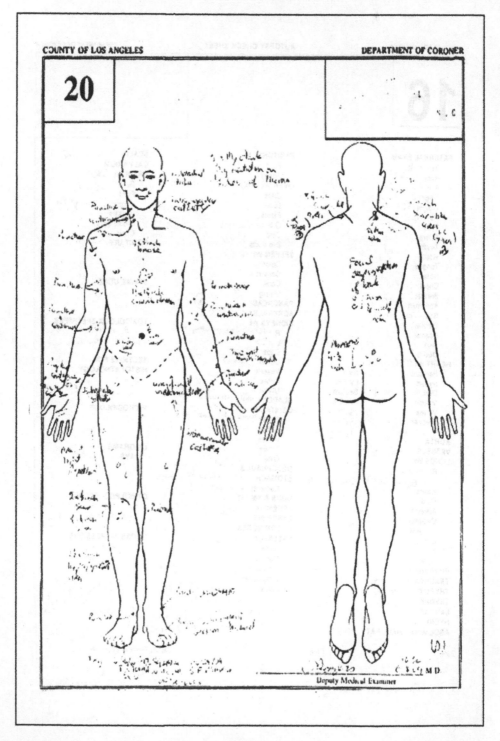

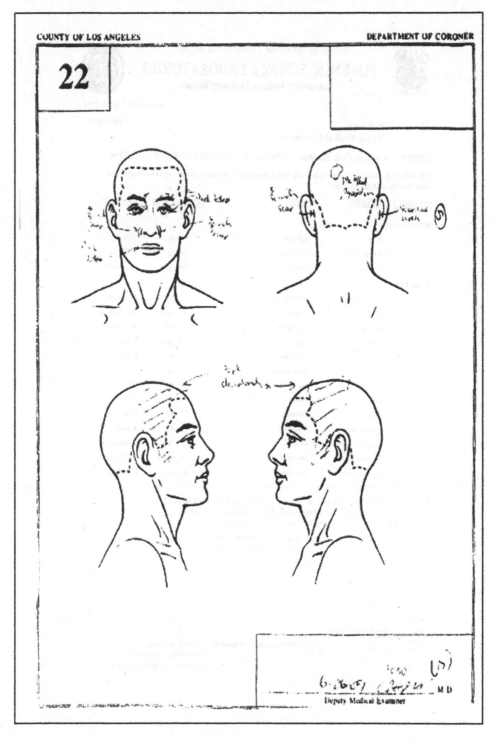

Deputy Medical Examiner

Department of Coroner, County of Los Angeles

FORENSIC SCIENCE LABORATORIES
Laboratory Analysis Summary Report

Wednesday, July 15, 2009

✓ Pending Tox

To: Dr. Rogers
        Deputy Medical Examiner

Subject: Coroner Case Number 2009-04415   JACKSON, MICHAEL JOSEPH

The following results have been technically and administratively reviewed and are the opinions and interpretations of the Analyst:

SPECIMEN	SERVICE	DRUG	LEVEL	UNITS	ANALYST
Blood, Femoral					
	Base	Lidocaine	0.84	ug/ml	E. Fu
	Benzodiazepine	Lorazepam	169	ng/ml	S. DeQuintana
	Propofol	Propofol	2.6	ug/ml	J. Lieberman
Blood, Heart					
	Acetaminophen	Acetaminophen		ND	J. Lieberman
	Alcohol	Ethanol		Negative	M. Schuchardt
	Barbiturate	Barbiturates		ND	D. Anderson
	Base	Lidocaine	0.68	ug/ml	E. Fu
	Base	Meperidine		ND	E. Fu
	Base	Normeperidine		ND	G. Fu
	Base	Nortriptyline		ND	E. Fu
	Base	Sertraline		ND	E. Fu
	Base	Trazodone		ND	E. Fu
	Benzodiazepine	Alprazolam		ND	R. Budd
	Benzodiazepine	Diazepam	<0.10	ug/ml	S. DeQuintana
	Benzodiazepine	Lorazepam	162	ng/ml	S. DeQuintana
	Benzodiazepine	Midazolam	4.6	ng/ml	R. Budd

NOTE: Hospital, Blood: Tube labeled "Trauma, Gershwin" drawn on 06/25-09 @ 1330 hours.
Urine*: Approximately 450 mls of urine collected from scene by Inv. E. Fleak.
*Done: See Form 13, Medical Evidence Analysis Summary Report.

Legend:

ug/g   Microgram per Gram
ug/ml   Microgram per Milliliter

%   of total Hgb
% Saturation
Done
mg   Milligram
ND   Not Detected
Negative
ng/ml   Nanogram per Milliliter
Present

Administratively reviewed by: Daniel T. Anderson
Supervising Criminalist II
FORENSIC LABORATORIES

Page 1 of 8

Department of Coroner, County of Los Angeles

FORENSIC SCIENCE LABORATORIES
Laboratory Analysis Summary Report

Wednesday, July 15, 2009

✔ Pending Tox

To: Dr. Rogers
Deputy Medical Examiner

Subject: Coroner Case Number 2009-04415   JACKSON, MICHAEL, JOSEPH

The following results have been technically and administratively reviewed and are the opinions and interpretations of the Analyst:

SPECIMEN	SERVICE	DRUG	LEVEL	UNITS	ANALYST
Benzodiazepines	Nordiazepam		~0.05	ug/ml	S. DeQuintana
Benzodiazepines	Zolpidem		ND		R. Budd
Carbon Monoxide	Carbon Monoxide		<10	% Saturation	D. Anderson
Cocaine	Cocaine and Metabolites		ND		D. Anderson
Cyanide	Cyanide		ND		M. Schuchardt
Fentanyl	Fentanyl		ND		D. Anderson
GC/MS	Tizanidine		ND		S. DeQuintana
Halogenated Hydrocarbons	Ethchlorvynol		ND		R. Budd
Halogenated Hydrocarbons	Trichloroethanol		ND		R. Budd
LC/MS	7-Aminoclonazepam		ND		J. Limcumpot
LC/MS	Clonazepam		ND		J. Limcumpot
LC/MS	Oxazepam		ND		J. Limcumpot
LC/MS	Temazepam		ND		J. Limcumpot
Marijuana	Carboxy-THC		ND		D. Anderson
Methamphetamine	Amphetamine		ND		O. Pletsar
Methamphetamine	Ephedrine		ND		O. Pletsar
Methamphetamine	Methamphetamine		ND		O. Pletsar
Neutrals	Propofol		Present		D. Anderson

NOTE: Hospital, Blood: Tube labeled "Trauma, Gershwin" drawn on 06/25/09 @ 1330 hours.
Urine*: Approximately 450 mls of urine collected from scene by Inv. E. Fleak.
*Done: See Form 13, Medical Evidence Analysis Summary Report.

Legend:

ug/g	Microgram per Gram
ug/ml	Microgram per Milliliter
%	mg/dl High
% Saturation	
Dose	
mg	Milligram
ND	Not Detected
Negative	
ng/ml	Nanogram per Milliliter
Present	

Administratively reviewed by: Daniel T. Anderson
Supervising Criminalist II
FORENSIC LABORATORIES

Page 2 of 8

Department of Coroner, County of Los Angeles

FORENSIC SCIENCE LABORATORIES
Laboratory Analysis Summary Report

Wednesday, July 15, 2009

☑ Pending Tox

To: Dr. Rogers
        Deputy Medical Examiner

Subject: **Coroner Case Number   2009-04415   JACKSON, MICHAEL JOSEPH**

The following results have been technically and administratively reviewed and are the opinions and interpretations of the Analyst:

SPECIMEN	SERVICE	DRUG	LEVEL	UNITS	ANALYST
	Opiates	Codeine		ND	D. Anderson
	Opiates	Hydrocodone		ND	D. Anderson
	Opiates	Hydromorphone		ND	D. Anderson
	Opiates	Morphine		ND	D Anderson
	Outside Test	Hemoglobin A1C	5.1	%	Quest Diagnostics
	Oxycodone	Oxycodone		ND	S. DeQuintana
	Phencyclidine	Phencyclidine		ND	D. Anderson
	Propofol	Propofol	3.2	ug/ml	J. Lintemoot
	Salicylate	Salicylate		ND	J. Lintemoot
Blood, Hospital					
	Acetaminophen	Acetaminophen		ND	J. Lintemoot
	Barbiturate	Barbiturate		ND	J. Lintemoot
	Bases	Diazepam		Present	E. Fu
	Bases	Lidocaine	0.51	ug/ml	E. Fu
	Bases	Meperidine		ND	E. Fu
	Bases	Normeperidine		ND	E. Fu
	Bases	Nortriptyline		ND	E. Fu
	Bases	Sertraline		ND	E. Fu

NOTE: Hospital, Blood: Tube labeled "Trauma, Gershwin" drawn on 06/25/09 @ 1330 hours.
Urine*: Approximately 450 mls of urine collected from scene by Inv. E. Fleak.
*Done: See Form 13, Medical Evidence Analysis Summary Report.

Legend:
                    ug/g   Microgram per Gram
                    ug ml   Microgram per Milliliter

%   at usual High
% Saturation
Draw
mg   Milligram
ND   Not Detected
Negative
ng/ml   Nanogram per Milliliter
Present

Administratively reviewed by: **Daniel T. Anderson**
                                Supervising Criminalist II
                                FORENSIC LABORATORIES

Page 1 of X

Department of Coroner, County of Los Angeles

FORENSIC SCIENCE LABORATORIES
Laboratory Analysis Summary Report

Wednesday, July 15, 2009

☑ PendingTox

To: Dr. Rogers
        Deputy Medical Examiner

Subject: **Coroner Case Number   2009-04415   JACKSON, MICHAEL JOSEPH**

The following results have been technically and administratively reviewed and are the opinions and interpretations of the Analyst:

SPECIMEN	SERVICE	DRUG	LEVEL	UNITS	ANALYST
	Bases	Trazodone	ND		E. Fu
	Cocaine	Cocaine and Metabolites	ND		J. Lintemoot
	Fentanyl	Fentanyl	ND		J. Lintemoot
	LC/MS	7-Aminoclonazepam	ND		J. Lintemoot
	LC/MS	Clonazepam	ND		J. Lintemoot
	LC/MS	Oxazepam	ND		J. Lintemoot
	LC/MS	Temazepam	ND		J. Lintemoot
	Marijuana	Carboxy-THC	ND		J. Lintemoot
	Methamphetamine	Methamphetamine	ND		J. Lintemoot
	Opiates	Codeine	ND		J. Lintemoot
	Opiates	Hydrocodone	ND		J. Lintemoot
	Opiates	Hydromorphone	ND		J. Lintemoot
	Opiates	Morphine	ND		J. Lintemoot
	Phencyclidine	Phencyclidine	ND		J. Lintemoot
	Propofol	Propofol	4.1	ug/ml	J. Lintemoot
	Salicylate	Salicylate	ND		J. Lintemoot
Liver					
	Bases	Lidocaine	0.45	ug/g	E. Fu

NOTE: Hospital, Blood: Tube labeled "Trauma, Gershwin" drawn on 06/25/09 @ 1330 hours.
Urine*: Approximately 450 mls of urine collected from scene by Inv. E. Fleak.
*Done: See Form 13, Medical Evidence Analysis Summary Report.

Legend:

	ug/g	Microgram per Gram
	ug/ml	Microgram per Milliliter
%	of total High	
*% Saturation		
Dose		
mg	Milligram	
ND	Not Detected	
Negative		
ng/ml	Nanogram per Milliliter	
Present		

Administratively reviewed by: Daniel T. Anderson
                               Supervising Criminalist II
                               FORENSIC LABORATORIES

Page 4 of 4

Department of Coroner, County of Los Angeles

FORENSIC SCIENCE LABORATORIES
Laboratory Analysis Summary Report

Wednesday, July 15, 2009

✔ PendingTox

To: **Dr. Rogers**
Deputy Medical Examiner

Subject: **Coroner Case Number 2009-04415 JACKSON, MICHAEL JOSEPH**

The following results have been technically and administratively reviewed and are the opinions and interpretations of the Analyst:

SPECIMEN	SERVICE	DRUG	LEVEL	UNITS	ANALYST
	Propofol	Propofol	0.2	ug/g	J. Linhslovt
Medical Evidence					
	Medical Evidence	.....	*	Done	J. Linlorvst
Stomach Contents					
	Basa	Lidocaine	1.6	mg	E. Fu
	Propofol	Propofol	0.13	mg	J. Linsenent
Urine					
	"Dipstick"	Glucose	Negative		J. Muto
	Acetaminophen	Acetaminophen	ND		J. Linhslovt
	Alcohol	Ethanol	Negative		M. Schschardt
	Barbiturate	Barbiturates	ND		D. Anderson
	Basa	Lidocaine	Present		E. Fu
	Bases	Meperidine	ND		E. Fu
	Bases	Normeperidine	ND		E. Fu
	Bases	Nortriptaline	ND		E. Fu
	Bases	Sertraline	ND		E. Fu
	Bases	Trazodone	ND		E. Fu
	Benzodiazepines	Alprazolam	ND		R. Gudd

NOTE: Hospital, Blood: Tube labeled "Trauma, Gershwin" drawn on 06/25/09 @ 1330 hours.
Urine*: Approximately 450 mls of urine collected from scene by Inv. E. Flenk.
*Done: See Form 13, Medical Evidence Analysis Summary Report.

Legend:
ug/g	Microgram per Gram
ug, ml	Microgram per Milliliter

%	of total High
*, Saturation	
Done	
mg	Milligram
ND	Not Detected
Negative	
ng, ml	Nanogram per Milliliter
Present	

Administratively reviewed by: **Daniel F. Anderson**
Supervising Criminalist II
FORENSIC LABORATORIES

Page 5 of 6

Department of Coroner, County of Los Angeles

FORENSIC SCIENCE LABORATORIES
Laboratory Analysis Summary Report

Wednesday, July 15, 2009

✔ PendingTox

To: Dr. Rogers
Deputy Medical Examiner

Subject: Coroner Case Number 2009-04415 JACKSON, MICHAEL JOSEPH

The following results have been technically and administratively reviewed and are the opinions and interpretations of the Analyst:

SPECIMEN	SERVICE	DRUG	LEVEL	UNITS	ANALYST
	Benzodiazepines	Midazolam	4.8	ug/ml	R. Budd
	Benzodiazepines	Zaleplon		ND	R. Budd
	Cocaine	Cocaine and Metabolites		ND	D. Anderson
	Fentanyl	Fentanyl		ND	D. Anderson
	Halogenated Hydrocarbons	Ethchlorvynol		ND	R. Budd
	Halogenated Hydrocarbons	Trichlorethanol		ND	R. Budd
	Marijuana	Carboxy-THC		ND	B. Watson
	Marijuana	Tetrahydrocannabinol (THC)		ND	B. Watson
	Methamphetamine	Amphetamine		ND	O. Pfeifer
	Methamphetamine	Ephedrine		Present	O. Pfeifer
	Methamphetamine	Methamphetamine		ND	O. Pfeifer
	Neutrals	Propofol		Present	D. Anderson
	Opiates	Codeine		ND	D. Anderson
	Opiates	Hydrocodone		ND	D. Anderson
	Opiates	Hydromorphone		ND	D. Anderson
	Opiates	Morphine		ND	D. Anderson
	Oxycodone	Oxycodone		ND	S. DiQuintana
	Phencyclidine	Phencyclidine		ND	D. Anderson

NOTE: Hospital, Blood: Tube labeled "Trauma, Gershwin" drawn on 06/25/09 @ 1330 hours.
Urine*: Approximately 450 mls of urine collected from scene by Inv. E. Fleak.
*Done: See Form 13, Medical Evidence Analysis Summary Report.

Legend:

ug/g	Micrograms per Gram
ug/ml	Micrograms per Milliliter
...	
%	of total High
% Saturated	
Dose	
mg	Milligram
ND	Not Detected
Negative	
ug/ml	Nanogram per Milliliter
Present	

Administratively reviewed by: Daniel T. Anderson
Supervising Criminalist II
FORENSIC LABORATORIES

Page 1 of 8

Department of Coroner, County of Los Angeles

FORENSIC SCIENCE LABORATORIES
Laboratory Analysis Summary Report

Wednesday, July 15, 2009

✓ Pending Tox

To: Dr. Rogers
Deputy Medical Examiner

Subject: **Coroner Case Number 2009-04415 JACKSON, MICHAEL JOSEPH**

The following results have been technically and administratively reviewed and are the opinions and interpretations of the Analyst:

SPECIMEN	SERVICE	DRUG	LEVEL	UNITS	ANALYST
	Propofol	Propofol	0.15	ug/ml	J. Lintermoot
	Salicylate	Salicylate	ND		J. Lintermoot
Urine*					
	"Dipstick"	Glucose	Negative		J. Motz
	Acetaminophen	Acetaminophen	ND		J. Linternoot
	Alcohol	Ethanol	Negative		M. Schrabach
	Barbiturate	Barbiturates	ND		D. Anderson
	Basas	Lidocaine	Present		E. Fu
	Basas	Meperidine	ND		E. Fu
	Basas	Normeperidine	ND		E. Fu
	Basas	Nonuroutine	ND		E. Fu
	Basas	Sertraline	ND		E. Fu
	Basas	Trazodone	ND		E. Fu
	Benzodiazepines	Alprazolam	ND		R. Budd
	Benzodiazepines	Midazolam	25	ng/ml	R. Budd
	Benzodiazepines	Zaleplon	ND		R. Budd
	Cocaine	Cocaine and Metabolites	ND		D. Anderson
	Fentanyl	Fentanyl	ND		D. Anderson

NOTE: Hospital, Blood: Tube labeled "Trauma, Gershwin" drawn on 06/25/09 @ 1330 hours.
Urine*: Approximately 450 mls of urine collected from scene by Inv. E. Fleak.
*Done: See Form 13, Medical Evidence Analysis Summary Report.

Legend:

	ng/g	Microgram per Gram
	ug/ml	Microgram per Milliliter
%	of total Hgb	
% Saturation		
Date		
mg	Milligram	
ND	Not Detected	
Negative		
ng/ml	Nanogram per Milliliter	
Present		

Administratively reviewed by: **Daniel T. Anderson**
Supervising Criminalist II
FORENSIC LABORATORIES

Page 2 of 8

Department of Coroner, County of Los Angeles

FORENSIC SCIENCE LABORATORIES
Laboratory Analysis Summary Report

Wednesday, July 15, 2009

✔ PendingTox

To: Dr. Rogers
Deputy Medical Examiner

Subject: Coroner Case Number 2009-04415 JACKSON, MICHAEL, JOSEPH

The following results have been technically and administratively reviewed and are the opinions and interpretations of the Analyst:

SPECIMEN	SERVICE	DRUG	LEVEL	UNITS	ANALYST
	Marijuana	Carboxy-THC		ND	B. Waters
	Marijuana	Tetrahydrocannabinol (THC)		ND	B. Waters
	Methamphetamine	Amphetamine		ND	O. Pletter
	Methamphetamine	Ephedrine		Present	O. Pletter
	Methamphetamine	Methamphetamine		ND	O. Pletter
	Opiates	Codeine		ND	D. Anderson
	Opiates	Hydrocodone		ND	D. Anderson
	Opiates	Hydromorphone		ND	D. Anderson
	Opiates	Morphine		ND	D. Anderson
	Oxycodone	Oxycodone		ND	S. DeQuintana
	Phencyclidine	Phencyclidine		ND	D. Anderson
	Propofol	Propofol	<0.10	ug/ml	J. Linscroat
	Salicylate	Salicylate		ND	O. Pletter
Vitreous					
	Propofol	Propofol	<0.40	ug/ml	J. Linscroat

NOTE: Hospital, Blood: Tube labeled "Trauma, Gershwin" drawn on 06/25/09 @ 1330 hours.
Urine*: Approximately 450 mls of urine collected from scene by Inv. E. Fleak.
*Done: See Form 13, Medical Evidence Analysis Summary Report.

Legend:

	ug/g Microgram per Gram
	ug/ml Microgram per Milliliter

%   of total high
% Saturation
Done
ug   Milligram
ND   Not Detected
Negative
ug/ml Nanogram per Milliliter
Present

Administratively reviewed by: Daniel T. Anderson
Supervising Criminalist II
FORENSIC LABORATORIES

Page 8 of 8

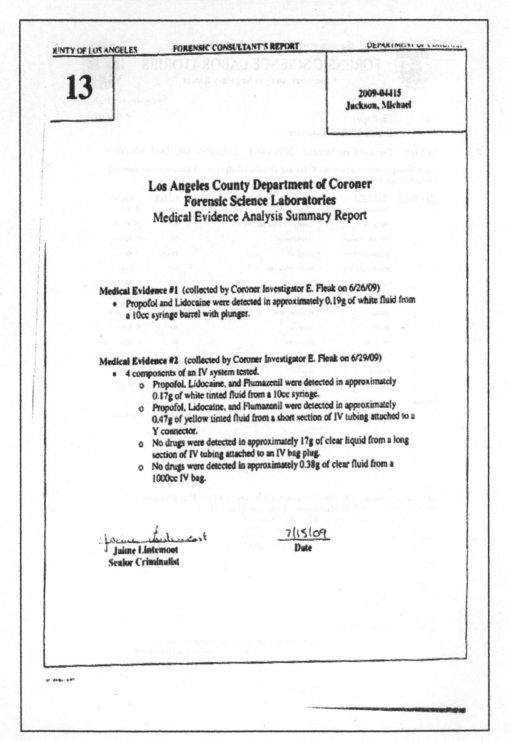

COUNTY OF LOS ANGELES   FORENSIC CONSULTANT'S REPORT   DEPARTMENT OF CORONER

13

2009-04415
Jackson, Michael

Los Angeles County Department of Coroner
Forensic Science Laboratories
Medical Evidence Analysis Summary Report

Medical Evidence #1 (collected by Coroner Investigator E. Fleak on 6/26/09)
- Propofol and Lidocaine were detected in approximately 0.19g of white fluid from a 10cc syringe barrel with plunger.

Medical Evidence #2 (collected by Coroner Investigator E. Fleak on 6/29/09)
- 4 components of an IV system tested.
    o Propofol, Lidocaine, and Flumazenil were detected in approximately 0.17g of white tinted fluid from a 10cc syringe.
    o Propofol, Lidocaine, and Flumazenil were detected in approximately 0.47g of yellow tinted fluid from a short section of IV tubing attached to a Y connector.
    o No drugs were detected in approximately 17g of clear liquid from a long section of IV tubing attached to an IV bag plug.
    o No drugs were detected in approximately 0.38g of clear fluid from a 1000cc IV bag.

Jaime Lintemoot   7/15/09
Jaime Lintemoot   **Date**
Senior Criminalist

SUMMARY of POSITIVE TOXICOLOGICAL FINDINGS
2009-04415 - Jackson, Michael Joseph

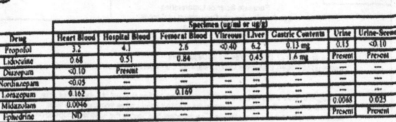

Drug	Specimen (ug/ml or ug/g)							
	Heart Blood	Hospital Blood	Femoral Blood	Vitreous	Liver	Gastric Contents	Urine	Urine-Scene
Propofol	3.2	4.1	2.6	<0.40	6.2	0.13 mg	0.15	<0.10
Lidocaine	0.68	0.51	0.84	---	0.45	1.6 mg	Present	Present
Diazepam	<0.10	Present	---	---	---	---	---	---
Nordiazepam	<0.05	---	---	---	---	---	---	---
Lorazepam	0.162	---	0.169	---	---	---	---	---
Midazolam	0.0046	---	---	---	---	---	0.0068	0.025
Ephedrine	ND	---	---	---	---	---	Present	Present

D. Anderson
Supervising Criminalist II
7/15/09

COUNTY OF LOS ANGELES   **FORENSIC CONSULTANT'S REPORT**   DEPARTMENT OF CORONER

13

2009-04415
Jackson, Michael

Forensic Science Laboratories
Los Angeles County Department of Coroner
Criminalist Report

Investigating Agency: Los Angeles Police Department
Investigating Officer: Detectives Orlando Martinez, Dan Myers, and Scott Smith

On August 6, 2009 at approximately 1300 hours, I was notified by Chief of Laboratories Joseph Muto that a Coroner Criminalist was requested to collect hair samples from the above listed decedent for potential toxicology testing. The decedent had been to the hospital, autopsied on two separate occasions, and handled by mortuary staff prior to my involvement. The decedent would be under the jurisdiction of the decedent's family and the mortuary during evidence collection.

Coroner Chief of Operations Craig Harvey, Forensic Technician II Jose Hernandez, and I arrived at the Glendale branch of Forest Lawn Memorial Park, Glendale at 1745 hours. Forest Lawn personnel, Darryl Drabing, escorted us to a waiting room while preparations were made for viewing the decedent. At 1835 hours we were permitted to view the decedent in a secured lobby area. Those present included Forest Lawn personnel D. Drabing and Scott Drolet, family member La Toya Jackson and her male companion, and the above mentioned coroner personnel.

At approximately 1840 hours I conducted a limited examination of a decedent supine in a yellow casket with blue lining. The majority of the decedent was covered with multiple white towels/sheets leaving only the hands and top of the head exposed. The top of the decedent's head was covered in a wig with long, dark apparent hair. Moving the wig revealed short, dark, curly, natural hair in the temporal regions measuring approximately one and a half inches in length. An unknown dark residue was present on the natural hair. The hair in the parietal region was sparse and covered in an unknown clear adhesive material. Hair samples were collected by plucking with gloved hands. Hernandez took photographs of the hair collection process.

The following items of evidence were collected at the mortuary:

    <u>Physical Evidence (PE)</u>
- Hair Samples (packaged in small PE envelope)
  - Hair Samples from Left Temporal Region (packaged in aluminum foil and paper bindle)
  - Hair Samples from Right Temporal Region (packaged in aluminum foil and paper bindle)

Evidence Collection was completed at the mortuary on August 6, 2009 at 1920 hours.

Evidence was sealed at the Forensic Science Center (FSC) on August 6, 2009 at 1950 hours and placed in a secured storage locker.

Jaime Lintemoot
Senior Criminalist

8/13/09
Date Written

9/9/09
Date Finalized

Brittany Murphy

Given Name: Brittany Anne Bertolotti
Born: November 10, 1977, Atlanta, Georgia
Died: December 20, 2009, Los Angeles, California
Cause of Death: Pneumonia

Actress Brittany Murphy appeared in several popular films including *Clueless* and *8 Mile*. Murphy died after collapsing in her Los Angeles home. The Los Angeles coroner who performed the autopsy concluded that the cause of death was pneumonia but that multiple drugs found in her system and anemia played a role in the actress's death.

COUNTY OF LOS ANGELES	DEPARTMENT OF CORONER

AUTOPSY REPORT

12

I performed an autopsy on the body of
the DEPARTMENT OF CORONER ➡

No.

2009-08735

MURPHY-MONJACK,
BRITTANY

at _____

Los Angeles, California _____ on DECEMBER 21, 2009 @ 0940 HOURS
(Date)　　　　　　(Time)

From the anatomic findings and pertinent history I ascribe the death to:

(A)　　COMMUNITY - ACQUIRED PNEUMONIA
DUE TO, OR AS A CONSEQUENCE OF

(B)
DUE TO, OR AS A CONSEQUENCE OF

(C)
DUE TO, OR AS A CONSEQUENCE OF

(D)
OTHER CONDITIONS CONTRIBUTING BUT NOT RELATED TO THE IMMEDIATE CAUSE OF DEATH

IRON DEFICIENCY ANEMIA, MULTIPLE DRUG INTOXICATION

Anatomical Summary:

    I.   No evidence of traumatic injury.

   II. Status post collapse at home followed by resuscitative efforts.

       A. Medical records: hypochromic microcytic anemia; thrombocytopenia; hyperkalemia and hypermagnesemia.

       B. All tubing in proper locations.

 III. Other findings:

       A. Pulmonary edema, moderate to severe, bilateral, with effusions.

       B. Gas distension of small bowel without obstruction.

       C. Generalized lymphadenopathy, moderate.

       D. Pallor consistent with anemia.

  IV. See additional reports:

       A. Toxicology

       B. Microscopic.

       C. Cultures.

       D. Radiology.

76AB90M Rev 6/84

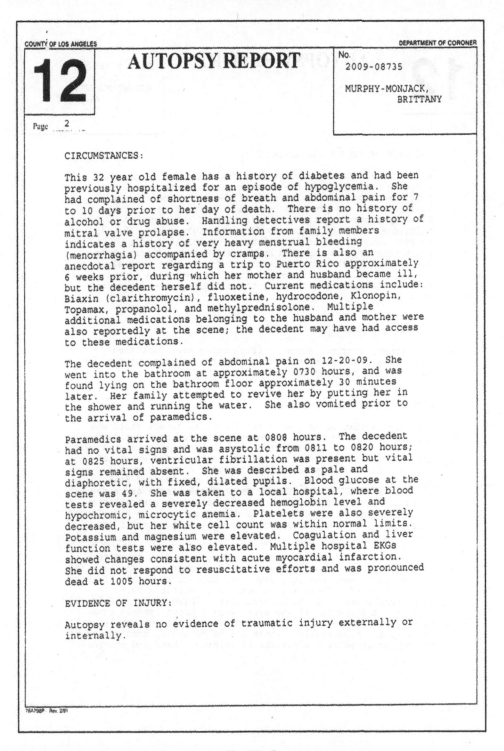

12

AUTOPSY REPORT

No.
2009-08735

MURPHY-MONJACK,
BRITTANY

Page   2

CIRCUMSTANCES:

This 32 year old female has a history of diabetes and had been previously hospitalized for an episode of hypoglycemia. She had complained of shortness of breath and abdominal pain for 7 to 10 days prior to her day of death. There is no history of alcohol or drug abuse. Handling detectives report a history of mitral valve prolapse. Information from family members indicates a history of very heavy menstrual bleeding (menorrhagia) accompanied by cramps. There is also an anecdotal report regarding a trip to Puerto Rico approximately 6 weeks prior, during which her mother and husband became ill, but the decedent herself did not. Current medications include: Biaxin (clarithromycin), fluoxetine, hydrocodone, Klonopin, Topamax, propanolol, and methylprednisolone. Multiple additional medications belonging to the husband and mother were also reportedly at the scene; the decedent may have had access to these medications.

The decedent complained of abdominal pain on 12-20-09. She went into the bathroom at approximately 0730 hours, and was found lying on the bathroom floor approximately 30 minutes later. Her family attempted to revive her by putting her in the shower and running the water. She also vomited prior to the arrival of paramedics.

Paramedics arrived at the scene at 0808 hours. The decedent had no vital signs and was asystolic from 0811 to 0820 hours; at 0825 hours, ventricular fibrillation was present but vital signs remained absent. She was described as pale and diaphoretic, with fixed, dilated pupils. Blood glucose at the scene was 49. She was taken to a local hospital, where blood tests revealed a severely decreased hemoglobin level and hypochromic, microcytic anemia. Platelets were also severely decreased, but her white cell count was within normal limits. Potassium and magnesium were elevated. Coagulation and liver function tests were also elevated. Multiple hospital EKGs showed changes consistent with acute myocardial infarction. She did not respond to resuscitative efforts and was pronounced dead at 1005 hours.

EVIDENCE OF INJURY:

Autopsy reveals no evidence of traumatic injury externally or internally.

78A798P Rev. 2/91

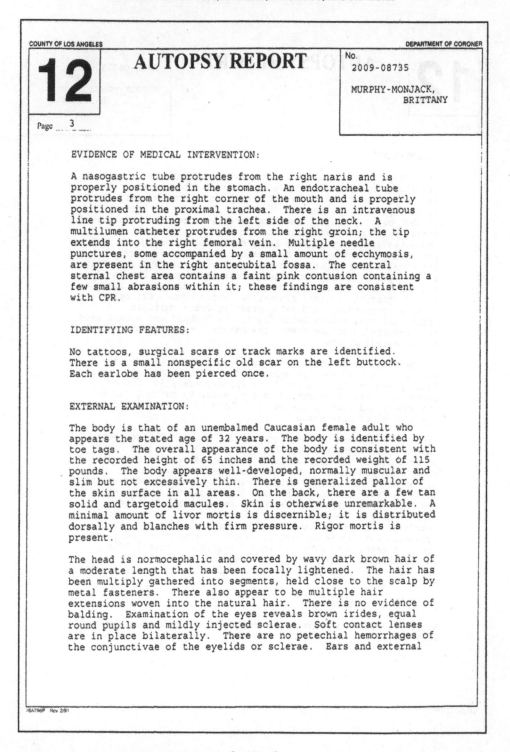

COUNTY OF LOS ANGELES

AUTOPSY REPORT

DEPARTMENT OF CORONER

12

No.
2009-08735

MURPHY-MONJACK,
BRITTANY

Page 3

EVIDENCE OF MEDICAL INTERVENTION:

A nasogastric tube protrudes from the right naris and is properly positioned in the stomach. An endotracheal tube protrudes from the right corner of the mouth and is properly positioned in the proximal trachea. There is an intravenous line tip protruding from the left side of the neck. A multilumen catheter protrudes from the right groin; the tip extends into the right femoral vein. Multiple needle punctures, some accompanied by a small amount of ecchymosis, are present in the right antecubital fossa. The central sternal chest area contains a faint pink contusion containing a few small abrasions within it; these findings are consistent with CPR.

IDENTIFYING FEATURES:

No tattoos, surgical scars or track marks are identified. There is a small nonspecific old scar on the left buttock. Each earlobe has been pierced once.

EXTERNAL EXAMINATION:

The body is that of an unembalmed Caucasian female adult who appears the stated age of 32 years. The body is identified by toe tags. The overall appearance of the body is consistent with the recorded height of 65 inches and the recorded weight of 115 pounds. The body appears well-developed, normally muscular and slim but not excessively thin. There is generalized pallor of the skin surface in all areas. On the back, there are a few tan solid and targetoid macules. Skin is otherwise unremarkable. A minimal amount of livor mortis is discernible; it is distributed dorsally and blanches with firm pressure. Rigor mortis is present.

The head is normocephalic and covered by wavy dark brown hair of a moderate length that has been focally lightened. The hair has been multiply gathered into segments, held close to the scalp by metal fasteners. There also appear to be multiple hair extensions woven into the natural hair. There is no evidence of balding. Examination of the eyes reveals brown irides, equal round pupils and mildly injected sclerae. Soft contact lenses are in place bilaterally. There are no petechial hemorrhages of the conjunctivae of the eyelids or sclerae. Ears and external

/6A79ebP Rev 2/91

COUNTY OF LOS ANGELES

12

AUTOPSY REPORT

DEPARTMENT OF CORONER

No.
2009-08735

MURPHY-MONJACK,
BRITTANY

Page   4

auditory canals are unremarkable. Oronasal passages are
unobstructed. There is a small amount of thin brown liquid at
the nares and mouth, but there is no evidence of oropharyngeal
obstruction. Dentition is natural. Mucous membranes are moist.
The neck is unremarkable. There is no appreciable chest
deformity or increased anterior-posterior chest diameter.
Breasts are symmetric and palpation reveals no masses or nipple
discharge. There are no scars of the chest or abdomen. The
lower abdomen appears mildly distended. The abdomen is otherwise
unremarkable. The genitalia are those of a normal adult female;
there is no evidence of trauma. The pubic hair has been partly
shaved peripherally and is only present centrally. The anus is
unremarkable and atraumatic; no hemorrhoids are identified. No
needle tracks are present. There are no needle punctures that do
not appear related to therapeutic procedures. There is no
appreciable edema of the extremities and no joint deformities are
present.

CLOTHING:

The body is unclothed. Clothing is examined separately and
consists of a single item. This is a pink-orange, floral
patterned shirt or pajama top, "Bed Head" brand, size Petite.
The garment has been previously cut. There is a moderate to
large amount of yellow to brown emesis on the left collar,
sleeve and front. Garment is otherwise unremarkable.

INITIAL INCISION:

The body cavities are entered through a Y-shaped incision.
Examination of the tongue, gingiva, lips and oral mucosa reveals
no lesions and no evidence of trauma. Examination of the oral
cavity reveals no abnormality of the tonsils or epiglottis.
There is a small amount of gastric material in the posterior
pharynx, without obstruction. The hyoid bone and larynx are
intact without fractures. There is no hemorrhage in the
adjacent throat organs or in the prevertebral fascia. Both
pleural cavities are free of adhesions. Each cavity contains up
to 200 cc of slightly cloudy serous fluid. There are no rib
fractures. Parietal pleurae are intact. There is no evidence
of pneumothorax. Both lungs appear fairly well-expanded. Soft
tissues of the thoracic and abdominal walls are well-preserved.
The subcutaneous fat of the abdominal wall measures 1.1 cm.
There is generalized pallor of the viscera and soft tissues.

76A798P Rev 2/91

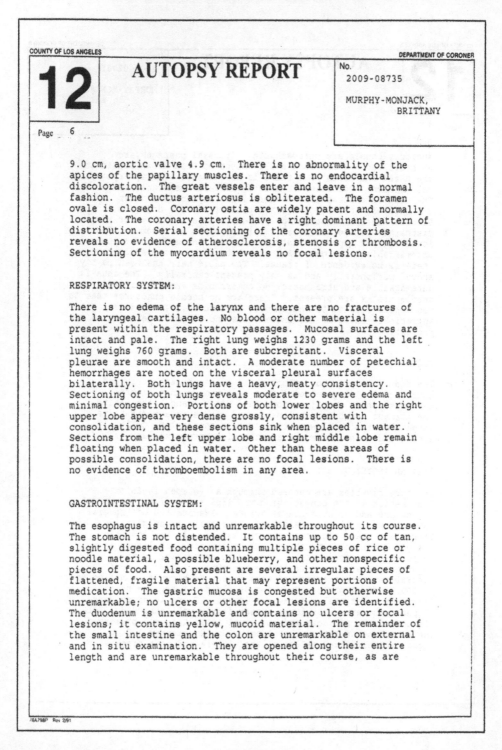

12

AUTOPSY REPORT

No.
2009-08735

MURPHY-MONJACK,
BRITTANY

Page 6

9.0 cm, aortic valve 4.9 cm. There is no abnormality of the apices of the papillary muscles. There is no endocardial discoloration. The great vessels enter and leave in a normal fashion. The ductus arteriosus is obliterated. The foramen ovale is closed. Coronary ostia are widely patent and normally located. The coronary arteries have a right dominant pattern of distribution. Serial sectioning of the coronary arteries reveals no evidence of atherosclerosis, stenosis or thrombosis. Sectioning of the myocardium reveals no focal lesions.

RESPIRATORY SYSTEM:

There is no edema of the larynx and there are no fractures of the laryngeal cartilages. No blood or other material is present within the respiratory passages. Mucosal surfaces are intact and pale. The right lung weighs 1230 grams and the left lung weighs 760 grams. Both are subcrepitant. Visceral pleurae are smooth and intact. A moderate number of petechial hemorrhages are noted on the visceral pleural surfaces bilaterally. Both lungs have a heavy, meaty consistency. Sectioning of both lungs reveals moderate to severe edema and minimal congestion. Portions of both lower lobes and the right upper lobe appear very dense grossly, consistent with consolidation, and these sections sink when placed in water. Sections from the left upper lobe and right middle lobe remain floating when placed in water. Other than these areas of possible consolidation, there are no focal lesions. There is no evidence of thromboembolism in any area.

GASTROINTESTINAL SYSTEM:

The esophagus is intact and unremarkable throughout its course. The stomach is not distended. It contains up to 50 cc of tan, slightly digested food containing multiple pieces of rice or noodle material, a possible blueberry, and other nonspecific pieces of food. Also present are several irregular pieces of flattened, fragile material that may represent portions of medication. The gastric mucosa is congested but otherwise unremarkable; no ulcers or other focal lesions are identified. The duodenum is unremarkable and contains no ulcers or focal lesions; it contains yellow, mucoid material. The remainder of the small intestine and the colon are unremarkable on external and in situ examination. They are opened along their entire length and are unremarkable throughout their course, as are

COUNTY OF LOS ANGELES

DEPARTMENT OF CORONER

12

AUTOPSY REPORT

No.
2009-08735

MURPHY-MONJACK,
BRITTANY

Page 7

their contents. There is focal erythema of the mucosa of the colon. The small bowel contains yellow, mucoid material throughout its course, with no evidence of blood or "coffee ground" material. The colon contains well-formed brown stool, showing no evidence of melena; there is no evidence of diarrhea. The appendix is present and is grossly unremarkable. The pancreas occupies a normal position. Sectioning reveals no parenchymal abnormality. Pancreatic ducts are not ectatic.

HEPATOBILIARY SYSTEM:

The liver weighs 1680 grams and is brown. The capsule is intact and unremarkable. The cut surface is smooth, has a normal consistency and shows no gross evidence of fatty change or fibrosis. The gallbladder has an edematous wall measuring between 0.5 and 0.6 cm, but the wall remains pliable. The gallbladder contains a small to moderate amount of bile; no stones are present. There is no obstruction or dilatation of the extrahepatic ducts. Periportal lymph nodes are moderately enlarged.

URINARY SYSTEM:

The right kidney weighs 170 grams and the left kidney weighs 220 grams. Both are normally situated and their capsules strip easily to reveal smooth cortical surfaces. Corticomedullary demarcation remains sharp. The relatively pale cortices sharply contrast with the congested medullary pyramids, giving them the appearance of "shock kidneys". No focal lesions are noted in any area. Peripelvic fat is not increased. Ureters show no evidence of dilatation or obstruction and pursue their normal course. The urinary bladder is unremarkable. It contains approximately 50 cc of cloudy yellow urine. Dipstick testing of the urine is negative for both glucose and ketones.

FEMALE GENITAL SYSTEM AND BREASTS:

Sectioning of the breast tissue reveals no cysts, masses or other focal lesions. The uterus is symmetrical and of appropriate size for age; the uterine cavity is not enlarged. The endometrium appears minimally hemorrhagic, and there is a minimal amount of bloody material at the cervical os; these findings are grossly consistent with menstruation. There are

76A798P Rev 2/91

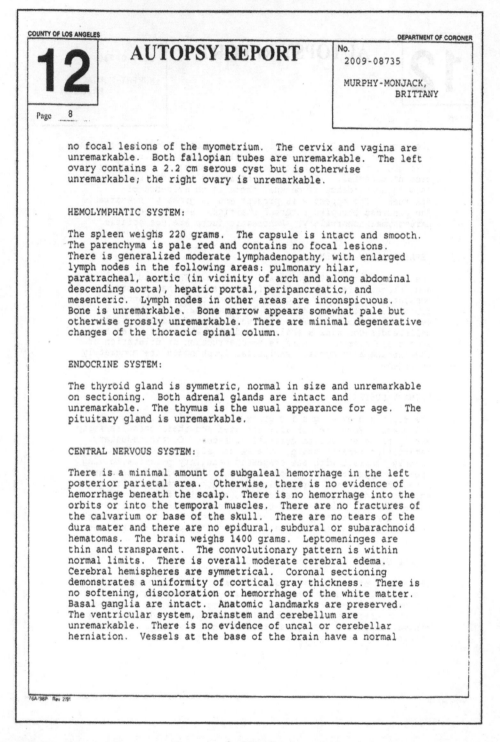

AUTOPSY REPORT

12

No.
2009-08735

MURPHY-MONJACK,
BRITTANY

Page   8

no focal lesions of the myometrium. The cervix and vagina are unremarkable. Both fallopian tubes are unremarkable. The left ovary contains a 2.2 cm serous cyst but is otherwise unremarkable; the right ovary is unremarkable.

HEMOLYMPHATIC SYSTEM:

The spleen weighs 220 grams. The capsule is intact and smooth. The parenchyma is pale red and contains no focal lesions. There is generalized moderate lymphadenopathy, with enlarged lymph nodes in the following areas: pulmonary hilar, paratracheal, aortic (in vicinity of arch and along abdominal descending aorta), hepatic portal, peripancreatic, and mesenteric. Lymph nodes in other areas are inconspicuous. Bone is unremarkable. Bone marrow appears somewhat pale but otherwise grossly unremarkable. There are minimal degenerative changes of the thoracic spinal column.

ENDOCRINE SYSTEM:

The thyroid gland is symmetric, normal in size and unremarkable on sectioning. Both adrenal glands are intact and unremarkable. The thymus is the usual appearance for age. The pituitary gland is unremarkable.

CENTRAL NERVOUS SYSTEM:

There is a minimal amount of subgaleal hemorrhage in the left posterior parietal area. Otherwise, there is no evidence of hemorrhage beneath the scalp. There is no hemorrhage into the orbits or into the temporal muscles. There are no fractures of the calvarium or base of the skull. There are no tears of the dura mater and there are no epidural, subdural or subarachnoid hematomas. The brain weighs 1400 grams. Leptomeninges are thin and transparent. The convolutionary pattern is within normal limits. There is overall moderate cerebral edema. Cerebral hemispheres are symmetrical. Coronal sectioning demonstrates a uniformity of cortical gray thickness. There is no softening, discoloration or hemorrhage of the white matter. Basal ganglia are intact. Anatomic landmarks are preserved. The ventricular system, brainstem and cerebellum are unremarkable. There is no evidence of uncal or cerebellar herniation. Vessels at the base of the brain have a normal

76A/98P Rev 2/91

COUNTY OF LOS ANGELES   DEPARTMENT OF CORONER

AUTOPSY REPORT

No.
2009-08735

MURPHY-MONJACK,
                BRITTANY

12

Page   9

pattern of distribution and are free of aneurysms and
atherosclerosis. The spinal cord is not dissected.

HISTOLOGIC SECTIONS:

Representative sections from various organs are preserved in
10% formalin and placed in a total of two storage jars.
Multiple sections from various organs have been submitted for
microscopic examination. The slide key is as follows:

1. Uterus, appendix (longitudinal and cross-sections of tip),
    clotted blood from heart
2. Left kidney, rectum, abdominal lymph nodes (2 sections)
3. Vertebral bone marrow
4. Right kidney, thyroid, pancreatic lymph node
5. Epiglottis, spleen
6. Liver, pancreas, gallbladder
7. Gastrointestinal tract (stomach, duodenum, jejunum, ileum,
    colon)
8. Left lung (3 sections)
9. Right lung (4 sections)
10. Heart: left ventricle (posterior), right ventricle
11. Heart: anterior-septal left ventricle, septum, right atrial
    appendage
12. Sinoatrial node area, Bundle of His area
13. Apical right atrium (septum with white material)
14. Septum with white material, subapical
15. Brain: frontal and occipital lobes
16. Cerebellum
17. Right basal ganglia

TOXICOLOGY:

Blood, bile, urine, liver tissue, vitreous humor, stomach
contents, and possible pill material from stomach have been
submitted to the laboratory. A complete drug screen has been
requested.

PHOTOGRAPHS:

Photographs have been taken prior to and during the course of
the autopsy.

76A79BP Rev 2/91

COUNTY OF LOS ANGELES

DEPARTMENT OF CORONER

12

AUTOPSY REPORT

No.
2009-08735

MURPHY-MONJACK,
BRITTANY

Page 10

RADIOLOGY:

The body has been fluoroscoped and a total of 14 x-rays have been taken.

DIAGRAMS USED:

Diagram 20 has been used in the preparation of this autopsy report. The diagram is not intended to be a facsimile, nor is it drawn to scale.

WITNESSES:

The following witnesses attended the autopsy: Los Angeles Police Department, Hollywood Division, Detectives C. Gable and S. Brandstetter; Dr. Lakshmanan (Chief Medical Examiner-Coroner).

OPINION:

Autopsy revealed a bilateral acute pneumonia consistent with a community-acquired infection. Blood cultures were positive for Oxacillin-Resistant Staphylococcus aureus, which is the most likely causative organism. Viral cultures were negative. Other cultures were positive for additional organisms, which may represent contaminants and/or minor pathogens.

Two additional factors cannot be ruled out as playing contributory roles. Blood tests at the hospital on the day of death revealed a severe hypochromic, microcytic anemia. Gross autopsy findings of pallor and decreased blood volume, as well as microscopic findings (see report) and decreased blood iron levels (see Toxicology report) are consistent with this finding. In a young woman with no history or evidence of gastrointestinal bleeding or trauma, the most common cause of this type of anemia is chronic iron deficiency. Her history of menorrhagia (heavy periods) is the most likely cause of this. The anemia would account for her recent complaints of tiredness, lightheadedness and shortness of breath. Chronic anemia leads to a weakened state of health and would increase her vulnerability to infection.

76A798P Rev 2/91

COUNTY OF LOS ANGELES

AUTOPSY REPORT

DEPARTMENT OF CORONER

12

No.
2009-08735

MURPHY-MONJACK,
BRITTANY

Page 11

The second contributory factor is multiple drug intoxication.
Multiple medications were present in the blood, with elevated
levels of hydrocodone, acetaminophen, and chlorpheniramine.
L-methamphetamine was also present.

It should be noted that the pattern of use of these medications
suggests treatment of symptoms of a cold or other respiratory
infection. Acetaminophen and hydrocodone are components of
Vicodin. Chlorpheniramine is the active ingredient in some
over-the-counter medications. L-methamphetamine is a component
of some inhalers.

It should be noted that L-methamphetamine is not an illegal
drug. Street methamphetamine is D-methamphetamine; none of this
or any other illegal drug was detected. L-methamphetamine is
not as active as the D-isomer, but still has physiological
effects.

The possible adverse physiological effects of elevated levels
of these medications cannot be discounted, especially in her
weakened state. Therefore the manner of death is Accident.

This case was discussed with Dr. Lakshmanan Sathyavagiswaran,
the Chief Medical Examiner-Coroner, who concurs with this
evaluation.

LISA A. SCHEININ, M.D.
DEPUTY MEDICAL EXAMINER

2/9/10
DATE

LAS:mtm:c
D-12/21/09
T-12/23/09

76A7MRP Rev 2/93

County of Los Angeles — **FORENSIC CONSULTANT'S REPORT** — Department of Coroner

13

RADIOLOGY CONSULT

CC#2009-08735
MURPHY-MONJACK, Brittany Anne

REQUEST:

32 year old Caucasian female with history of diabetes, found unresponsive by responding para-medics at home and taken to a local hospital and pronounced. Please evaluate for ante mortem pathology/trauma.

FILMS:

1. Skull—AP and lateral
2. Chest
3. Abdomen
4. Pelvis
5. Shoulders

FINDINGS:

Incidently noted is degenerative spondylosis of the C5/6 and C 6/7 cervical disc spaces. There are no visible skeletal fractures or other significant skeletal pathology.

The lateral view of the skull demonstrates a horizontal air-fluid level within a maxillary sinus, consistent with sinusitis or other sinus fluid. No facial fracture is identified.

Iatrogenic endotracheal tube, nasogastric tube and right femoral intravascular catheter are in place.

There is diffuse moderate, gaseous distension of the bowel, but there is no evidence of pneumoperitoneum or pneumothorax.

There is diffuse pulmonary opacity consistent with atelectasis, consolidation or pulmonary edema.

IMPRESSION:

1. There are no visible skeletal fractures or recent post traumatic skeletal pathology.
2. There is evidence of maxillary sinus fluid on the lateral view of the skull.
3. There is moderate air/gas bowel distension, opacification of the lungs secondary to consolidation/atelectasis or edema.
4. Multiple iatrogenic tubes/lines are present.

DONALD C. BOGER, M.D.   Date   12/22/09
RADIOLOGY CONSULTANT

DCB/ecl
hw 12/21/09

COUNTY OF LOS ANGELES   **FORENSIC CONSULTANT'S REPORT**   DEPARTMENT OF CORONER

13

CC#2009-08735
Murphy, Brittany

Criminalist Report

Investigating agency: LAPD - Hollywood
Investigating officer: Detective Berndt
Date written: 12-21-09

At 0830 hours on December 21, 2009, Supervising Criminalist II D. Anderson notified me that evidence needed to be collected from the decedent at the Forensic Science Center (FSC).

At 0847 hours, I observed a nude female (covered by a white sheet) in room S-6 with Supervising Criminalist II Anderson present. Medical apparatus was present in the decedent's nose, mouth, and along the left side of her neck. Autopsy Technician II D. Dominguez washed and photographed the decedent prior to my involvement.

I collected the following items of evidence at the FSC:

- Hair kit
  - Head hair
    - bindle of decedent's natural hair
    - bindle of hair from a weave/extension
  - Facial hair
  - Arm hair

The following evidence was collected by me for toxicology purposes and submitted to the toxicology laboratory

- Hair kit (toxicology)
- Pubic hair kit (toxicology)

I completed evidence collection at 0935 hours on December 21, 2009.

Eucen L. Fu, Senior Criminalist   _1-20-10_   Page 1 of 1
                                          Date

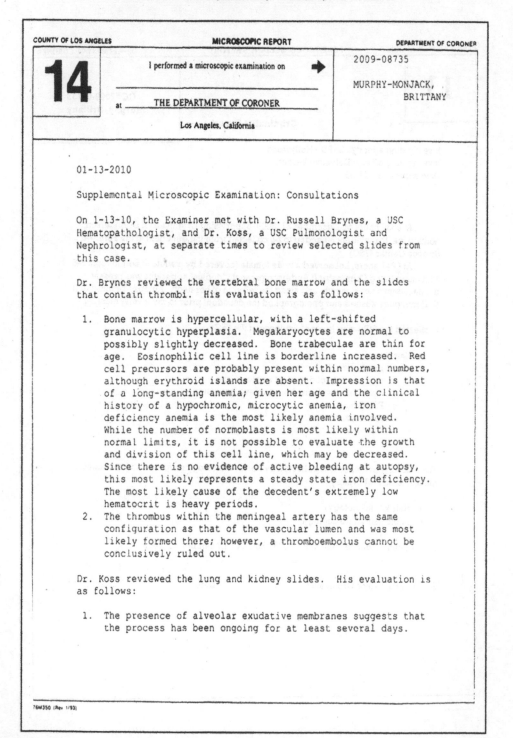

COUNTY OF LOS ANGELES   **MICROSCOPIC REPORT**   DEPARTMENT OF CORONER

14

I performed a microscopic examination on   ➡

at _____ THE DEPARTMENT OF CORONER _____

Los Angeles, California

2009-08735

MURPHY-MONJACK,
BRITTANY

01-13-2010

Supplemental Microscopic Examination: Consultations

On 1-13-10, the Examiner met with Dr. Russell Brynes, a USC
Hematopathologist, and Dr. Koss, a USC Pulmonologist and
Nephrologist, at separate times to review selected slides from
this case.

Dr. Brynes reviewed the vertebral bone marrow and the slides
that contain thrombi. His evaluation is as follows:

1. Bone marrow is hypercellular, with a left-shifted
   granulocytic hyperplasia. Megakaryocytes are normal to
   possibly slightly decreased. Bone trabeculae are thin for
   age. Eosinophilic cell line is borderline increased. Red
   cell precursors are probably present within normal numbers,
   although erythroid islands are absent. Impression is that
   of a long-standing anemia; given her age and the clinical
   history of a hypochromic, microcytic anemia, iron
   deficiency anemia is the most likely anemia involved.
   While the number of normoblasts is most likely within
   normal limits, it is not possible to evaluate the growth
   and division of this cell line, which may be decreased.
   Since there is no evidence of active bleeding at autopsy,
   this most likely represents a steady state iron deficiency.
   The most likely cause of the decedent's extremely low
   hematocrit is heavy periods.
2. The thrombus within the meningeal artery has the same
   configuration as that of the vascular lumen and was most
   likely formed there; however, a thromboembolus cannot be
   conclusively ruled out.

Dr. Koss reviewed the lung and kidney slides. His evaluation is
as follows:

1. The presence of alveolar exudative membranes suggests that
   the process has been ongoing for at least several days.

76M350 (Rev 1/93)

14

2009-08735

MURPHY-MONJACK,
                                BRITTANY

Page   2

2. The acute bronchopneumonia is well-developed.
3. Bacteria seen in routine and gram-stained sections most
   likely represent postmortem overgrowth.
4. In renal slides, the cells of the proximal tubules have
   irregularly placed nuclei in addition to being somewhat
   flattened. This suggests some element of acute tubular
   damage.

_____   ___2/3/10___
LISA A. SCHEININ, M.D.   DATE
DEPUTY MEDICAL EXAMINER

LAS:mtm:c
D-1/14/10
T-1/25/10

COUNTY OF LOS ANGELES   **MICROSCOPIC REPORT**   DEPARTMENT OF CORONER

14

I performed a microscopic examination on ➡

at   THE DEPARTMENT OF CORONER

Los Angeles, California

2009-08735

MURPHY-MONJACK,
BRITTANY

01/06/2010

Supplemental Microscopic Report: Special stains

Sections submitted:
- Iron stain on vertebral bone marrow (slide 3)
- Tissue gram stains on slides 1,9,13 and 15

Iron stain: Iron stain on bone marrow is completely negative, showing no evidence of iron deposition either extracellularly or intracellularly.

Gram stain: Gram stains on the right ventricular apex and its adherent thrombus (slide #13), the cardiac thrombus (slide 1), and cerebral hemispheres (slide 15) are negative. Gram stain on right lung (slide 9) shows apparent mixed gram-positive flora, both cocci and bacilli, within alveoli. Distribution is suggestive of postmortem overgrowth. The possible bacterial cocci seen within a blood vessel in the routinely stained section are not identified in this section.

LISA A. SCHEININ, M.D.
DEPUTY MEDICAL EXAMINER

2/3/10
DATE

LAS:mtm:c
D-1/14/10
T-1/25/10

76M350 (Rev 1/93)

COUNTY OF LOS ANGELES   **MICROSCOPIC REPORT**   DEPARTMENT OF CORONER

14

I performed a microscopic examination on
12/30/09

➡

2009-08735

MURPHY-MONJACK,
BRITTANY

at   THE DEPARTMENT OF CORONER

Los Angeles, California

MICROSCOPIC DESCRIPTION

Sections submitted:
1. Appendix (cross and longitudinal sections), uterus, thrombus from heart
2. Abdominal lymph nodes (2 sections), rectum, left kidney
3. Vertebral bone marrow
4. Right kidney, pancreatic lymph nodes (2 sections), thyroid
5. Spleen, epiglottis
6. Liver, pancreas, gallbladder
7. Gastrointestinal tract, random sections (stomach, duodenum, jejunum, ileum, colon)
8. Left lung (3 sections)
9. Right lung (4 sections)
10. Heart: right ventricle, posterior left ventricle
11. Heart: septum, anterior-septal left ventricle, left atrial appendage
12. Sinoatrial node area, Bundle of His area
13. Apical right ventricle
14. Apical right ventricle
15. Frontal and occipital cerebral cortex
16. Right basal ganglia
17. Cerebellum

Heart: Right ventricle, septum, posterior left ventricle, anterior-septal left ventricle and the sinoatrial node area are all unremarkable except for mild to moderate interstitial edema; sinoatrial node area also shows mild fatty infiltration. The myocardium in the vicinity of the Bundle of His shows minimal focal basophilic degeneration of a few septal myocytes, but is otherwise unremarkable. A portion of the mitral valve attached to this section shows no vegetations; the valve itself is mildly fibrotic.

Section of the left atrial appendage shows unremarkable myocardium with a thrombus interdigitating with the endocardium but not adherent to it. The thrombus itself contains a large number of erythrocytes and neutrophils, which appear to form separate layers; it appears to be antemortem.

76M350 (Rev 1/93)

COUNTY OF LOS ANGELES　　　　　MICROSCOPIC REPORT　　　　　DEPARTMENT OF CORONER

14

2009-08735

MURPHY-MONJACK,
BRITTANY

Page.　3

suggestive of postmortem overgrowth. However, sheets of what
appear to be bacterial cocci are noted in one small blood vessel
within the right lung.

Epiglottis: Small number of submucosal lymphocytes; otherwise
unremarkable.

Liver: Fatty change is absent. A few hepatocytes show
erythrophagia. There is mild to moderate hepatocellular
cholestasis. Mild vacuolization of hepatocytes is noted.
Portal areas are unremarkable.

Gallbladder: Gallbladder wall is diffusely and severely
autolyzed; no abnormality is identified.

Pancreas: Sections reveal interstitial edema and minimal fatty
infiltration. Exocrine and endocrine portions are unremarkable.

Stomach: Basilar lamina propria contains a few lymphocytes,
plasma cells and rare eosinophils. Section is otherwise
unremarkable.

Small bowel: The duodenum, jejunum and ileum all contain mild
to moderate infiltrates of neutrophils in the basilar lamina
propria; jejunum and ileum also contain foci of mildly to
moderately elevated eosinophils.

Colon: Lamina propria contains a moderate to focally severe
increase in eosinophils; neutrophils are present but very rare.
There is occasional prominent vascular dilatation and congestion.

Appendix: Essentially unremarkable; few eosinophils in lamina
propria.

Kidneys: Both kidneys show similar findings. Medullary areas
show vascular congestion. Cortical areas show abundant
flocculent material within tubular lumina and the glomerular
space. The proximal tubular cells appear somewhat flattened.
Glomeruli and blood vessels are unremarkable.

14

2009-08735

MURPHY-MONJACK,
BRITTANY

Page   4

Spleen: There is a borderline to mild increase in neutrophils in several areas. Parenchymal erythrocytes are decreased.

Lymph nodes: Abdominal lymph nodes show mild sinus histiocytosis. One of two abdominal lymph nodes contains foci in which neutrophils are mildly increased. Pancreatic lymph nodes contain numerous active-appearing germinal centers. A mild increase in neutrophils is noted in interfollicular areas.

Vertebral bone marrow: Bone marrow is hypercellular, and there is prominent granulocytic hyperplasia. Myelocytes are abundant, indicating a mild shift to the left. Megakaryocytes appear adequate, although many appear somewhat small. Erythroid precursors are present and appear adequate in numbers, although erythroid elements are rather scattered throughout the bone marrow and do not form well-defined erythropoietic islands. The myeloid/erythroid ratio appears within normal limits in most areas; in rare areas, it appears very mildly increased.

The eosinophilic cell line is present in normal to mildly increased numbers. A few macrophages contain phagocytosed erythrocytes. Bony trabeculae appear somewhat thin for age. A rare small lymphoid aggregate is present within the bone marrow.

Thyroid gland: Lymphoid follicles are unremarkable. A few small lymphoid aggregates are present, one containing a germinal center. There is focal, mild interstitial fibrosis towards the periphery of the gland.

Uterus: There are no myometrial lesions. Vascular dilatation and congestion is noted in both the myometrium and endometrium. Within the endometrium, there are a few spiral glands; surface endometrium is largely absent. There are a few small foci of hemorrhage within the superficial stroma. Stroma also contains a few lightly pigmented macrophages.

Central nervous system: Sections from right basal ganglia and cerebellum are unremarkable. Sections from frontal and occipital lobes reveal an essentially unremarkable cerebral cortex. A few

COUNTY OF LOS ANGELES   MICROSCOPIC REPORT   DEPARTMENT OF CORONER

14

2009-08735

MURPHY-MONJACK,
BRITTANY

Page   5

small parenchymal and meningeal blood vessels contain fibrin
thrombi, and one small meningeal artery contains a nonadherent
thrombus consisting of erythrocytes, neutrophils and fibrin.

DIAGNOSES:

1. Acute bronchopneumonia, moderate to severe, bilateral.
2. Adult Respiratory Distress Syndrome with diffuse alveolar
   damage, moderate, multifocal, right and left lungs.
3. Acute duodenitis, jejunitis, and ileitis, mild to moderate.
4. Acute splenitis and lymphadenitis, mild.
5. Hypercellular bone marrow with granulocytic hyperplasia and
   absence of well-defined erythropoietic islands (see note).
6. Antemortem thrombi, left atrial appendage, right ventricular
   apex, cerebral leptomeninges (see note).
7. Possible menstrual endometrium.
8. Fibrosis, mild, mitral valve.

NOTES:

1. The absence of well-defined erythropoietic islands in the
   bone marrow is suggestive of a decrease in cell division
   and proliferation of this cell line.
2. No definite infectious organisms are identified; organisms
   noted in lungs may represent postmortem bacterial
   overgrowth. Special stains have been requested; please
   refer to separate report.
3. It is not possible to determine whether the thrombus in the
   cerebral meninges represents a thromboembolus, or whether
   it was formed locally.

LISA A. SCHEININ, M.D.   2/3/10
DEPUTY MEDICAL EXAMINER   DATE

LAS:mtm:c
D-1/14/10
T-1/22/10

01/14/2010 10:07 FAX 3232267076   MICROBIOLOGY LAB   @002

Microbiology Results   Page 1 of 1

ATT : Denms

Time of report: 01/14/2010 09:58

MURPHY,BRITTANY (CC-200908735)   Hospital ID: LAC
Date of birth: 11/10/1977 (32Y)   Sex: F   Location: CC
SSN:

T448332   Collection D/T: 12/21/2009 1130   Receive D/T:
                                                  PUNBX: 12/22/2009 0809

Transport Time: UNKNOWN hours
Requisition No:
                                          Order Location: CC
AD Diagnosis:

AD Comment:
Attending Phys: UNK
   FUNGAL CULTURE, BIOPSY
     SETUP D/T: 12/22/2009 11:38   (100206)
     SPECIMEN DESCRIPTION   AUTOPSY   (100206) (LA)
     SPECIAL REQUESTS   HEART   (100206) (LA)
     DIRECT EXAM   **KOH PREP** No fungi seen   (100206) (LA)
     CULTURE   Rhodotorula mucilaginosa   (100977) (LA)
                                Candida parapsilosis
     REPORT STATUS   PENDING

END OF REPORT

01/27/2010 07:54 FAX 3232267076   MICROBIOLOGY LAB   → CORONER'S   ☒002

LAC + USC Medical Center
1200 N. State St., Los Angeles, CA 90033
Ira A. Shulman, M.D., Director, Laboratories & Pathology
01/27/2010 07:00

Page: 1

T448332   COLL: 12/21/2009 1130   REC: 12/22/2009 0809 PHYS: UNKNOWN, PHYSICIAN
FUNGAL CULTURE, BIOP   FINAL 01/26/2010
MICRO LAB SETUP: 12222009 1138
          SPECIMEN DESCRIPTION: AUTOPSY
          SPECIAL REQUESTS: HEART

          DIRECT EXAM: **KOH PREP** No fungi seen

          CULTURE: Rhodotorula mucilaginosa
                          Candida parapsilosis

DEPARTMENT OF
CORONER DOCUMENT

END OF REPORT

ACCOUNT #: 9068

MURPHY, BRITTANY
CC-200908735
CC CORONERS CASE
F 11/10/1977

C O N F I D E N T I A L
SUMMARY REPORT

12/25/2009 07:49 FAX 3232267076   MICROBIOLOGY LAB   › CORONER'S   @008

LAC + USC Medical Center
1200 N. State St., Los Angeles, CA 90033
Ira A. Shulman, M.D., Director, Laboratories & Pathology
12/25/2009 07:00

Page: 1

M298928   COLL: 12/21/2009 1130   REC: 12/21/2009 2101 PHYS: UNKNOWN, PHYSICIAN
BIOPSY CULTURE   FINAL 12/24/2009
MICRO LAB SETUP: UNKNOWN UNKNOWN
                 SPECIMEN DESCRIPTION: AUTOPSY
                 SPECIAL REQUESTS: HEART

        GRAM STAIN: <1+ POLYMORPHONUCLEAR LEUKOCYTES
                         <1+ GRAM NEGATIVE RODS

        CULTURE: 2+ Escherichia coli
                         2+ Staphylococcus aureus - Oxacillin Resistant
                         (ORSA)
                         1+ Streptococcus agalactiae (Group B)

SUSCEPTIBILITY (KB)
2+ Staphylococcus aureus - Oxacillin Resistant (ORSA)
ANTIBIOTIC   INTERPRETATION
----------   --------------

Oxacillin   Resistant

T448306   COLL: 12/21/2009 1000   REC: 12/22/2009 2028 PHYS: UNKNOWN, PHYSICIAN
RESPIRATORY PNL, VIR   FINAL 12/24/2009
MICRO LAB SETUP: UNKNOWN UNKNOWN
                 SPECIMEN DESCRIPTION: NASAL
                 SPECIAL REQUESTS: SPECIMEN RECEIVED ON ICE.

        CULTURE: NO VIRUS ISOLATED IN TISSUE CULTURE.
                         Interpret results with caution if specimen is not
                         received on ice.

M298901   COLL: 12/21/2009 0940   REC: 12/21/2009 2056 PHYS: UNKNOWN, PHYSICIAN
BLOOD CULTURE - AERO   FINAL 12/24/2009
MICRO LAB SETUP: 12212009 2058
                 SPECIMEN DESCRIPTION: BLOOD
                 SPECIAL REQUESTS: NONE

        CULTURE: Staphylococcus aureus - Oxacillin Resistant (ORSA)
                         Diphtheroids

    << CONTINUED ON NEXT PAGE >>

                              CONTINUED

                              MURPHY, BRITTANY
ACCOUNT #: 9068   CC-200908735
                              CC CORONERS CASE
C O N F I D E N T I A L   F 11/10/1977
SUMMARY REPORT

12/25/2009 07:49 FAX 3232267076   MICROBIOLOGY LAB   → CORONER'S   @009

LAC + USC Medical Center
1200 N. State St., Los Angeles, CA 90033
Ira A. Shulman, M.D., Director, Laboratories & Pathology
12/25/2009 07:00

Page: 2

<< ACC. NO: M298901 - CONTINUED FROM PREVIOUS PAGE >>

M298901 COLL: 12/21/2009 0940   REC: 12/21/2009 2056 PHYS: UNKNOWN, PHYSICIAN
BLOOD CULTURE - AERO   FINAL 12/24/2009
MICRO LAB SETUP: 12212009 2058
        SPECIMEN DESCRIPTION: BLOOD
        SPECIAL REQUESTS: NONE

SUSCEPTIBILITY (KB)
Staphylococcus aureus - Oxacillin Resistant (ORSA)
ANTIBIOTIC   INTERPRETATION
-----------   --------------

Oxacillin   Resistant

M298902 COLL: 12/21/2009 0940   REC: 12/21/2009 2056 PHYS: UNKNOWN, PHYSICIAN
BLOOD CULTURE - ANAE   FINAL 12/24/2009
MICRO LAB SETUP: 12212009 2058
        SPECIMEN DESCRIPTION: BLOOD
        SPECIAL REQUESTS: NONE

        CULTURE: Diphtheroids

M298932 COLL: 12/21/2009 0930   REC: 12/21/2009 2106 PHYS: UNKNOWN, PHYSICIAN
WOUND CULT, AEROBIC   *** PRELIMINARY ***
MICRO LAB SETUP: UNKNOWN UNKNOWN
        SPECIMEN DESCRIPTION: AUTOPSY
        SPECIAL REQUESTS: PLEURA

        GRAM STAIN: Cell debris
                    NO ORGANISMS SEEN

        CULTURE: Specimen received. Culture in progress.

DEPARTMENT OF
CORONER

END OF REPORT

MURPHY,BRITTANY
ACCOUNT #: 9068   CC-200908735
                                   CC CORONERS CASE
C O N F I D E N T I A L   F 11/10/1977
SUMMARY REPORT

_Jr 12/25/09_

12/26/2009 07:56 FAX 3232267076   MICROBIOLOGY LAB   › CORONER'S   @002

LAC + USC Medical Center
1200 N. State St., Los Angeles, CA 90033
Ira A. Shulman, M.D., Director, Laboratories & Pathology
12/26/2009 07:00

Page: 1

T448332 COLL: 12/21/2009 1130   REC: 12/22/2009 0809 PHYS: UNKNOWN, PHYSICIAN
FUNGAL CULTURE, BIOP   *** PRELIMINARY ***
MICRO LAB SETUP: 12222009 1138
        SPECIMEN DESCRIPTION: AUTOPSY
        SPECIAL REQUESTS: HEART

        DIRECT EXAM: **KOH PREP** No fungi seen

        CULTURE: YEAST - Identification to follow

M298901 COLL: 12/21/2009 0940   REC: 12/21/2009 2056 PHYS: UNKNOWN, PHYSICIAN
BLOOD CULTURE - AERO   FINAL 12/25/2009
MICRO LAB SETUP: 12212009 2058
        SPECIMEN DESCRIPTION: BLOOD
        SPECIAL REQUESTS: NONE

        CULTURE: Staphylococcus aureus - Oxacillin Resistant (ORSA)
                    Lactobacillus species CORRECTED ON 12/25 AT 1131:
                    PREVIOUSLY REPORTED AS Diphtheroids

SUSCEPTIBILITY (KB)
Staphylococcus aureus - Oxacillin Resistant (ORSA)
ANTIBIOTIC   INTERPRETATION
-----------   --------------

Oxacillin   Resistant

M298902 COLL: 12/21/2009 0940   REC: 12/21/2009 2056 PHYS: UNKNOWN, PHYSICIAN
BLOOD CULTURE - ANAE   FINAL 12/25/2009
MICRO LAB SETUP: 12212009 2058
        SPECIMEN DESCRIPTION: BLOOD
        SPECIAL REQUESTS: NONE

        CULTURE: Lactobacillus species CORRECTED ON 12/25 AT 1132:
                    PREVIOUSLY REPORTED AS Diphtheroids

DEPARTMENT OF
CORONER DOCUMENT

CONTINUED

ACCOUNT #: 9068

CONFIDENTIAL
SUMMARY REPORT

MURPHY, BRITTANY
CC-200908735
CC CORONERS CASE
F 11/10/1977

12/25/09

12/26/2009 07:56 FAX 3232267076   MICROBIOLOGY LAB   → CORONER'S   ☒003

LAC + USC Medical Center
1200 N. State St., Los Angeles, CA 90033
Ira A. Shulman, M.D., Director, Laboratories & Pathology
12/26/2009 07:00
                                                        Page: 2
M298932   COLL: 12/21/2009 0930   REC: 12/21/2009 2106 PHYS: UNKNOWN, PHYSICIAN
WOUND CULT, AEROBIC   *** PRELIMINARY ***
MICRO LAB SETUP: UNKNOWN UNKNOWN
        SPECIMEN DESCRIPTION: AUTOPSY
        SPECIAL REQUESTS: PLEURA

        GRAM STAIN: Cell debris
                       NO ORGANISMS SEEN

        CULTURE: GRAM POSITIVE RODS - Identification to follow

DEPARTMENT OF

END OF REPORT

                                        MURPHY, BRITTANY
ACCOUNT #: 9068   CC-200908735
                                        CC CORONERS CASE
C O N F I D E N T I A L   F 11/10/1977
SUMMARY REPORT

12/25/09

LAC + USC Medical Center
1200 N. State St., Los Angeles, CA 90033
Ira A. Shulman, M.D., Director, Laboratories & Pathology
12/27/2009 07:00

Page: 1

M299049 COLL: 12/21/2009 1035   REC: 12/21/2009 2201 PHYS: UNKNOWN, PHYSICIAN
STOOL CULTURE   FINAL 12/26/2009
MICRO LAB SETUP: UNKNOWN UNKNOWN
        SPECIMEN DESCRIPTION: STOOL
        SPECIAL REQUESTS: NONE

        CULTURE: NO SALMONELLA, SHIGELLA, YERSINIA, OR
                         CAMPYLOBACTER ISOLATED.

M298932 COLL: 12/21/2009 0930   REC: 12/21/2009 2106 PHYS: UNKNOWN, PHYSICIAN
WOUND CULT, AEROBIC   FINAL 12/26/2009
MICRO LAB SETUP: UNKNOWN UNKNOWN
        SPECIMEN DESCRIPTION: AUTOPSY
        SPECIAL REQUESTS: PLEURA

        GRAM STAIN: Cell debris
                    NO ORGANISMS SEEN

        CULTURE: Lactobacillus species - Susceptibility routinely
                 NOT done

END OF REPORT

                           MURPHY, BRITTANY
ACCOUNT #: 9068   CC-200908735
                           CC CORONERS CASE
C O N F I D E N T I A L   F 11/10/1977
SUMMARY REPORT

H 12/28/09

01/06/2010 13:13 FAX 3232267076   MICROBIOLOGY LAB   · CORONER'S   ☑004

LAC + USC Medical Center
1200 N. State St., Los Angeles, CA 90033
Ira A. Shulman, M.D., Director, Laboratories & Pathology
01/06/2010 07:00

Page: 1

T451610   Coll: 12/21/2009 10:40 Rec: 12/22/2009 13:11 Phys: ILLEGIBLE, PHYSICIAN
                        Result   Reference Range   Units

Viral Culture and Identific
  Specimen Description
              STOOL ENTVC,ADEVC
              CORRECTED ON 12/22 AT 1321: PREVIOUSLY REPORTED AS STOOL CORRECTED ON
              12/22 AT 1319: PREVIOUSLY REPORTED AS STOOL[AEDVC CORRECTED ON 12/22 AT
              1315: PREVIOUSLY REPORTED AS STOOL
  Status   PRELIMINARY
  Culture and Identification
              NO VIRUS ISOLATED
              (NOTE)

      Performed at Focus Diagnostics, 5785 Corporate Avenue,
      Cypress, CA
      90630, Dr. Alfred Lui, MD., Director, CLIA 05D0644251

DEPARTMENT OF
CORONER DOCUMENT

END OF REPORT

                                          MURPHY,BRITTANY
ACCOUNT #: 9068   CC-200908735
                                          CC CORONERS CASE
C O N F I D E N T I A L   F 11/10/1977
SUMMARY REPORT

                          Schleuder

12/31/2009 08:10 FAX 3232267076   MICROBIOLOGY LAB   › CORONER'S   ☒001

LAC + USC Medical Center
1200 N. State St., Los Angeles, CA 90033
Ira A. Shulman, M.D., Director, Laboratories & Pathology
12/31/2009 07:00

Page: 1

T448297   Coll: 12/21/2009 10:35 Rec: 12/22/2009 08:06 Phys: UNKNOWN, PHYSICIAN
                    Result   Reference Range   Units

Ova and Parasites, Stool Co
  Trichrome (1)   SEE NOTE   {Q3}
                               (NOTE)
      OVA AND PARASITES, STOOL CONC AND PERM SMEAR

      MICRO NUMBER: 91625194
      TEST STATUS: FINAL
      SPECIMEN SOURCE: STOOL
      SPECIMEN COMMENTS: ADEQUATE
      CONCENTRATION 1:   NO OVA OR PARASITES SEEN
      TRICHROME 1:   NO OVA OR PARASITES SEEN

      Test performed at QUEST DIAGNOSTICS-WEST HILLS
      8401 FALLBROOK AVENUE
      WEST HILLS, CA 91304-3226
      Director: LEE H. HILBORNE, MD
  Concentrate (1)   PENDING

{Q3} = Performed by: Quest Diagnostics, 8401 Fallbrook Ave., West Hills, CA
      91304; Lee H. Hilborne, MD, Director

DEPARTMENT OF
CORONER DOCUMENT

END OF REPORT

                                    MURPHY, BRITTANY
ACCOUNT #: 9068   CC-200908735
                                    CC CORONERS CASE
C O N F I D E N T I A L   F 11/10/1977
SUMMARY REPORT

12/23/2009 08:01 FAX 3232267076   MICROBIOLOGY LAB   → CORONER'S   @010

LAC + USC Medical Center
1200 N. State St., Los Angeles, CA 90033
Ira A. Shulman, M.D., Director, Laboratories & Pathology
12/23/2009 07:00

Page: 2

M299699 COLL: 12/21/2009 1040   REC: 12/21/2009 1957 PHYS: UNKNOWN, PHYSICIAN
ROTAVIRUS ANTIGEN   FINAL 12/22/2009
MICRO LAB SETUP: UNKNOWN UNKNOWN
          SPECIMEN DESCRIPTION: STOOL
          SPECIAL REQUESTS: SPECIMEN RECEIVED ON ICE.

          RESULT: Rotavirus Antigen not detected.

M298901 COLL: 12/21/2009 0940   REC: 12/21/2009 2056 PHYS: UNKNOWN, PHYSICIAN
BLOOD CULTURE · AERO   *** PRELIMINARY ***
MICRO LAB SETUP: 12212009 2056
          SPECIMEN DESCRIPTION: BLOOD
          SPECIAL REQUESTS: NONE

          CULTURE: GRAM POSITIVE COCCI - Identification to follow
                         GRAM POSITIVE RODS - Identification to follow

M298902 COLL: 12/21/2009 0940   REC: 12/21/2009 2056 PHYS: UNKNOWN, PHYSICIAN
BLOOD CULTURE - ANAE   *** PRELIMINARY ***
MICRO LAB SETUP: 12212009 2056
          SPECIMEN DESCRIPTION: BLOOD
          SPECIAL REQUESTS: NONE

          CULTURE: GRAM POSITIVE RODS - Identification to follow

M298932 COLL: 12/21/2009 0930   REC: 12/21/2009 2106 PHYS: UNKNOWN, PHYSICIAN
WOUND CULT, AEROBIC   *** PRELIMINARY ***
MICRO LAB SETUP: UNKNOWN UNKNOWN
          SPECIMEN DESCRIPTION: AUTOPSY
          SPECIAL REQUESTS: PLEURA

          GRAM STAIN: Cell debris
                         NO ORGANISMS SEEN

          CULTURE: NO GROWTH AT 24 HRS.

DEPARTMENT OF
CORONER DOCUMENT

END OF REPORT

                                        MURPHY, BRITTANY
ACCOUNT #: 9068   CC-200908735
                                        CC CORONERS CASE
C O N F I D E N T I A L   F 11/10/1977
SUMMARY REPORT

```
12/23/2009 08:00 FAX 3232267076        MICROBIOLOGY LAB        ; CORONER'S        ☑009
```

LAC + USC Medical Center
1200 N. State St., Los Angeles, CA 90033
Ira A. Shulman, M.D., Director, Laboratories & Pathology
12/23/2009 07:00

Page: 1

```
M298928  COLL: 12/21/2009  1130    REC: 12/21/2009  2101  PHYS: UNKNOWN, PHYSICIAN
BIOPSY CULTURE                                              *** PRELIMINARY ***
MICRO LAB SETUP: UNKNOWN UNKNOWN
              SPECIMEN DESCRIPTION:    AUTOPSY
              SPECIAL REQUESTS:        HEART

      GRAM STAIN:    <1+ POLYMORPHONUCLEAR LEUKOCYTES
                     <1+ GRAM NEGATIVE RODS

      CULTURE:       2+ GRAM NEGATIVE RODS - Identification to follow
                     2+ Staphylococcus species - Identification to
                     follow
```

```
T448101  COLL: 12/21/2009  1130    REC: 12/22/2009  0744  PHYS: UNKNOWN, PHYSICIAN
AFB CULTURE, WOUND                                          *** PRELIMINARY ***
MICRO LAB SETUP: 12222009 1420
              SPECIMEN DESCRIPTION:    HEART
              SPECIAL REQUESTS:        SWAB

      AFB STAIN:    **AURAMINE-RHODAMINE STAIN** No acid fast
                    bacilli seen
                    Negative results obtained from specimens
                    submitted on swabs are not reliable.

      CULTURE:      PENDING
```

```
T448332  COLL: 12/21/2009  1130    REC: 12/22/2009  0809  PHYS: UNKNOWN, PHYSICIAN
FUNGAL CULTURE, BIOP                                        *** PRELIMINARY ***
MICRO LAB SETUP: 12222009 1138
              SPECIMEN DESCRIPTION:    AUTOPSY
              SPECIAL REQUESTS:        HEART

      DIRECT EXAM:  **KOH PREP** No fungi seen

      CULTURE:      PENDING
```

DEPARTMENT OF
CORONER DOCUMENT

CONTINUED

MURPHY, BRITTANY
CC-200908735
CC CORONERS CASE
F 11/10/1977

ACCOUNT #: 9068

C O N F I D E N T I A L
SUMMARY REPORT

LAC + USC Medical Center
1200 N. State St., Los Angeles, CA 90033
Ira A. Shulman, M.D., Director, Laboratories & Pathology
01/12/2010 07:00

Page: 1

T448101   COLL: 12/21/2009 1130   REC: 12/22/2009 0744 PHYS: UNKNOWN, PHYSICIAN
AFB CULTURE, WOUND   *** PRELIMINARY ***
MICRO LAB SETUP: 12222009 1420
          SPECIMEN DESCRIPTION: HEART
          SPECIAL REQUESTS: SWAB

     AFB STAIN: **AURAMINE-RHODAMINE STAIN** No acid fast
                    bacilli seen
                    Negative results obtained from specimens
                    submitted on swabs are not reliable.

     CULTURE: NO ACID FAST BACILLI ISOLATED AFTER 2 WEEKS

END OF REPORT

ACCOUNT #: 9068   MURPHY, BRITTANY
                                         CC-200908735
C O N F I D E N T I A L   CC CORONERS CASE
SUMMARY REPORT   F 11/10/1977

Ira A. Shulman, M.D., Director, Laboratories & Pathology
01/13/2010 07:00

Page: 1

T451610   Coll: 12/21/2009 10:40 Rec: 12/22/2009 13:11 Phys: ILLEGIBLE, PHYSICIAN
Result   Reference Range   Units

Viral Culture and Identific
  Specimen Description
                STOOL ENTVC,ADEVC
                CORRECTED ON 12/22 AT 1321: PREVIOUSLY REPORTED AS STOOL CORRECTED ON
                12/22 AT 1319: PREVIOUSLY REPORTED AS STOOL[AEDVC CORRECTED ON 12/22 AT
                1315: PREVIOUSLY REPORTED AS STOOL
  Status   FINAL
                CORRECTED ON 01/12 AT 1649: PREVIOUSLY REPORTED AS PRELIMINARY
  Culture and Identification
                NO VIRUS ISOLATED
                (NOTE)

        Performed at Focus Diagnostics, 5785 Corporate Avenue,
        Cypress, CA
        90630, Dr. Alfred Lui, MD., Director, CLIA 05D0644251

DEPARTMENT OF
CORONER DOCUMENT

END OF REPORT

                                    MURPHY,BRITTANY
ACCOUNT #: 9068   CC-200908735
                                    CC CORONERS CASE
C O N F I D E N T I A L   F 11/10/1977
SUMMARY REPORT

                                        Schenin

12/22/2009 05:15 FAX 3232267076   MICROBIOLOGY LAB   · CORONER'S   ✉012

LAC · USC Medical Center
1200 N. State St., Los Angeles, CA 90033
Ira A. Shulman, M.D., Director, Laboratories & Pathology
12/22/2009 07:00

Page: 1

M298928 COLL: 12/21/2009 1130   REC: 12/21/2009 2101 PHYS: UNKNOWN, PHYSICIAN
BIOPSY CULTURES   *** PRELIMINARY ***
MICRO LAB SETUP: UNKNOWN UNKNOWN
       SPECIMEN DESCRIPTION: AUTOPSY
       SPECIAL REQUESTS: HEART

       GRAM STAIN: <1+ POLYMORPHONUCLEAR LEUKOCYTES
                       <1+ GRAM NEGATIVE RODS

       CULTURE: PENDING

M298931 COLL: 12/21/2009 1030   REC: 12/21/2009 2038 PHYS: ILLEGIBLE, PHYSICIAN
INFLUENZA A&B ANTIGEN   FINAL 12/21/2009
MICRO LAB SETUP: UNKNOWN UNKNOWN
       SPECIMEN DESCRIPTION: NASAL
       SPECIAL REQUESTS: SPECIMEN RECEIVED ON ICE.

       RESULT: Influenza A and B Antigens not detected. The
                      published sensitivity of this test for
                      Influenza A virus is 80% for seasonal H1N1,
                      80% for seasonal H3N2, and 69% for novel
                      H1N1 strains. Therefore, patient management
                      decision should be made on clinical grounds
                      rather than on the results of the antigen
                      test alone.
                      Respiratory viral cultures will be set up
                      automatically for ICU patients whose rapid
                      antigen test results are negative.
                      RESPIRATORY VIRAL CULTURE FOR ALL OTHER
                      INPATIENTS AND OUTPATIENTS MAY BE ORDERED ON
                      SPECIMENS WITH NEGATIVE RESULTS BY CALLING
                      X97012.

M298933 COLL: 12/21/2009 0930   REC: 12/21/2009 2106 PHYS: UNKNOWN, PHYSICIAN
WOUND CULT, AEROBIC   *** PRELIMINARY ***
MICRO LAB SETUP: UNKNOWN UNKNOWN
       SPECIMEN DESCRIPTION: AUTOPSY
       SPECIAL REQUESTS: PLEURA

       GRAM STAIN: Cell debris
                      NO ORGANISMS SEEN

   << CONTINUED ON NEXT PAGE >>

                                        CONTINUED

                                        MURPHY, BRITTANY
ACCOUNT #: 9068   CC-200908735
                                        CC CORONERS CASE
C O N F I D E N T I A L   F 11/10/1977
SUMMARY REPORT

12/22/2009 08:15 FAX 3232267076   MICROBIOLOGY LAB   • CORONER'S   @013

LAC • USC Medical Center
1200 N. State St., Los Angeles, CA 90033
Ira A. Shulman, M.D., Director, Laboratories & Pathology
12/22/2009 07:00

Page: 2

<< ACC. NO: M298932 - CONTINUED FROM PREVIOUS PAGE >>

M298932   COLL: 12/21/2009 0930   REC: 12/21/2009 2106   PHYS: UNKNOWN, PHYSICIAN
WOUND CULT, AEROBIC   *** PRELIMINARY ***
MICRO LAB SETUP: UNKNOWN UNKNOWN
        SPECIMEN DESCRIPTION: AUTOPSY
        SPECIAL REQUESTS: PLEURA

        CULTURE: PENDING

END OF REPORT

ACCOUNT #: 9068

C O N F I D E N T I A L
SUMMARY REPORT

MURPHY, BRITTANY
CC-200908735
CC CORONERS CASE
F 11/10/1977

COUNTY OF LOS ANGELES — **MEDICAL REPORT** — **DEPARTMENT OF CORONER**

15

AUTOPSY CLASS: ☒ A ☐ B ☐ C ☐ Examination Only D

☐ FAMILY OBJECTION TO AUTOPSY

Date: 12/21/09 Time: 0940 Dr. SCHERNIN *(Print)*

FINAL ON: 2/3/10 By: SCHERNIN *(Print)*

APPROXIMATE INTERVAL BETWEEN ONSET AND DEATH

DEATH WAS CAUSED BY: (Enter only one cause per line for A, B, C, and D)

IMMEDIATE CAUSE:

(A) Community-Acquired Pneumonia   Unk

DUE TO, OR AS A CONSEQUENCE OF:

(B)

DUE TO, OR AS A CONSEQUENCE OF:

(C)

DUE TO, OR AS A CONSEQUENCE OF:

(D)

OTHER CONDITIONS CONTRIBUTING BUT NOT RELATED TO THE IMMEDIATE CAUSE OF DEATH:

Iron Deficiency Anemia, Multiple Drug Intoxication

☐ NATURAL ☐ SUICIDE ☐ HOMICIDE

☒ ACCIDENT ☐ COULD NOT BE DETERMINED

If other than natural causes,
HOW DID INJURY OCCUR?

Drug intake ♯ 2/3/10
~~ingestion & probable inhalation~~

WAS OPERATION PERFORMED FOR ANY CONDITION STATED ABOVE: ☐ YES ☒ NO

TYPE OF SURGERY: _____ DATE: _____

☐ ORGAN PROCUREMENT ☐ TECHNICIAN: L. Bivens

PREGNANCY IN LAST YEAR ☐ YES ☒ NO ☐ UNK ☐ NOT APPLICABLE

☐ WITNESS TO AUTOPSY ☐ EVIDENCE RECOVERED AT AUTOPSY
LAPD Hollywood   Item Description:
Det. S. Brandstetter •
Det. C. Gable;
Dr. Lakshmanan

32 C F collapsed @ home 12/20/09. At hosp, Hgb 3.0,
MCV 64.4, plts 36, wbc 8.5, K 8.6, Mg 9.8,
EtOH ND.
Exam - No trauma, Heavy lungs. At GI bleed.
Perd - Tox, slides, CXS, consistent reports.

RESIDENT X _____

DME _____

SEC

Age 32   Gender   Male   ⓕ Female

PRIOR EXAMINATION REVIEW BY DME

☒ BODY TAG   ☐ CLOTHING
☐ X-RAY (No. _____)   ☐ FLUORO
☐ SPECIAL PROCESSING TAG   ☐ MED. RECORDS
☐ AT SCENE PHOTOS (No.   )   1

CASE CIRCUMSTANCES

☐ EMBALMED
☐ DECOMPOSED
☐ > 24 HRS IN HOSPITAL
☐ OTHER: _____ Person

TYPING SPECIMEN

TYPING SPECIMEN TAKEN BY: LS
SOURCE: heart

TOXICOLOGY SPECIMEN

COLLECTED BY: LS + LB
☒ HEART BLOOD   ☒ STOMACH CONTENTS
☒ FEMORAL BLOOD   ☒ VITREOUS
TECHNIQUE: _____
☐ _____ BLOOD   ☐ SPLEEN
☐ _____ BLOOD   ☐ KIDNEY
☒ BILE   ☒ pills from
☒ LIVER   stomach
☒ URINE   ☒ cultures

URINE GLUCOSE DIPST-CX REBUL: 4+ 3+ 2+ 1+ ⓞ
TOX SPECIMEN RECONCILIATION BY:

HISTOLOGY

☒ Regular (No. 2)   ☐ Oversize (No. _____)
Histopath Cut: ☒ Autopsy ☐ Lab

TOXICOLOGY REQUESTS

FORM 3A: ☒ YES ☐ NO
☐ NO TOXICOLOGY REQUESTED
SCREEN ☒ C ☐ H ☐ T ☐ S ☐ D
☐ ALCOHOL ONLY
☐ CARBON MONOXIDE
☒ OTHER (Specify drug and tissue)
Please ID possible pill
material (if possible)
Fluoxetine

REQUESTED MATERIAL ON PENDING CASES

☐ POLICE REPORT   ☐ MED HISTORY
☐ TOX FOR COD   ☒ HISTOLOGY
☒ TOX FOR R/O   ☐ INVESTIGATIONS
☒ MICROBIOLOGY   ☐ EYE PATH. CONS.
☒ RADIOLOGY CONS.
☐ CONSULT ON:
☐ BRAIN SUBMITTED
☐ NEURO CONSULT   ☐ DME TO CUT
☐ CRIMINALISTICS
☐ GSR ☐ SEXUAL ASSAULT ☐ OTHER

WHITE - File Copy   CANARY - Forensic Lab   PINK - Certification   GOLDENROD - DME   Rev 04-06

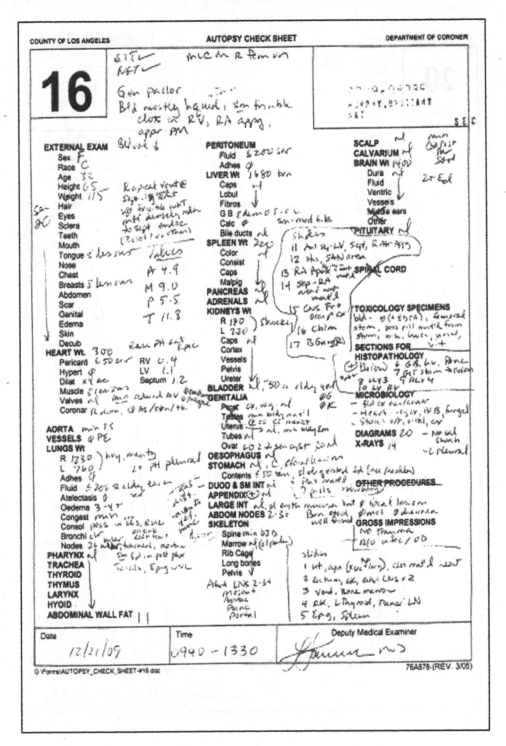

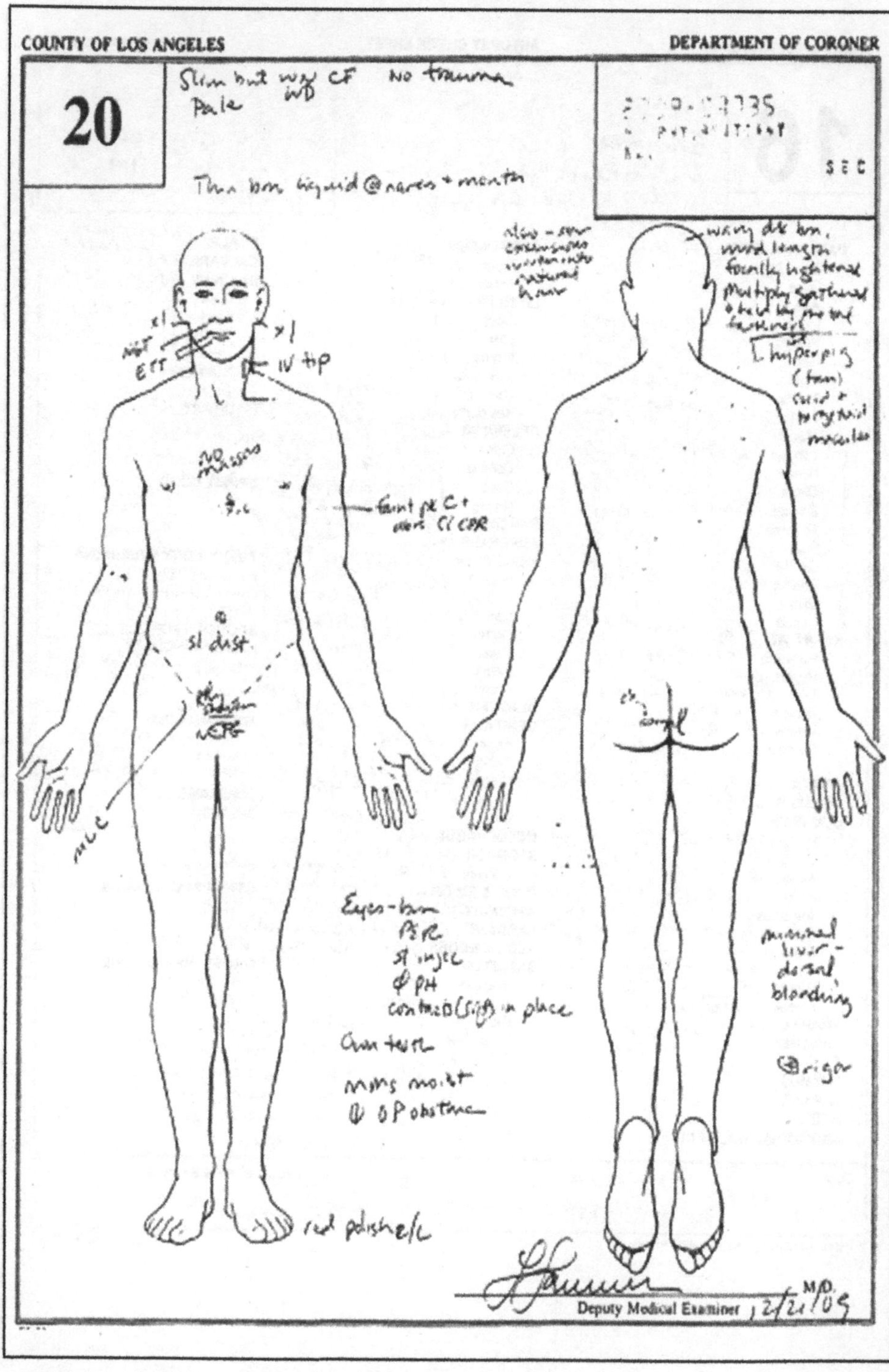
COUNTY OF LOS ANGELES
DEPARTMENT OF CORONER
20
Deputy Medical Examiner
M.D.
2/21/09

COUNTY OF LOS ANGELES   MEDICAL EVIDENCE   DEPARTMENT OF CORONER

3A

CASE #: 2009-08735
DECEDENT'S NAME: MURPHY-MONJACK, BRITTANY
DOD: 12/20/2009
INCOMING MODE:

Page 1 of 1

Drug Name	Rx Number	Date of Issue	Number Issued	Number Remaining	Form	Dosage	Rx Directions	Physician	Pharmacy Phone/ Comments
BIAXIN	1039946	9/17/2007	30	30	TABLET	500MG	2CD	DR. KROOP	RITE AID 323-876-4466
CLARITHROMYCIN	1185602	11/18/2008	14	14	TABLET	500MG	2CC	DR. KROOP	RITE AID 323-876-4466
FLUOXETINE	1271533	11/17/2009	44	27	CAPSULE	20MG	2QAM	DR. KROOP	RITE AID 323-876-4466
HYDROCODONE	0784527	12/9/2009	120	11	TABLET	7.5/750MG	4QID	DR. COHEN	WALGREENS 310-273-2117
KLONOPIN	1271053	12/15/2009	60	18	TABLET	.5MG	18D	DR. KROOP	RITE AID 323-876-4466
METHYLPREDNISOLO NE	1252010	9/10/2009	21	3	TABLET	4MG	N/A	DR. KROOP	RITE AID 323-876-4466
PROPRANOLOL	1233034	9/14/2009	100	97	TABLET	10MG	1QAH	DR. KROOP	RITE AID 323-876-4466
TOPAMAX	1006133	3/18/2007	180	153	TABLET	25MG	10D	DR. COHEN	RITE AID 323-876-4466

Paraphernalia Description

(24) EMPTY PRESCRIPTION MEDICATION BOTTLES FOR THE FOLLOWING MEDICATIONS: PREVACID, CLONAZEPAM, PROPRANOLOL, VICODIN, ZOLPIDEM, CARBAMAZEPINE, KLONOPIN, ATIVAN, AND HYDROCODONE/VICODIN. MISC UNKNOWN VITAMINS.

Investigator: JAMES BLACKLOCK (534037)

Date: 12/21/2009

EVIDENCE LOG (side 1 of 2) Los Angeles County Department of Coroner

2009 - O8735

CC#: 2009 - O8735	Inv. Agency: LAPO - HOLLYWOOD
Decedent: MURPHY-MONJACK, BRITTANY	Agency File #:
Mode: NATURAL	Agency DR #:
HOLD initiated by: ___/___/2009	Inv. Officer/Detective: BERNDT # 23627
on ___/___/2009 HOLD release date: ___/___/2009	

EVIDENCE COLLECTED

Item Description	By	Date	Time
Decedent Clothing (itemized by _____)			
Hair Kit			
Fingernail Kit			
GSR Kit #			
Bullet(s) _____			
Medical Evidence envelopes	BERNDT	12/22/09	1145

RECEIVED INTO EVIDENCE

By	Date	Time

EVIDENCE RELEASED

To	Badge#	Agency	By	Date	Time

(Rev 12/08)

Department of Coroner, County of Los Angeles

FORENSIC SCIENCE LABORATORIES
Laboratory Analysis Summary Report

To: Dr. Scheinin   ☑ PendingTox
Deputy Medical Examiner

The following results have been technically and administratively reviewed and are the opinions and interpretations of the Analyst:

Coroner Case Number: 2009-08735 **Decedent:** MURPHY-MONJACK, BRITTANY ANNE

SPECIMEN	SERVICE	DRUG	LEVEL	UNITS	ANALYST
Blood, Femoral					
	Bases	Chlorpheniramine	0.31	ug/ml	S. DeQuintana
	Bases	Fluoxetine	0.16	ug/ml	S. DeQuintana
	Bases	Norfluoxetine	0.55	ug/ml	S. DeQuintana
	Bases	Propranolol	<0.10	ug/ml	S. DeQuintana
	Benzodiazepines	Chlordiazepoxide	0.37	ug/ml	S. DeQuintana
	Benzodiazepines	Diazepam	<0.10	ug/ml	S. DeQuintana
	Benzodiazepines	Nordiazepam	0.22	ug/ml	S. DeQuintana
	Methamphetamines	Amphetamine	ND		D. Pickar
	Methamphetamines	Methamphetamine	0.09	ug/ml	D. Pickar
	Opiates	Codeine, Free	ND		D. Anderson
	Opiates	Hydrocodone, Free	0.04	ug/ml	D. Anderson
	Opiates	Morphine, Free	ND		D. Anderson
Blood, Heart					
	Acetaminophen	Acetaminophen	63	ug/ml	D. Pickar
	Alcohol	Ethanol	Negative		S. Brooks
	Barbiturates	Barbiturate	ND		J. Linterneat
	Bases	Chlorpheniramine	0.43	ug/ml	S. DeQuintana
	Bases	Dextromethorphan	<0.10	ug/ml	S. DeQuintana
	Bases	Fluoxetine	0.30	ug/ml	S. DeQuintana
	Bases	Hydrocodone	Present		S. DeQuintana
	Bases	Nordiazepam	Present		S. DeQuintana
	Bases	Norfluoxetine	0.89	ug/ml	S. DeQuintana
	Bases	Phenylpropanolamine	Present		S. DeQuintana
	Bases	Propranolol	0.20	ug/ml	S. DeQuintana
	Bases	Zolpidem	ND		S. DeQuintana
	Benzodiazepines	7-Aminoclonazepam	38	ng/ml	S. Brooks
	Benzodiazepines	Chlordiazepoxide	0.26	ug/ml	S. DeQuintana
	Benzodiazepines	Clonazepam	ND		S. Brooks

Date Printed: Tuesday, February 02, 2010   Page 1 of 3

Coroner Case Number: 2009-08735 **Decedent:** MURPHY-MONJACK, BRITTANY ANNE

SPECIMEN	SERVICE	DRUG	LEVEL	UNITS	ANALYST
	Benzodiazepines	Diazepam	0.06	ug/ml	S. DeQuintana
	Benzodiazepines	Lorazepam	14	ng/ml	S. DeQuintana
	Benzodiazepines	Nordiazepam	0.25	ug/ml	S. DeQuintana
	Cocaine	Cocaine and Metabolites	ND		J. Limeroos
	Fentanyl	Fentanyl	ND		J. Limeroos
	Methamphetamine	Amphetamine	ND		O. Plotor
	Methamphetamine	Methamphetamine	0.12	ug/ml	O. Plotor
	Neutrals	Carbamazepine	ND		O. Plotor
	Neutrals	Ibuprofen	20	ug/ml	O. Plotor
	Neutrals	Topiramate	ND		O. Plotor
	Opiates	Codeine, Free	ND		D. Anderson
	Opiates	Hydrocodone, Free	0.66	ug/ml	D. Anderson
	Opiates	Morphine, Free	ND		D. Anderson
	Outside Test	HIV	Done		B. Waters
	Outside Test	Lead	ND		NMS Labs, Inc.
	Outside Test	Methamphetamine	* Done		NMS Labs, Inc.
	Phencyclidine	Phencyclidine	ND		O. Plotor
	Salicylate	Salicylate	54	ug/ml	O. Plotor

Blood, Hospital

	Methamphetamine	Amphetamine	ND		O. Plotor
	Methamphetamine	Methamphetamine	0.11	ug/ml	O. Plotor

Pills

	Medical Evidence	.....	** ND		D. Anderson

Serum, Hospital

	Outside Test	***	Done		Quest Diagnostics

Stomach Contents

	Bases	Chlorpheniramine	<1.0	mg	S. DeQuintana
	Bases	Dextromethorphan	<1.0	mg	S. DeQuintana
	Bases	Fluoxetine	<1.0	mg	S. DeQuintana
	Bases	Phenazopyridine	Present		S. DeQuintana
	Bases	Propranolol	<1.0	mg	S. DeQuintana
	Opiates	Hydrocodone	<1.0	mg	D. Anderson

Urine

	Methamphetamine	Amphetamine	0.36	ug/ml	O. Plotor
	Methamphetamine	Methamphetamine	>2.0	ug/ml	O. Plotor
	Phencyclidine	Phencyclidine	ND		O. Plotor

Coroner Case Number: 2009-08735 **Decedent:** MURPHY-MONJACK, BRITTANY ANNE

SPECIMEN	SERVICE	DRUG	LEVEL	UNITS	ANALYST

NOTE: *The Methamphetamine reported in the Heart Blood was detected as the L-isomer form and does NOT indicate use of an illegal drug.   **No drugs detected in the 0.538g of white pill fragments removed by the Deputy Medical Examiner from the stomach contents.   ***Iron & Iron Binding Capacity performed on Serum, Hospital drawn 12/20/09 @ 1100 hours.   Blood, Hospital drawn 12/20/09 @ 0924 hours.

Legend:

%	of total Hgb	ND	Not Detected
g%	gram percent (g/100ml)	ng/ml	Nanogram per Milliliter
mg	Milligram	ug/g	Microgram per Gram
mg/dL	milligrams per deciliter	ug/ml	Microgram per Milliliter

Administratively reviewed by: Daniel T. Anderson
Supervising Criminalist II
TOXICOLOGY

▲ NMS

NMS Labs

CONFIDENTIAL

3701 Welsh Road, PO Box 433A, Willow Grove, PA 19090-0437
Phone: (215) 657-4900 Fax: (215) 657-2972
e-mail: nms@nmslabs.com
Robert A. Middleberg, PhD, DABFT, DABCC-TC, Laboratory Director

Toxicology Report

Report Issued   12/25/2009 11:00

To: 10139
Los Angeles County Coroner Medical Examiner
Attn: Joseph Muto
1104 N. Mission Road
Los Angeles, CA 90033

Patient Name	DOE, JANE
Patient ID	2009-08735
Chain	11110608
Age	Not Given
Gender	Female
Workorder	09282532

Page 1 of 2

Positive Findings:

None Detected

See Detailed Findings section for additional information

Testing Requested:

Analysis Code	Description
2492B	Lead, Blood

Specimens Received:

ID	Tube/Container	Volume/ Mass	Collection Date/Time	Matrix Source	Miscellaneous Information
001	Clear Vial	1 mL	12/23/2009 06:00	Cardiac Blood	

All sample volumes/weights are approximations.
Specimens received on 12/24/2009

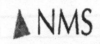

CONFIDENTIAL

Workorder	09282532
Chain	11110608
Patient ID	2009-08735

Page 2 of 2

Detailed Findings:

Examination of the specimen(s) submitted did not reveal any positive findings of toxicological significance by procedures outlined in the accompanying Analysis Summary.

Chain of custody documentation has been maintained for the analyses performed by NMS Labs.

Unless alternate arrangements are made by you, the remainder of the submitted specimens will be discarded six (6) weeks from the date of this report; and generated data will be discarded five (5) years from the date the analyses were performed

Analysis Summary and Reporting Limits:

Acode 24928 - Lead, Blood - Cardiac Blood

-Analysis by Inductively Coupled Plasma/Mass Spectrometry (ICP/MS) for:

Compound	Rpt. Limit	Compound	Rpt. Limit
Lead	1.1 mcg/dL		

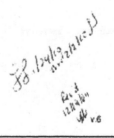

Quest Diagnostics

QUEST DIAGNOSTICS INCORPORATED
CLIENT SERVICE 800.877.7515

SPECIMEN INFORMATION
SPECIMEN: EN6253418
REQUISITION: (8443664)

Hosp #1 Blood - Red Top Serum 12/29/09 1100

COLLECTED: 12/29/2009 12:00 PT
RECEIVED: 12/29/2009 23:23 PT
REPORTED: 12/30/2009 08:14 PT

PATIENT INFORMATION
DOE, JANE

DOB: AGE:
GENDER: FASTING: U

ID: 2009-08735
PHONE:

REPORT STATUS **FINAL**

ORDERING PHYSICIAN

CLIENT INFORMATION
W90033076   TZ24000
EXAMINER OFFICE (CORONER)
FORENSIC LABORATORY
1104 N MISSION RD
LOS ANGELES, CA 90033-1017

Test Name	In Range	Out of Range	Reference Range	Lab
IRON AND TOTAL IRON				EN
BINDING CAPACITY				
IRON, TOTAL		21 L	40-170 mcg/dL	
IRON BINDING CAPACITY		232 L	250-450 mcg/dL	
% SATURATION		9 L	15-50 % (calc)	

PERFORMING LABORATORY INFORMATION

EN QUEST DIAGNOSTICS-WEST HILLS, 8401 FALLBROOK AVENUE, WEST HILLS, CA 91304-3226, Laboratory Director: LEE H. HILBORNE, MD
CLIA: 05D0643827

DOE, JANE - EN6253418   Page 1 - End of Report

▲ **NMS**

NMS Labs

CONFIDENTIAL

3701 Welsh Road, PO Box 433A, Willow Grove, PA 19090-0437
Phone: (215) 657-4900 Fax: (215) 657-2972
e-mail: nms@nmslabs.com
Robert A. Middleberg, PhD, DABFT, DABCC-TC, Laboratory Director

Toxicology Report

Report Issued 02/02/2010 11:00

To: 10139
Los Angeles County Coroner Medical Examiner
Attn: Joseph Muto
1104 N. Mission Road
Los Angeles, CA 90033

Patient Name	DOE, JANE
Patient ID	2009-08735
Chain	11110641
Age	Not Given
Gender	Not Given
Workorder	10021586

Page 1 of 2

Positive Findings:

Compound	Result	Units	Matrix Source
D/L Methamphetamine Ratio	BEE COMMENT		Cardiac Blood

See Detailed Findings section for additional information

Testing Requested:

Analysis Code	Description
0329B	Amphetamines (D/L Ratio), Blood

Specimens Received:

ID	Tube/Container	Volume/ Mass	Collection Date/Time	Matrix Source	Miscellaneous Information
001	Clear Vial	3.5 mL	01/27/2010 08:00	Cardiac Blood	

All sample volumes/weights are approximations.

Specimens received on 01/28/2010.

▲NMS

CONFIDENTIAL

Workorder	10021586
Chain	11110641
Patient ID	2009-08735

Page 2 of 2

Detailed Findings:

Analysis and Comments	Result	Units	Rpt. Limit	Specimen Source	Analysis By
D/L Methamphetamine Ratio	SEE COMMENT			001 - Cardiac Blood	GC/MS

Present in I-form only.

Other than the above findings, examination of the specimen(s) submitted did not reveal any positive findings of toxicological significance by procedures outlined in the accompanying Analysis Summary.

Reference Comments:

1. D/L Methamphetamine Ratio - Cardiac Blood:

    If the D/L Methamphetamine ratio is greater than 0.13, the Methamphetamine found is probably the result of the use of the DEA Schedule II CNS stimulant (d-methamphetamine).

Chain of custody documentation has been maintained for the analyses performed by NMS Labs.

Unless alternate arrangements are made by you, the remainder of the submitted specimens will be discarded six (6) weeks from the date of this report; and generated data will be discarded five (5) years from the date the analyses were performed.

Workorder 10021586 was electronically signed on 02/02/2010 10:43 by:

Laura M. Labay, Ph.D., DABFT
Forensic Toxicologist

Analysis Summary and Reporting Limits:

Acode 03296 - Amphetamines (D/L Ratio), Blood - Cardiac Blood

-Analysis by Gas Chromatography/Mass Spectrometry (GC/MS) for:

Compound	Rpt. Limit	Compound	Rpt. Limit
D/L Amphetamine Ratio	N/A	D/L Methamphetamine Ratio	N/A

CASE REPORT

COUNTY OF LOS ANGELES

DEPARTMENT OF CORONER

1

APPARENT MODE
NATURAL

CASE NO
2009-08735

SPECIAL CIRCUMSTANCES
Celebrity, Media Interest

CHART
SEC

LAST FIRST MIDDLE
MURPHY-MONJACK, BRITTANY ANNE

AKA: 0

ADDRESS

CITY

STATE

ZIP

SEX	RACE APPEARS	DOB	AGE	HGT	WGT	EYES	HAIR	TEETH	FACIAL HAIR NONE	ID NUM	CONDITION
FEMALE	CAUCASIAN	11/08/1977	32	63 in	115 lbs	BROWN	BROWN	ALL NATURAL TEETH		Yes	FAIR

MARK TYPE   MARK LOCATION   MARK DESCRIPTION

NOK

ADDRESS

CITY

STATE

ZIP

RELATIONSHIP
HUSBAND

PHONE

NOTIFIED BY
BY HOSPITAL PERSONNEL

DATE
12/20/2009

TIME
10:15

SEX

D.L. ID

STATE
CA

VIEWED BY

O METHOD
CALIFORNIA DRIVER'S LICENSE

LIC #

MARK #

DL #

SID #

MILITARY #

FBI #

CERTIFIED BY NAME/PRINT
PHOTO COMPARISON W/CDL

RELATIONSHIP

PHONE

DATE
12/20/2009

TIME

PLACE OF DEATH / PLACE FOUND
HOSPITAL
CEDARS-SINAI MEDICAL CENTER

ADDRESS OR LOCATION
8700 BEVERLY BLVD.

CITY
LOS ANGELES

ZIP
90048

PLACE OF INJURY

AT WORK
No

DATE

TIME

LOCATION/OR ADDRESS

ZIP

DOD
12/20/2009

TIME
10:05

FOUND OR PRONOUNCED BY
DR. CASEY

OTHER AGENCY INV. OFFICER
LAPD HOLLYWOOD - DET. BERNDT #23627

PHONE
(213) 972-2910

REPORT NO

NOTIFIED BY

ID

TRANSPORTED BY
JULIE M. BISHOP

TO
LOS ANGELES FSC

DATE
12/20/2009

TIME
14:45

FINGERPRINTED	Yes	CLOTHING	Yes	PAINT	No	MORTUARY	
VISD EV	Yes	INVEST PHOTO #	25	BOX TYPE	NOT SEALED	HOSP RPT	Yes
PHYS EV	No	EVIDENCE LIST	Yes	PROPERTY	No	HOSP CHART	Yes
SUICIDE NOTE	No	OSB NO		RPT NO	244723	FF NO	000081802

SYNOPSIS
THE DECEDENT IS A 32-YEAR-OLD WHITE FEMALE WHO WAS DISCOVERED UNRESPONSIVE IN HER BATHROOM BY FAMILY MEMBERS ON 12/20/09. 911 WAS CALLED AND THE DECEDENT WAS TRANSPORTED TO CEDARS-SINAI MEDICAL CENTER WHERE SHE WAS PRONOUNCED DEAD AT 1005 HOURS BY DR. CASEY. THE DECEDENT HAD A MEDICAL HISTORY OF HYPOGLYCEMIA AND MORE RECENTLY COMPLAINTS OF SHORTNESS OF BREATH AND ABDOMINAL PAINS. NO OBVIOUS SIGNS OF EXTERNAL TRAUMA WERE NOTED AND FOUL PLAY IS NOT SUSPECTED

JAMES BLACKLOCK
530357

DATE
12/20/2009

TIME
21:34

REVIEWED BY

DATE
12/26/09

INVESTIGATOR

FORM #3 NARRATIVE TO FOLLOW? ☑

County of Los Angeles, Department of Coroner
Investigator's Narrative

Case Number: 2009-08736   Decedent: MURPHY-MONJACK, BRITTANY ANNE

Information Sources:

1. Medical Records –   Cedars-Sinai Medical Center, 8700 Beverly
   Boulevard, Los Angeles, CA 90048.

2. Detective Berndt #23627, Los Angeles Police Department – Hollywood Homicide Bureau,
   (213) 972-2910.

3.   . Decedent's husband,

Investigation:

On 12/20/09 at 1117 hours, Registered Nurse Dallas Pofenroth of the Cedars-Sinai Medical
Center called to report this apparent natural death to Sandra Espinoza. Acting Supervisor Selena
Barros assigned me this death to investigate at 1230 hours. I responded from the Forensic
Science Center and conducted an investigation at the hospital and subsequently at the
decedent's residence. I concluded my investigation and departed the scene at 1710 hours.
Forensic Attendants Julie Bishop and Ramiro Gonzalez transported the decedent to the Forensic
Science Center on 12/20/09 at 1445 hours.

Location:

Location of Incidence: Residence

Location of Death: Cedars-Sinai Medical Center, 8700 Beverly Boulevard, Los Angeles, CA
90048.

Informant/Witness Statements:

Upon my arrival at Cedar-Sinai Medical Center I made contact with hospital staff and obtained the
decedent's medical records and admission blood. According to the provided medical records, on
12/20/09 at 0800 hours Los Angeles City Fire Department personnel were dispatched the location
of incidence on report of an unresponsive female. Upon arrival, RA 41 paramedics found the
decedent in her residence bathroom without signs of life. ALS was initiated and the decedent
was transported to the hospital via rescue ambulance. The decedent presented to the
emergency room at approximately 0838 hours in full cardiac arrest. Despite all attempts to
resuscitate the decedent by the emergency room staff, the decedent was pronounced dead at
1005 hours by Dr. Casey. The decedent had a reported medical history of diabetes. A cause of
death was not noted.

I responded to the decedent's residence and made contact with Detective Berndt and she related
the following statement. On 12/20/09 Los Angeles Police Department detectives were dispatched
to the location of incidence regarding a death investigation. Contact was made with the
decedent's husband,   , and her mother.   They advised that on
12/20/09 the decedent had been complaining of shortness of breath and severe abdominal pain.
At approximately 0730 hours the decedent walked in to her bathroom and closed the door. After
approximately 30 minutes the decedent's mother went in to the bathroom and discovered the
decedent lying on the floor unresponsive. She yelled for help and the decedent's husband
entered the bathroom. She called 911 and the decedent's husband attempted to revive the
decedent by placing her in the shower and running the water. The decedent remained
unresponsive and purged her stomach contents prior to the arrival of paramedics. They were
later advised by hospital staff of the decedent's death. The decedent had a medical history of
hypoglycemia and more recently complaints of shortness of breath and abdominal pain. Based
on the initial police investigation, foul play is not suspected.

I made contact with the decedent's husband,   , while at the scene and he related
the following statement. On 12/20/09 at approximately 0730 hours the decedent complained of
severe abdominal pain and went to the bathroom. He remained in bed until he heard the

Notorious B.I.G.

Given Name: Christopher George Latore Wallace
Born: May 21, 1972, Brooklyn, New York
Died: March 9, 1997, Los Angeles, California
Cause of Death: Shooting

Christopher Wallace had a short recording career. Before his death, he released just one rap album, *Ready to Die*. That record became one of the most influential rap albums of all time. His music caused a resurgence of the East Coast rap scene. Modern rappers list Notorious B.I.G (a.k.a. Biggie Smalls) as one of the greatest MCs of all time. Before the release of his second album, he was shot in a drive by shooting in Los Angeles. Some believe his murder was a result of his ongoing feud with Tupac Shakur, but the murder remains unsolved. His posthumous album sold ten million copies and was the highest selling rap album ever at the time. The 2009 movie *Notorious* was based on his life. His autopsy was released to the public in 2012, fifteen years after his death.

1

COUNTY OF LOS ANGELES

CASE REPORT MAR 10 1997

DEPARTMENT OF CORONER

CASE NO. 97-01812

APPARENT MODE: NAT ACC SUI [HOMI]

☐ STATE HOSP   ☐ O.I.S.   ☐ AUTOPSY WAIVER   ☐ CLOSELY WATCHED   ☐ DOMESTIC VIOLENCE
☐ IN CUSTODY   ☐ AT WORK   ☐ LAW ENFORCEMENT RELATED   ☒ VICTIMS OF CRIME   ☒ GANG RELATED

SPECIAL CIRCUMSTANCES: DRIVE-BY

MULTIPLE GSW's

CRYPT: 111

LAST, FIRST, MIDDLE: WALLACE, CHRISTOPHER GEORGE LATORE

AKA:

☐ JOHN   ☐ JANE   ☐ UND   N/A

ADDRESS: 5 ELLIOT COURT   CITY: TEANECK, N.J.   STATE   ZIP

SEX	RACE APPEARS	DOB	AGE	HGT	WGT	EYES	HAIR	TEETH	ID VIEW	CONDITION	☐ EMBALMED
M	B	5-21-72	24	74	395	BRO	BLK	OWN	(YES) NO	VIEWABLE	

BEARD ☐Y ☒N
MUSTACHE ☒Y ☐N (VERY SPARSE)
UNSHAVEN ☐Y ☒N

SCARS (DESCRIBE)

MARKS

TATTOOS (DESCRIBE): ®INSIDE FOREARM

AMPUTATIONS

PIERCINGS: "THE LORD IS MY LIGHT AND MY SALVATION..."

DEFORMITIES

NOK   ADDRESS   CITY   STATE   #BXL-127   A-7112

RELATIONSHIP   PHONE   NOTIFIED BY ☒YES ☐NO   PRESENT @ HOSP.   DATE   TIME

SSN   MULT. ☐   DL ID NONE   STATE   PENDING BY: N/A

ID BY: ☒VISUAL (SEE BELOW)   ☐ LAPD PRINTS   ☐ DOJ PRINTS
☐ FAMILY @ HOSPITAL   ☐ LASD PRINTS   ☐ CAL ID PRINTS
☐ DL/ID   ☐ FBI PRINTS

By WIFE & MOTHER   NCIC PRINT CLASS √-310-...

A #   MAIN #   CII #   FBI # 774795MA6   MILITARY #   POB: NY

NAME (PRINT)   SIGNATURE   RELATIONSHIP   PHONE

I HAVE PERSONALLY SEEN THE DECEASED OR A PHOTOGRAPH AND CONFIRM THE IDENTIFICATION

PLACE OF DEATH/PLACE FOUND   ADDRESS OR LOCATION   CITY   ZIP

CEDARS-SINAI MEDICAL CENTER
8700 BEVERLY BLVD., LA 90048

PLACE OF INJURY: VEHICLE   AT WORK ☐YES ☒NO   DATE 3.9.97   TIME 0030   LOCATION OR ADDRESS: N/B FAIRFAX @ WILSHIRE   LOS ANGELES, CA 90048

DOD 3-9-97   ROD   TIME 0115   FOUND BY (PRON. BY) DR. PAUL SILKA

OTHER AGENCY & INV. OFFICER: LAPD/WILSHIRE DET.'S SCOTT & COOPER   PHONE   REPORT NO.   NOTIFIED BY   NO

TRANSPORTED BY: CARLOS GARCIA / GREG MYERS

TO: FSC ☒   AVRO ☐   SCVRO ☐   DATE 3-9-97   TIME 0830

	YES	NO		YES	NO	PA RPT ☐ YES ☐ NO
PRINTS	☒	☐	CLOTHING	☐	☒	MEC SEAL PA SEAL (NOT SEALED) MORTUARY
MED. EV.	☐	☒	INVEST. PHOTO #	☐	☐	HOSP. RPT. YES ☒ NO ☐
PHYS. EV.	☒	☐	EVIDENCE LOG	☐	☐	PROP: YES ☐ NO ☒
SUICIDE NOTE	☐	☒	GSR NO A9117			RCPT. NO. 144609 HOSP. CHART YES ☒ NO ☐ PF NO. 966265

SYNOPSIS: PER DET. FELIX AND FAMILY, DECEDENT WAS A PASSEN-
GER, ® FRONT SEAT OF A SUBURBAN TRAV. N/B FAIRFAX,
DRIVEN BY DEC'DS COUSIN DAMION BUTLER. THE VEH STOPPED
AT THE LIGHT AT THE I/S WITH WILSHIRE BLVD. AND AN UNK
VEH DROVE UP ON THE ® SIDE AND OPENED FIRE. DEC'D
WAS IMMEDIATELY DRIVEN TO HOSPITAL AND LATER PRONOUNCED.

Cheryl L. Godman #411487   INVESTIGATOR   DATE 3-9-97   TIME   REVIEWED BY   DATE   TIME

FORM #3 NARRATIVE TO FOLLOW? ☐ YES ☒ NO

FORENSIC SCIENCE CENTER
COUNTY OF LOS ANGELES

GSR DATA SHEET

DEPARTMENT OF CORONER

82

☐ Accident
☒ Homicide
☐ Suicide
☐ Questionable Accident/Homicide
☐ Questionable Accident/Suicide
☐ Questionable Suicide/Homicide
☐ Investigator Requests Rush

Kit #

A·9117

97-01812
WALLACE,CHRISTOPHER

HOMICIDE   111
LAPD/WILSHIRE

INFORMATION ABOUT DECEDENT/SHOOTING

☐ Right Handed   ☐ Left Handed   ☒ Unknown   ☒ Male ☐ Female

Occupation _____ ☒ Unknown

Activity Prior to Shooting *RIDING IN FT PASS SEAT OF VEH*

Have the decedent's hands been touched by anyone prior to taking the GSR sample? ☒ Yes ☐ No ☐ Unknown
If yes, by whom? ☐ Paramedics   ☐ Family   ☐ Police   ☒ Hospital Personnel
☐ Other _____

Was the weapon found in the decedent's hand?   ☐ Yes ☒ No ☐ Unknown – Moved prior arrival
If yes, which one? ☐ Right   ☐ Left
If no, describe weapon's location in relationship to decedent _____

Shooting Occurred: ☐ Indoors   ☒ Outdoors   ☐ Unknown *FROM VEH*

Location of Body: ☐ Indoors   ☐ Outdoors   ☐ Automobile   ☒ Hospital
Other _____

Number of Shots Fired: *MULTIPLE*

Date *3-9-97* and Time *0030* of Shooting

Date *3·9·97* and Time *0900* GSR samples were taken.

GSR evidence collected ☐ At Scene ☒ At FSC ☐ At Hospital
☐ Other _____ By: *CARLOS GARCIA #233798*

Body transported to FSC via ☒ Coroner ☐ Contractor _____

FIREARM

☐ Revolver   ☐ Semi-automatic/automatic   ☐ Rifle   ☐ Shotgun

☐ Other _____

Make/Model _____ Caliber _____

AMMUNITION

Brand of Ammunition _____ Caliber of Ammunition _____

Bullet Configuration: ☐ Round Nose   ☐ Hollow Point   ☐ Wad Cutter   ☐ Pointed

Other _____

Bullet Surface: ☐ Jacketed   ☐ Semi-jacketed   ☐ Bare Lead   ☐ Plated

Comments: _____

_____ *3-9-97*
Investigator   Date

————— Do not write below this line —————

RESULTS:

White: Medical file
Pink: Laboratory Copy
Yellow: Laboratory Copy

76GR (Rev 1/93) P1/93

COUNTY OF LOS ANGELES

DEPARTMENT OF CORONER

12

AUTOPSY REPORT

I performed an autopsy on the body of

at _____

the DEPARTMENT OF CORONER

No.

97-01812

WALLACE, CHRISTOPHER

Los Angeles, California _____ on **MARCH 10, 1997 @ 1030 HOURS**
(Date) (Time)

From the anatomic findings and pertinent history I ascribe the death to:

(A) GUNSHOT WOUND TO ABDOMEN-CHEST
DUE TO, OR AS A CONSEQUENCE OF

(B) _____
DUE TO, OR AS A CONSEQUENCE OF

(C) _____
DUE TO, OR AS A CONSEQUENCE OF

(D) _____
OTHER CONDITIONS CONTRIBUTING BUT NOT RELATED TO THE IMMEDIATE CAUSE OF DEATH
MULTIPLE NONFATAL GUNSHOT WOUNDS

Anatomical Summary:

I. Multiple gunshot wounds.

    A. Gunshot wound #1 to left forearm, penetrating, nonfatal; soft tissue injury only; bullet recovered.

    B. Gunshot wound #2 to soft tissue of back, perforating, nonfatal; no projectile recovered.

    C. Gunshot wound #3 to soft tissue of left thigh, perforating; superficial laceration of scrotum; nonfatal, no projectile recovered.

    D. Gunshot wound #4 to abdomen-chest, penetrating, fatal; perforating injuries to ascending colon, liver, right hemidiaphragm, pericardium, heart and upper lobe of left lung; bullet recovered from anterior left shoulder area.

II. Other findings.

    A. Morbid obesity (395 pounds).

        1. Cardiomegaly (660 grams) with biventricular hypertrophy.

        2. Hepatosplenomegaly (liver 2280 grams, spleen 260 grams).

        3. Thyroidomegaly (120 grams).

76A890M--Rev 8/94

COUNTY OF LOS ANGELES

12

Page ___2___

AUTOPSY REPORT

No.

97-01812

WALLACE, CHRISTOPHER

DEPARTMENT OF CORONER

B. Pulmonary edema, moderate.

C. Cerebral edema, mild to moderate.

D. Cholelithiasis (cholesterol type stones).

E. Status post left femoral fracture with placement of orthopedic rod, remote.

F. Status post emergent medical and surgical intervention.

    1. Clinical history of hemothorax and hemopericardium.

III. See Toxicology report.

CIRCUMSTANCES:

The following information is obtained from Coroner's Forms 1 and 18 as well as medical records. This 24-year-old male was a passenger in a vehicle when he was shot in a drive-by incident at approximately 0030 hours on 3-9-97. He was taken to Cedars-Sinai Hospital, arriving in the emergency room at approximately 0048 hours in full arrest and with agonal rhythm. An emergency thoracotomy revealed a large amount of blood and in the chest and in the pericardium, all of which was evacuated. Intracardiac massage and internal defibrillations were performed, with no response, and he was officially pronounced dead at 0115 hours.

Medical records indicate that a bullet was found at the hospital when the body was turned over after pronouncement of death; according to records, this was given to the police. According to LAPD Wilshire Division Detectives Chavez and Balderrama, two bullets were recovered from the hospital, each of which was found on the gurney on which the decedent was lying. The same detectives also reported to the examiner that the bullets passed through a car door before striking the decedent.

EVIDENCE OF INJURY:

The gunshot wounds are arbitrarily numbered for the convenience of the examiner and do not indicate a sequence of injury. No

76A798P—Rev 2/91

COUNTY OF LOS ANGELES

AUTOPSY REPORT

DEPARTMENT OF CORONER

12

Page ___3___

No.

97-01812

WALLACE, CHRISTOPHER

soot or stippling is noted in association with any of the entrance gunshot wounds.

Gunshot wound #1:

The entrance wound is located on the dorsal left forearm close to the olecranon process (point of the elbow), 14-1/4 inches from the apex of the shoulder and 5/8 inch distal to the olecranon process. The slightly irregular, ovoid defect measures 15/16 x 1/4 inch and is abraded on all but its most distal aspect. Abrasion rim is largest proximally (3/16 inch maximal width) and at the ulnar aspect (1/4 inch maximal width).

The projectile follows a proximal to distal, slightly dorsal to volar and minimally radial trajectory through the soft tissue of the forearm, passing through soft tissue and muscle. There is no evident fracture of the ulna. The projectile comes to rest approximately 10-1/2 inches distal to the entrance defect in the ulnar aspect of the distal forearm close to the wrist. The projectile is located volar to the ulna. The track is explored and/or probed from beginning to end, showing a mild to moderate amount of hemorrhage along it. There is no evident injury to the ulnar artery.

The bullet is recovered from the above location at 1058 hours. It is a medium caliber lead bullet with a full copper jacket open at the base. The bullet appears slightly compressed. The base is marked with "LS" for identification purposes, and it is placed into evidence envelope #1. A small piece of dark fabric, present at the edge of the entrance wound, is recovered and placed in the same evidence envelope.

This is a nonfatal wound since it involves only injury to soft tissue and muscle, with no major vascular involvement.

Gunshot wound #2:

The entry wound is located on the back, 20-3/8 inches from the top of the head and 3-1/2 inches left of midline. The ovoid defect measures 1/4 x 5/16 inch and is abraded on inferior-medial aspect only, to a maximal width of 5/16 inch. The projectile follows a back to front, right to left and upward

76A798P—Rev 2/91

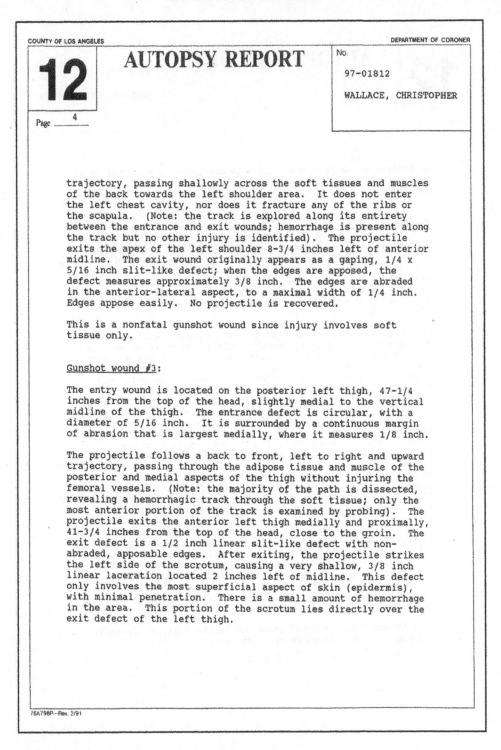

COUNTY OF LOS ANGELES

DEPARTMENT OF CORONER

AUTOPSY REPORT

12

Page ___4___

No.

97-01812

WALLACE, CHRISTOPHER

trajectory, passing shallowly across the soft tissues and muscles of the back towards the left shoulder area. It does not enter the left chest cavity, nor does it fracture any of the ribs or the scapula. (Note: the track is explored along its entirety between the entrance and exit wounds; hemorrhage is present along the track but no other injury is identified). The projectile exits the apex of the left shoulder 8-3/4 inches left of anterior midline. The exit wound originally appears as a gaping, 1/4 x 5/16 inch slit-like defect; when the edges are apposed, the defect measures approximately 3/8 inch. The edges are abraded in the anterior-lateral aspect, to a maximal width of 1/4 inch. Edges appose easily. No projectile is recovered.

This is a nonfatal gunshot wound since injury involves soft tissue only.

Gunshot wound #3:

The entry wound is located on the posterior left thigh, 47-1/4 inches from the top of the head, slightly medial to the vertical midline of the thigh. The entrance defect is circular, with a diameter of 5/16 inch. It is surrounded by a continuous margin of abrasion that is largest medially, where it measures 1/8 inch.

The projectile follows a back to front, left to right and upward trajectory, passing through the adipose tissue and muscle of the posterior and medial aspects of the thigh without injuring the femoral vessels. (Note: the majority of the path is dissected, revealing a hemorrhagic track through the soft tissue; only the most anterior portion of the track is examined by probing). The projectile exits the anterior left thigh medially and proximally, 41-3/4 inches from the top of the head, close to the groin. The exit defect is a 1/2 inch linear slit-like defect with non-abraded, apposable edges. After exiting, the projectile strikes the left side of the scrotum, causing a very shallow, 3/8 inch linear laceration located 2 inches left of midline. This defect only involves the most superficial aspect of skin (epidermis), with minimal penetration. There is a small amount of hemorrhage in the area. This portion of the scrotum lies directly over the exit defect of the left thigh.

76A798P—Rev. 2/91

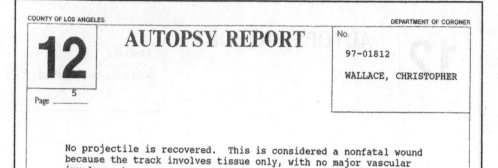

COUNTY OF LOS ANGELES

AUTOPSY REPORT

12

Page ___5___

DEPARTMENT OF CORONER

No.
97-01812

WALLACE, CHRISTOPHER

No projectile is recovered. This is considered a nonfatal wound because the track involves tissue only, with no major vascular involvement.

<u>Gunshot wound #4</u>:

The entrance wound is located on the anterolateral right hip, 30 inches from the top of the head and 12 inches right of anterior midline. It is a slightly irregular, ovoid defect measuring 1/2 x 5/16 inch. It is surrounded by a continuous, slightly irregular margin of abrasion that is minimal posteriorly and largest in the anterior-inferior aspect, where it has a maximal width of 1/4 inch.

The projectile follows a right to left, slightly back to front and upward trajectory through the abdomen and chest areas. It initially passes through the soft tissue of the right hip area, with no injury to the pelvis, entering the peritoneum in the right lower quadrant. It perforates the ascending colon and the liver, entering the liver inferiorly and exiting it superiorly. It then perforates the right hemidiaphragm and the overlying basilar pericardium. It perforates the heart, entering it at the right atrium near the inferior vena cava, perforating the ventricular septum in the subvalvular area, then exiting the anterior left ventricular wall. The projectile then re-perforates the pericardium and perforates the medial aspect of the upper lobe of the left lung. It then exits the left chest cavity anteriorly by passing through the 3rd rib, which is fractured. It then perforates the soft tissue and muscle of the left pectoral area, passing through the axillary area to come to rest subcutaneously in the anterior left shoulder area.

The projectile is recovered in the anterior left shoulder area, 14-1/4 inches from the top of the head and 9-3/4 inches left of midline, with the subcutaneous adipose tissue, at 1150 hours. It is a medium caliber lead bullet with a full copper jacket that remains open at the base. The bullet appears deformed (flattened) at the nose. The base is marked "LS" for identification purposes, and the bullet is placed into evidence envelope #2.

This is considered a fatal wound due to the multiple visceral injuries (colon, liver, heart, left lung).

76A798P—Rev. 2/91

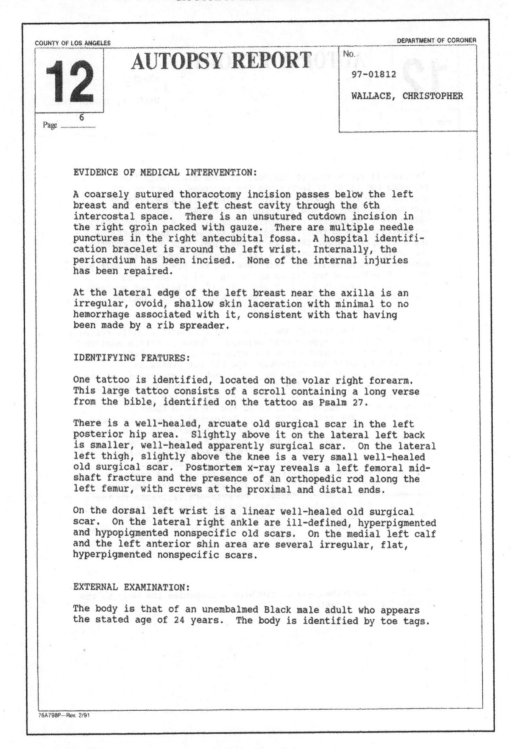

COUNTY OF LOS ANGELES

DEPARTMENT OF CORONER

AUTOPSY REPORT

12

Page 6

No.

97-01812

WALLACE, CHRISTOPHER

EVIDENCE OF MEDICAL INTERVENTION:

A coarsely sutured thoracotomy incision passes below the left breast and enters the left chest cavity through the 6th intercostal space. There is an unsutured cutdown incision in the right groin packed with gauze. There are multiple needle punctures in the right antecubital fossa. A hospital identification bracelet is around the left wrist. Internally, the pericardium has been incised. None of the internal injuries has been repaired.

At the lateral edge of the left breast near the axilla is an irregular, ovoid, shallow skin laceration with minimal to no hemorrhage associated with it, consistent with that having been made by a rib spreader.

IDENTIFYING FEATURES:

One tattoo is identified, located on the volar right forearm. This large tattoo consists of a scroll containing a long verse from the bible, identified on the tattoo as Psalm 27.

There is a well-healed, arcuate old surgical scar in the left posterior hip area. Slightly above it on the lateral left back is smaller, well-healed apparently surgical scar. On the lateral left thigh, slightly above the knee is a very small well-healed old surgical scar. Postmortem x-ray reveals a left femoral mid-shaft fracture and the presence of an orthopedic rod along the left femur, with screws at the proximal and distal ends.

On the dorsal left wrist is a linear well-healed old surgical scar. On the lateral right ankle are ill-defined, hyperpigmented and hypopigmented nonspecific old scars. On the medial left calf and the left anterior shin area are several irregular, flat, hyperpigmented nonspecific scars.

EXTERNAL EXAMINATION:

The body is that of an unembalmed Black male adult who appears the stated age of 24 years. The body is identified by toe tags.

76A798P—Rev. 2/91

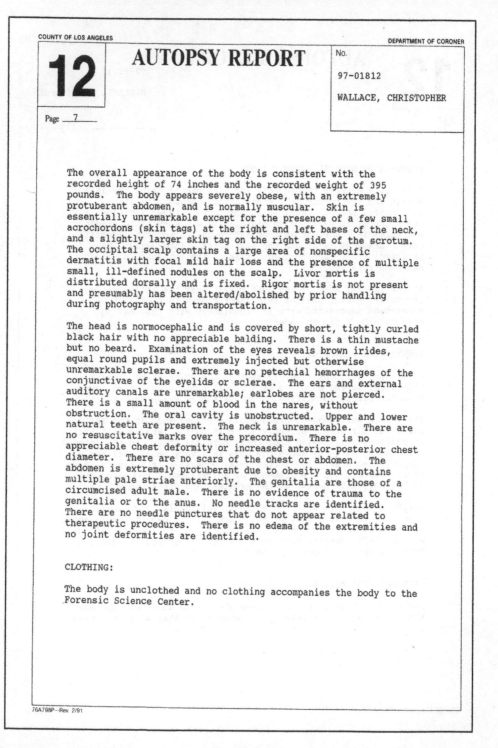

COUNTY OF LOS ANGELES

AUTOPSY REPORT

12

Page 7

DEPARTMENT OF CORONER

No.

97-01812

WALLACE, CHRISTOPHER

The overall appearance of the body is consistent with the recorded height of 74 inches and the recorded weight of 395 pounds. The body appears severely obese, with an extremely protuberant abdomen, and is normally muscular. Skin is essentially unremarkable except for the presence of a few small acrochordons (skin tags) at the right and left bases of the neck, and a slightly larger skin tag on the right side of the scrotum. The occipital scalp contains a large area of nonspecific dermatitis with focal mild hair loss and the presence of multiple small, ill-defined nodules on the scalp. Livor mortis is distributed dorsally and is fixed. Rigor mortis is not present and presumably has been altered/abolished by prior handling during photography and transportation.

The head is normocephalic and is covered by short, tightly curled black hair with no appreciable balding. There is a thin mustache but no beard. Examination of the eyes reveals brown irides, equal round pupils and extremely injected but otherwise unremarkable sclerae. There are no petechial hemorrhages of the conjunctivae of the eyelids or sclerae. The ears and external auditory canals are unremarkable; earlobes are not pierced. There is a small amount of blood in the nares, without obstruction. The oral cavity is unobstructed. Upper and lower natural teeth are present. The neck is unremarkable. There are no resuscitative marks over the precordium. There is no appreciable chest deformity or increased anterior-posterior chest diameter. There are no scars of the chest or abdomen. The abdomen is extremely protuberant due to obesity and contains multiple pale striae anteriorly. The genitalia are those of a circumcised adult male. There is no evidence of trauma to the genitalia or to the anus. No needle tracks are identified. There are no needle punctures that do not appear related to therapeutic procedures. There is no edema of the extremities and no joint deformities are identified.

CLOTHING:

The body is unclothed and no clothing accompanies the body to the Forensic Science Center.

76A798P—Rev. 2/91

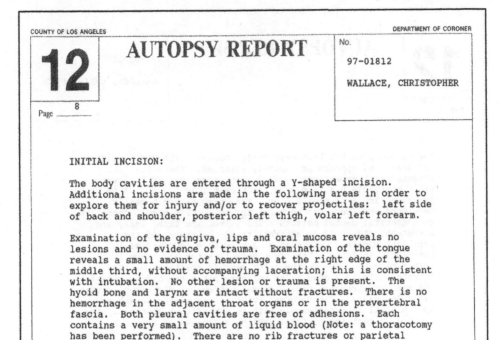

COUNTY OF LOS ANGELES

DEPARTMENT OF CORONER

12

AUTOPSY REPORT

No.

97-01812

WALLACE, CHRISTOPHER

Page   8

INITIAL INCISION:

The body cavities are entered through a Y-shaped incision.
Additional incisions are made in the following areas in order to
explore them for injury and/or to recover projectiles: left side
of back and shoulder, posterior left thigh, volar left forearm.

Examination of the gingiva, lips and oral mucosa reveals no
lesions and no evidence of trauma. Examination of the tongue
reveals a small amount of hemorrhage at the right edge of the
middle third, without accompanying laceration; this is consistent
with intubation. No other lesion or trauma is present. The
hyoid bone and larynx are intact without fractures. There is no
hemorrhage in the adjacent throat organs or in the prevertebral
fascia. Both pleural cavities are free of adhesions. Each
contains a very small amount of liquid blood (Note: a thoracotomy
has been performed). There are no rib fractures or parietal
pleural defects other than those previously described in
association with the gunshot injury and the therapeutic
thoracotomy. There is no evidence of pneumothorax. The lungs
appear fairly well expanded. Soft tissues of the thoracic and
abdominal walls are well-preserved. The organs of the abdominal
cavity have a normal arrangement. None is absent. There is a
small amount of blood in the abdominal cavity (visually estimated
at no greater than 50 cc, liquid with small clots). There is no
evidence of peritonitis and there are no peritoneal adhesions.

SYSTEMIC AND ORGAN REVIEW

The following observations are limited to findings other than the
injuries and/or changes described above.

CARDIOVASCULAR SYSTEM:

The aorta is elastic and of even caliber throughout with vessels
distributed normally from it. No aneurysms are present. The
intimal surface shows moderate fatty streaking and mild diffuse
hemoglobin staining, the latter consistent with very early
decompositional change.

76A798P—Rev 2/91

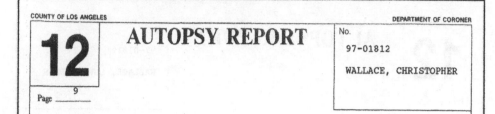

12

AUTOPSY REPORT

No.

97-01812

WALLACE, CHRISTOPHER

Page ___ 9

The pericardium has been previously incised. The heart weighs 660 grams and appears prominently enlarged. There is biventricular hypertrophy. Wall thicknesses are as follows: right ventricle 0.4 to 0.6 cm, left ventricle 1.7 to 2.1 cm, interventricular septum 2.0 cm. The chambers are normally developed and there are no mural thrombi within them. There are no congenital septal defects. The valves are thin, leafy and competent. There is no abnormality of the apices of the papillary muscles. There is no appreciable endocardial hemoglobin staining. The great vessels enter and leave in a normal fashion. The ductus arteriosus is obliterated. The foramen ovale is closed. The coronary ostia are widely patent. The coronary arteries have a normal pattern of distribution with right dominance. The coronary arteries are widely patent and show minimal atherosclerosis with no significant stenosis. The myocardium contains no focal lesions exclusive of trauma.

RESPIRATORY SYSTEM:

There is no edema of the larynx and there are no fractures of the laryngeal cartilages. The posterior pharynx contains moderately prominent pharyngeal tonsils bilaterally. There is no blood or other material within the trachea or major bronchi. The mucosal surfaces of the respiratory passages are intact and unremarkable. The right lung weighs 690 grams and the left lung weighs 600 grams. Both are subcrepitant. Visceral pleurae are smooth and intact (exclusive of the gunshot injuries on the left). Sectioning reveals moderate edema and congestion bilaterally. There is no evidence of consolidation and there are no focal lesions exclusive of trauma. There is no evidence of thrombo-embolism within the pulmonary vasculature.

GASTROINTESTINAL SYSTEM:

The esophagus is intact throughout and is grossly unremarkable. The stomach is not distended. It contains up to 50 cc of thin, green-brown liquid. No residual medication or capsular material is identified. The gastric mucosa is unremarkable. The small intestine and colon are unremarkable on external and in-situ examination (exclusive of the gunshot injury to the ascending colon, previously described). The small intestine and colon are opened along their entire length and are unremarkable throughout.

76A798P—Rev. 2/91

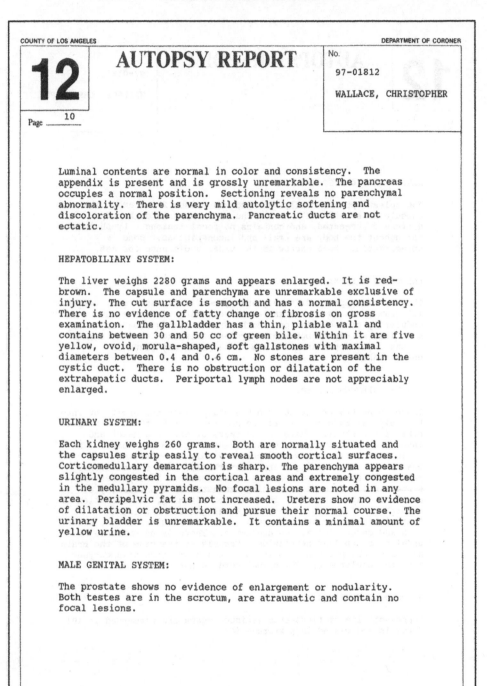

COUNTY OF LOS ANGELES

12

AUTOPSY REPORT

Page _____ 10

DEPARTMENT OF CORONER

No.

97-01812

WALLACE, CHRISTOPHER

Luminal contents are normal in color and consistency. The appendix is present and is grossly unremarkable. The pancreas occupies a normal position. Sectioning reveals no parenchymal abnormality. There is very mild autolytic softening and discoloration of the parenchyma. Pancreatic ducts are not ectatic.

HEPATOBILIARY SYSTEM:

The liver weighs 2280 grams and appears enlarged. It is red-brown. The capsule and parenchyma are unremarkable exclusive of injury. The cut surface is smooth and has a normal consistency. There is no evidence of fatty change or fibrosis on gross examination. The gallbladder has a thin, pliable wall and contains between 30 and 50 cc of green bile. Within it are five yellow, ovoid, morula-shaped, soft gallstones with maximal diameters between 0.4 and 0.6 cm. No stones are present in the cystic duct. There is no obstruction or dilatation of the extrahepatic ducts. Periportal lymph nodes are not appreciably enlarged.

URINARY SYSTEM:

Each kidney weighs 260 grams. Both are normally situated and the capsules strip easily to reveal smooth cortical surfaces. Corticomedullary demarcation is sharp. The parenchyma appears slightly congested in the cortical areas and extremely congested in the medullary pyramids. No focal lesions are noted in any area. Peripelvic fat is not increased. Ureters show no evidence of dilatation or obstruction and pursue their normal course. The urinary bladder is unremarkable. It contains a minimal amount of yellow urine.

MALE GENITAL SYSTEM:

The prostate shows no evidence of enlargement or nodularity. Both testes are in the scrotum, are atraumatic and contain no focal lesions.

76A798P—Rev. 2/91

COUNTY OF LOS ANGELES

12

AUTOPSY REPORT

Page _____11_____

DEPARTMENT OF CORONER

No.

97-01812

WALLACE, CHRISTOPHER

HEMOLYMPHATIC SYSTEM:

The spleen appears mildly enlarged and weighs 260 grams. The capsule is smooth and intact. The parenchyma is dark red, diffusely congested, and contains no focal lesions. Lymph nodes throughout the body are small and inconspicuous. Bone is unremarkable. Bone marrow is the usual appearance for age.

ENDOCRINE SYSTEM:

The thyroid appears diffusely and symmetrically enlarged, weighs 120 grams, and is unremarkable on sectioning with no evidence of nodularity or focal lesion. Both adrenal glands show very early medullary autolysis but are otherwise unremarkable. The thymus is the usual appearance for age. The pituitary gland is unremarkable.

CENTRAL NERVOUS SYSTEM:

There is no hemorrhage beneath the scalp, into the orbits or into the temporal muscles. There are no fractures of the calvarium or base of the skull. There are no tears of the dura mater and there are no epidural, subdural or subarachnoid hematomas. The brain weighs 1490 grams and appears mildly to moderately edematous. Leptomeninges are unremarkable. The convolutionary pattern is within normal limits. The cerebral hemispheres are symmetrical. Coronal sectioning demonstrates a uniformity of cortical gray thickness. There is no softening, discoloration or hemorrhage of the white matter. Basal ganglia are intact. Anatomic landmarks are preserved. The ventricular system, brain stem and cerebellum are unremarkable. There is no evidence of uncal or cerebellar herniation. Vessels at the base of the brain have a normal pattern of distribution and are free of aneurysms and atherosclerosis. The spinal cord is not dissected.

HISTOLOGIC SECTIONS:

Representative sections from various organs are preserved in 10% formalin and placed in a storage jar.

76A798P—Rev. 2/91

AUTOPSY REPORT

12

Page _____ 12

No.

97-01812

WALLACE, CHRISTOPHER

TOXICOLOGY:

Blood, bile, minimal urine, liver tissue and stomach contents
have been submitted to the laboratory. A homicide screen has
been requested.

PHOTOGRAPHS:

Photographs have been taken prior to and during the course of the
autopsy.

RADIOLOGY:

The body has been fluoroscoped and 9 x-rays have been taken.

DIAGRAMS USED:

Diagrams 20 (3 sets) and 21 have been used in the preparation of
this autopsy report.

WITNESSES:

LAPD Wilshire Division Detectives Balderrama and Chavez were
present at the autopsy.

OPINION:

The cause of death is a penetrating gunshot wound to the abdomen
and chest, causing multiple visceral injuries (gunshot wound #4).
In addition, the decedent received 3 gunshot wounds (left
forearm, left thigh and back) that were not considered fatal
wounds due to the absence of visceral or major vascular
involvement. The mode of death is homicide.

LISA SCHEININ, M.D.
DEPUTY MEDICAL EXAMINER

04/07/97
DATE

LS:rs:c
T-3/19/97

76A798P—Rev. 2/91

COUNTY OF LOS ANGELES — MEDICAL REPORT — FORENSIC SCIENCE CENTER — DEPARTMENT OF CORONER

15

AUTOPSY CLASS: ☒ A ☐ B ☐ C
☐ EXAMINATION ONLY (0)

Date 3/10/97 Time 1030 Dr. SCHEININ (PRINT NAME)

☐ PENDING ☒ FINAL ON. 3/10/97
☐ TOX ☐ NEURO ☐ LAW ENF. REPORT
☐ HISTO ☐ MED HIST. ☐ OTHER

HOMICIDE
LAPD/WILSHIRE

22. DEATH WAS CAUSED BY: (ENTER ONLY ONE CAUSE PER LINE FOR A, B, C AND D) IMMEDIATE CAUSE — APPROXIMATE INTERVAL BETWEEN ONSET AND DEATH

(A) Gunshot Wound to Abdomen - Chest — up to 45 min

DUE TO, OR AS A CONSEQUENCE OF
(B)

DUE TO, OR AS A CONSEQUENCE OF
(C)

DUE TO, OR AS A CONSEQUENCE OF
(D)

Other conditions contributing but not related to the immediate cause of death:
Multiple nonfatal gunshot wounds

☐ NATURAL ☐ ACCIDENT ☐ SUICIDE ☒ HOMICIDE ☐ UNDETERMINED

If other than natural causes HOW DID INJURY OCCUR? Shot by assailant(s)

WAS OPERATION PERFORMED FOR ANY CONDITION STATED ABOVE? ☒ Yes ☐ No

TYPE SURGERY Thoracotomy DATE 3-9-97

☐ ORGAN PROCUREMENT ∅

☒ WITNESSES TO AUTOPSY: LAPD Wilshire Dets. Chavez + Balderrama

☒ EVIDENCE RECOVERED AT AUTOPSY
Item Description: Two medium caliber lead bullets with copper jackets; piece of dark fabric

☒ PERTINENT COMMENTS: 1-18-MR— 24 BM psgr in vehicle, shot in drive-by incident ~0030 hrs 3-9-97. Taken to ER of Cedars-Sinai Hosp. Thoracotomy + defib done, no response. Pronounced dead at 0115. Bullet found @ hosp. when body turned over p̄ pronouncement + given to police. (Arrived full arrest + agonal rhythm. Tcut → lg amt bld chest + pericardium - all evacuated)
Per above Dets., two bullets recov. from hospital - on gurney
GSW ① Ⓡ elbow → wrist ⊕ bullet, not fatal
② Back → L shoulder, no projec (T+T), not fatal
③ L thigh, T+T, not fatal
④ R hip → L shoulder, ⊕ bullet, FATAL
Morbid obesity (395 lbs)

______ M.D. (RESIDENT) — [signature] M.D. (DEPUTY MEDICAL EXAMINER)

DEATH CERTIFICATE ISSUED
☒ FINAL DATE ISSUED ______ ISSUED BY ______
☐ PENDING DATE ISSUED ______ ISSUED BY ______

REQUEST
☐ Police Report
☐ Med. History
☐ Consultation
☐ Investigations
☐ Criminalistics
☐ GSR ☐ Other

☐ HISTOPATH CUT: ☐ AUTOPSY ☐ LAB
☐ MICROBIOLOGY:
☐ NEUROPATHOLOGY

TOXICOLOGICAL SPECIMENS COLLECTED
☒ YES, by MJ/LS
☒ BLOOD: ☒ HEART ☐ OTHER
☒ BILE ☐ BRAIN
☒ LIVER ☐ SPLEEN
☒ URINE minimal ☐ KIDNEY
☒ STOMACH CONTENTS ☐ VITREOUS
☒ femoral bld
☐ NO BLOOD
☐ EMBALMED
☐ > 24 HR. IN HOSPITAL
☐ NOT INDICATED
☐ OTHER ______ REASON

TOXICOLOGICAL ANALYSES ORDERED
SCREEN: ☐ C ☒ H ☐ T ☐ S
☐ ALCOHOL ONLY
☐ CARBON MONOXIDE
☐ NO TOXICOLOGY REQUESTED
☐ OTHER (SPECIFY DRUG AND TISSUE)

☒ STORAGE JARS (No. 1)

Typing Blood Taken by MJ/LS
☒ HEART ☐ OTHER

PRIOR EXAMINATION REVIEW BY DME
☒ BODY TAG ☒ MED. RECORD brief ER
☐ CLOTHING none ☐ AT SCENE PHOTO (NO. ...)
☐ SPECIAL PROCESSING TAG ☒ X-RAY (NO. 9)
☐ FLUORO

WHITE - FILE COPY
CANARY - FORENSIC LAB COPY
PINK - INVESTIGATION COPY
GOLDENROD - MEDICAL EXAMINER COPY

COUNTY OF LOS ANGELES   **AUTOPSY CHECK SHEET**   **DEPARTMENT OF CORONER**

16

Thoracot 6 ics (L)

EXTERNAL EXAM
Sex M
Race B
Age 24
Height 74
Weight 395
Hair — see 20
Eyes
Sclera
Teeth
Mouth
Tongue — H R edg mid ½ s lac
Nose
Chest
Breasts
Abdomen
Scar
Genital
Edema
Skin
Decub 660 ↑

HEART Wt 660 ↑
Pericard bld, incised
(+) Hypert R 0.4-0.6 L 1.7-2.1 S 2.0
Dilat ∅
Muscle s̄ fox lesion (nl EoT)
Valves nl
Coronar min AS, no signif sten
AORTA mild ES, High stag.
VESSELS nl

LUNGS Wt
R 690
L 600
Adhes ∅
Fluid sm bld
Atelectasis ∅
Oedema 2+
Congest 2+
Consol ∅
Bronchi nl
Nodes nl

PERITONEUM
Fluid sm bld ≤ 50cc lg clots
Adhes ∅
LIVER Wt 2280 r-br ↑
Caps nl EoT
Lobul
Fibros nl
GB 30-50cc, ∅ng'd ∅ thk
Calc 5 yel munda soft ov. 0.4-0.6
Bile ducts nl
SPLEEN Wt 260 slt ↑ c
Color nl
Consist
Caps
Malpig nl Early ant.
PANCREAS nl Early ant. (mod)
ADRENALS nl Early ant. (mod)
KIDNEYS Wt 260 Each slt C
Caps nl Very C medullae
Cortex
Vessels
Pelvis
Ureter
BLADDER nl, min urine
GENITALIA
Prost nl
Testes nl s̄ trauma
Uterus
Tubes
Ovar
OESOPHAGUS nl
STOMACH nl, ≤50cc thin grn-br fl.
DUOB & SM INT nl
APPENDIX (+)
LARGE INT nl EoT
ABDOM NODES nl
SKELETON nl
Spine
Marrow

PHARYNX nl — Mod prom pharyng. tons
TRACHEA nl
THYROID — Symm. enlargt Wt 120 g no nodules
THYMUS nl

BRAIN Wt 1490
Dura nl — mild mod
Fluid
Ventric
Vessels ↓ 2
Ears
Nasal Sin
PITUITARY nl

Forms 20 (3)
91

TOXICOLOGY
bld untl (min) bile
Sm bld liver stom

SECTIONS ∅
XR -9
fluoro of ST neg
src 2 bullets LUE

GROSS IMPRESSION
Morbid obesity
Cmeg c̄ BiVH
Hmeg Smeg
S/P ortho rod, fem fx (L)
Cholelithiasis
Pulm E

GSW (x 4)
① L forearm, NF, (+) bullet
② Back, NF, No projec
③ Post o med L thigh, NF No projec
★ ④ R hip → L shldr Fatal, (+) bullet

S/P Thoracot + med/surg intervention

N/B Dets. Chavez + Balderrama present
They say 2 bullets recov. from gurney at hosp.

Tech - M Johnson

te	Time	Deputy Medical Examiner
03-10-97	1030 - 1320	(signature) M.D.

7B-(REV. 8/91)

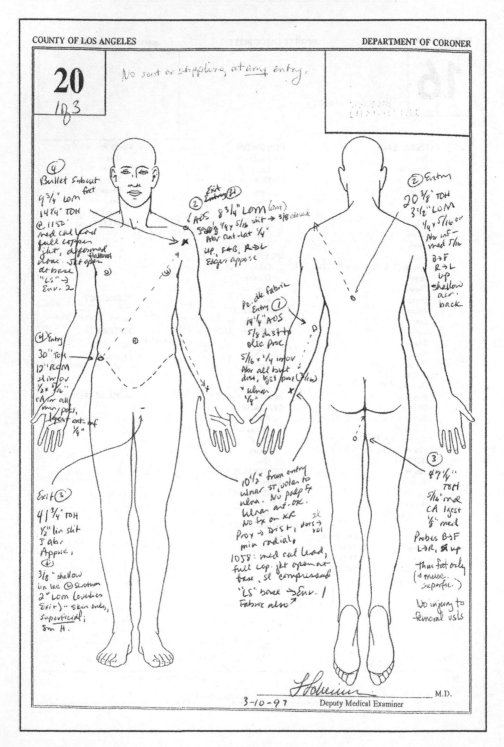

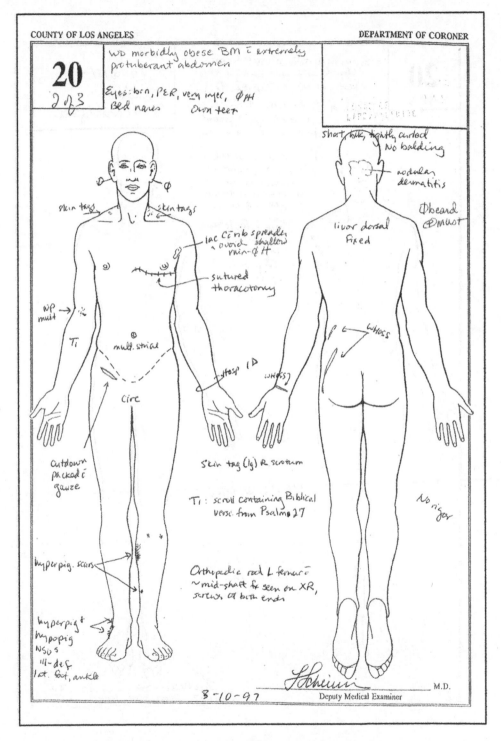

COUNTY OF LOS ANGELES · DEPARTMENT OF CORONER

20
3]3

Entire track of ② dissected from entry to exit. No entry to Chest, no rib or scapular fx.

Track of ③ dissected through post. ⓛ thigh + probed to anterior exit wound.

Track of ① dissected + probed along entire ln. No evident fx ulna + no obvious injury to ulnar artery.

Track of ④ followed via visceral injuries. Trajectory photo taken.

97-01812
Wallace,
Christopher

H along all tracks.

Incisions (extra)
• ⓛ back / shoulder
• post ⓛ thigh
• volar ⓛ forearm

3/10/97 Deputy Medical Examiner M.D.

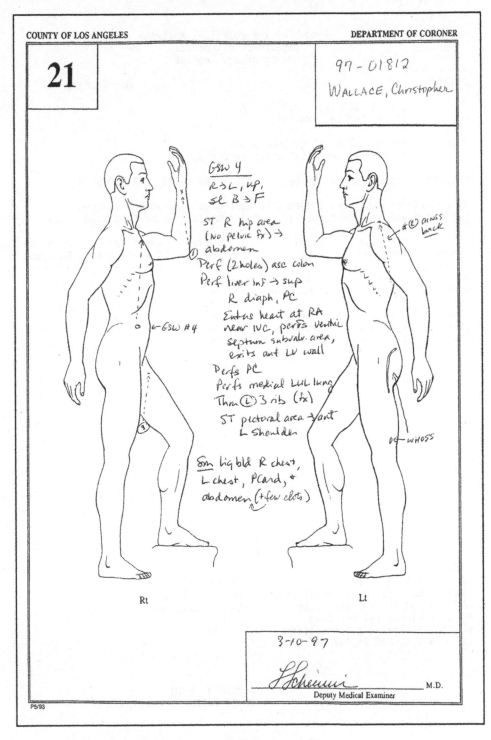

Report of Toxicological Analyses
Department of Coroner
County of Los Angeles

03/25/97   Non-Pending

TO: Lisa A. Scheinin, M.D.
           Deputy Medical Examiner

FROM: Forensic Toxicology Laboratory
           Forensic Science Laboratories Division

SUBJECT: Coroner's Case Number 97-01812 SWALLACE, CHRISTOPHE R

In accordance with your request, toxicological analyses have been
performed and are now completed on the subject case as tabulated below:

Tissue	Analyses Requested	Drugs Analyzed	Level Found	Assigned Toxicologist	Date Analyzed
Blood	Alcohols	Alcohols	Negative	J. Park	03/12/97
Blood	Cocaine	Cocaine and Metabolites	ND	M. Schuchardt	03/17/97
Blood	Narcotics	Codeine	ND	M. Schuchardt	03/17/97
Blood	Narcotics	Morphine	ND	M. Schuchardt	03/17/97
Blood	Phencyclidine	Phencyclidine	ND	M. Schuchardt	03/17/97
Blood	Methamphetamine	Methamphetamine	ND	S. Winter	03/21/97

LEGEND:
MG/L = Milligram per Liter   G% = Gram Percent
UG/ML = Micrograms per Milliliter   ND = Not Detected
QNS   = Quanity Not Sufficent   MG = Milligrams
UG/G = Micrograms per Gram
MG/DL = Milligram per Deciliter
TNP   = Test Not Performed

                        JOSEPH J. MUTO
                        CHIEF FORENSIC TOXICOLOGIST

Taken "3-9-97 0450   Can 8947

COUNTY OF LOS ANGELES 3-9-97 0450   **CASE REPORTED**   DEPARTMENT OF CORONER

1B

POST MORTEM AT:
☒ MEC/FSC
☐ MORTUARY
☐ OTHER FACILITY

REPORTED AS: ☐ OIS/LER

☐ Natural ☐ Accident ☐ Suicide ☒ Homicide
☐ At Work ☐ Nursing Home ☐ In Custody ☐ State Hosp.

CASE NO. **97-01812**

DECEDENT IDENTIFIED BY:
LAST NAME _Wallace_
FIRST _Christopher_ MIDDLE _—_
Age _XXX_ DOB _5-21-72_ MALE ☒ FEMALE ☐

CROSS REFERENCE TO: RACE APPEARS _BLK_

PLACE OF DEATH - NAME OF FACILITY _CEDAR SANI._   STREET ADDRESS   ZIP CODE

DATE OF DEATH - Month, Day, Year _3-9-97_ HOUR _0115_ FOUND OR PRONOUNCED BY _S. LKA_   SCENE PHONE ( )   ZIP CODE

Usual Residence _UNK_

Reported by _BERCHEM_   Agency _LAPD/WILSHIRE HOM_ Phone (213) 485-4033

Reported to M.E.C. _OOfen_   Date/Time _3-10-97_ 0430   847-3990

Investigating Agency _(RH)_   Officer _____ 3-9-97 DATE TIME

Next of Kin: _____   Relationship

Street Address _____   Phone

City _____   State   6345 ZIP CODE

Notified by _By Agency_   DATE TIME

DESCRIBE TERMINAL EPISODE AND OTHER PERTINENT INFORMATION: _MULT- GSW_

FAIRFAX & WILSHIRE 3-8-97 2300 HRS

✱ NOTE ✱ DECEDENT 400+ LBS ✱

✱ DECEDENT MAY BE RAP SINGER ✱

EVIDENCE REQUESTED: HAIR ☐ FINGERNAIL ☐ GSR ☐ OTHER ☐ _____

Hospital paperwork ready Date/Time _3-9-97 0745_ Per _Monson_ POLICE REPORT #

THIS SECTION FOR INQUIRY ONLY

Attending Physician   Phone

Address   LAST DATE ATTENDED

	107 DEATH WAS CAUSED BY: (ENTER ONLY ONE CAUSE PER LINE FOR A, B, C, AND D)	TIME INTERVAL BETWEEN ONSET AND DEATH	108 DEATH REPORTED TO CORONER ☐ YES ☐ NO REFERRAL NUMBER
	IMMEDIATE CAUSE (A)		
CAUSE	DUE TO (B)		109. BIOPSY PERFORMED ☐ YES ☐ NO
OF	DUE TO (C)		110. AUTOPSY PERFORMED ☐ YES ☐ NO
DEATH	DUE TO (D)		111. USED IN DETERMINING CAUSE ☐ YES ☐ NO
	112. OTHER SIGNIFICANT CONDITIONS CONTRIBUTING TO DEATH BUT NOT RELATED TO CAUSE GIVEN IN 107		
	113. WAS OPERATION PERFORMED FOR ANY CONDITION IN ITEM 107 OR 112? IF YES, LIST TYPE OF OPERATION AND DATE		

Discussed With _____ , M.D. By _____ Deputy

Date & Time Mortuary Notified

SUPPLEMENTAL INFORMATION BY: _____ Approved

78C100F-1-78 (Rev. 3/84)   **Original Jurisdictional Determination Record — DO NOT DISCARD**

#97-01812

COUNTY OF LOS ANGELES
Department of Coroner

HOSPITAL AND NURSING
CARE FACILITY REPORT

1104 NORTH MISSION ROAD
LOS ANGELES, CALIF. 90033

18

TO REPORT A DEATH--PHONE (213) 343-0711
COMPLETE ALL LINES. USE INK, IF UNKNOWN OR NOT APPLICABLE,
SO STATE.
CEDARS-SINAI MEDICAL CENTER
NAME OF FACILITY

001/000966265
WALLACE, CHRISTOPHER
M/99/99/999

ADDRESS _8700 Beverly Blvd._ PHONE (213) 855-5452

NAME OF DECEDENT _WALLACE, CHRISTOPHER_ DOS 03/09/97

DATE OF DEATH _3-9-97_ TIME _0115Am_ ER 00239 AGE SEX _M_ RACE _BLK_
999/999/999 E EM

PRONOUNCED BY _DR. PAUL SILKA_ HOSP. OR I.D.NO. _000966265_

☑ EMERGENCY ROOM PATIENT

ORGAN/TISSUE DONATION INFORMATION
WAS THE NEXT-OF-KIN APPROACHED REGARDING ORGAN/TISSUE DONATION?

☐ HOSPITAL IN PATIENT   NO ☐ YES ☐ IF YES WHAT WAS THEIR RESPONSE? ___

DATE ADMITTED _3/9/97_ TIME _0115_

TO HOSPITAL BY: ☐ POLICE ☐ RELATIVES ☑ FRIENDS ☐ SELF ☐ AMBULANCE (Name or R.A. #) ___

FROM ___
(STATE WHETHER HOME, HOSPITAL OR OTHER)   GIVE ADDRESS   (IF HOSPITAL ATTACH THEIR HISTORY)

ADMITTED BY ___ M.D.   ATTENDING PHYSICIAN ___ M.D.

INJURIES _3/9/97_ _0045_ PLACE ___ CAUSE ___
DATE TIME (TRAFFIC, FALL, ETC.)

DESCRIBE INJURIES:

CLINICAL HISTORY:

SURGICAL PROCEDURES: STATE TYPE, DATE, TIME AND RESULTS OF ANY OPERATION OR AMPUTATION PERFORMED

unknown kind & bullett fire to
police officer McKinney Badge # 27422

WAS A BULLET OR OTHER FOREIGN OBJECT RECOVERED? SPECIFY

LABORATORY: SPECIFY SPECIMENS TAKEN ___ DATE & TIME _3/9/97_ _0115Am_
LABORATORY RESULTS:

RETAIN LABORATORY SPECIMENS

X-RAY REPORT:

REMARKS: ESPECIALLY SYMPTOMS PRECEDING AND DURING TERMINAL EPISODE _CARDIOPULMONARY ARREST_
MULTIPLE GUNSHOT WOUNDS

IN MY OPINION, THE IMMEDIATE CAUSE OF DEATH IS: _PERICARDIAL TAMPONADE_

BY _Paul A. Silka_ M.D.   —OR— ___
OTHER OFFICIAL

76H655

THE BODY WILL NOT BE REMOVED BY THE CORONER WITHOUT THIS REPORT

River Phoenix

Given Name: River June Bottom
Born: August 23, 1970, Metolius, Oregon
Died: October 31, 1993, West Hollywood, California
Cause of Death: Drug-Induced Heart Failure

River Phoenix started his acting career when he was a child with roles in TV movies and after-school specials. By the mid eighties he was a star in major motion pictures including *Stand by Me* and *Running on Empty*, for which he was nominated for an Academy Award in 1988. He died from an overdose of cocaine and heroin after collapsing outside the Viper Room in Hollywood.

COUNTY OF LOS ANGELES   DEPARTMENT OF CORONER

12   AUTOPSY REPORT

No. 93-10011

I performed an autopsy on the body of   ➡   PHOENIX, RIVER J.

the DEPARTMENT OF CORONER

at _____

Los Angeles, California   on   NOVEMBER 1, 1993 @ 1000 HOURS
                                   (Date)   (Time)

From the anatomic findings and pertinent history I ascribe the death to:

(A)   **ACUTE MULTIPLE DRUG INTOXICATION**

DUE TO OR AS A CONSEQUENCE OF

(B)

DUE TO OR AS A CONSEQUENCE OF

(C)

OTHER SIGNIFICANT CONDITIONS —

Anatomical Summary:

1. History of cocaine, heroin and diazepam use.

2. Abrasions of hand.

3. Contusion of shin.

4. Evidence of therapy.

     a. Intravenous catheters of neck, subclavian region, arm and hand.

     b. Resuscitation mark on chest.

     c. Foley catheter.

12   AUTOPSY REPORT   No 93-10011

PHOENIX, RIVER J.

Page 2

CIRCUMSTANCES:

On 10/30/93, the decedent reportedly went to a nightclub.
He was allegedly speedballing, as well as receiving Valium.
Early the next morning, he was found by paramedics just
outside the front door of the club in cardiac arrest. He
was taken to Cedars-Sinai Medical Center, where he was
pronounced dead shortly after arrival. Drug screen at the
hospital was presumptively positive for benzodiazepine,
cannabinoids, cocaine metabolite, propoxyphene and opiates.
Ethanol was not detected.

EXTERNAL EXAMINATION:

The body is that of an unembalmed Caucasian young adult male
who appears the stated age of 23 years. The body is identified
by toe tags. The body weighs 159 pounds, measures 70 inches in
length and is well-built, muscular and fairly well-nourished.
There is no abnormal skin coloring or pigmentation. No tattoos
are present. Rigor mortis is well-developed in the limbs and
jaw. Livor mortis is fixed and distributed over the posterior
surface of the body as well as the palms of the hands. The
are small abrasions on the knuckles of the right index finger
and the right thumb. The right shin shows a red-purple
contusion. The head, which is normocephalic is covered by
brown hair. There is no balding. Examination of the eyes
reveals pupils with green irides and sclerae that show no
injection or jaundice. There are no petechial hemorrhages
of the conjunctivae of the lids or the sclerae. The oronasal
passages are unobstructed. The nasal septum is intact and without
inflammation. Upper and lower teeth are present. The neck is
unremarkable. Resuscitative marks are present over the precordium.
There is no chest deformity. There is no increase in the anterior-
posterior diameter of the chest. There are no scars of the chest
or abdomen. The abdomen is flat. The genitalia are those of
a circumcised adult male. A Foley catheter is present. There
is no anal or genital trauma. There are no needle tracks
identified on the arms or neck. There are fresh venipunctures
of the right neck, left subclavian region, right antecubital
region and left hand which are related to therapeutic procedures.
Edema of the extremities is not present. Joint deformities,
crepitance and abnormal mobility are not present.

COUNTY OF LOS ANGELES

12

AUTOPSY REPORT

No 93-10011

PHOENIX, RIVER J.

DEPARTMENT OF CORONER

Page ___3___

CLOTHING:

The body is unclothed when received. Accompanying the body
are the following items:

1. A pair of brown long pants with dark stripes. The label
   says "split" size M-Long.

2. A pair of white and black high top tennis shoes with the
   label "ALL STAR" size 10 1/2.

3. A pair of socks.

INITIAL INCISION:

The body cavities are entered through a Y-shaped incision.
No foreign material is present in the mouth or upper airway.
No lesions are present nor is trauma of the gingiva, lips or
oral mucosa demonstrated. Both hyoid bone and larynx are
intact without fractures. No hemorrhage present in the
adjacent throat organs. There are no prevertebral fascial
hemorrhages. The pleural cavities contains a small quantity
of straw-colored fluid. Rib fractures are not present. The
parietal pleurae are intact. The lungs are well-expanded.
Soft tissues of the thoracic and abdominal walls are well-
preserved. There is no recent evidence of injury to the
chest and abdominal walls other than the resuscitation mark
and liver temperature mark. The organs of the abdominal cavity
have a normal arrangement. None is absent. There is no fluid
collection of the abdomen. The peritoneal cavity is without
evidence of peritonitis. There are no adhesions.

SYSTEMIC AND ORGAN REVIEW

CARDIOVASCULAR SYSTEM:

The aorta is elastic and of even caliber throughout with vessels
distributed normally from it. It shows a minimal lipid streaking.
There is no tortuosity, widening or aneurysm of the aorta.

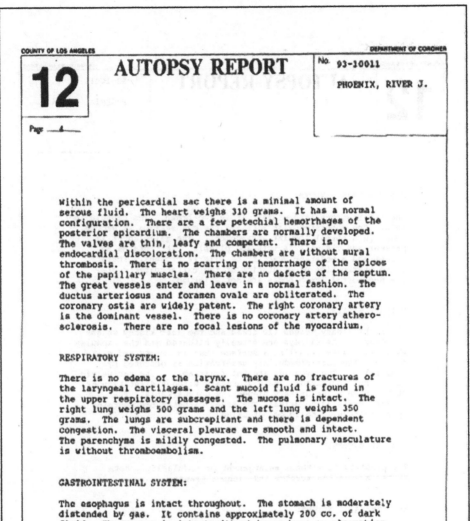

COUNTY OF LOS ANGELES

DEPARTMENT OF CORONER

AUTOPSY REPORT

No. 93-10011

PHOENIX, RIVER J.

12

Page ____4____

Within the pericardial sac there is a minimal amount of
serous fluid. The heart weighs 310 grams. It has a normal
configuration. There are a few petechial hemorrhages of the
posterior epicardium. The chambers are normally developed.
The valves are thin, leafy and competent. There is no
endocardial discoloration. The chambers are without mural
thrombosis. There is no scarring or hemorrhage of the apices
of the papillary muscles. There are no defects of the septum.
The great vessels enter and leave in a normal fashion. The
ductus arteriosus and foramen ovale are obliterated. The
coronary ostia are widely patent. The right coronary artery
is the dominant vessel. There is no coronary artery atherosclerosis. There are no focal lesions of the myocardium.

RESPIRATORY SYSTEM:

There is no edema of the larynx. There are no fractures of
the laryngeal cartilages. Scant mucoid fluid is found in
the upper respiratory passages. The mucosa is intact. The
right lung weighs 500 grams and the left lung weighs 350
grams. The lungs are subcrepitant and there is dependent
congestion. The visceral pleurae are smooth and intact.
The parenchyma is mildly congested. The pulmonary vasculature
is without thromboembolism.

GASTROINTESTINAL SYSTEM:

The esophagus is intact throughout. The stomach is moderately
distended by gas. It contains approximately 200 cc. of dark
fluid. The mucosa is intact without hemorrhage or ulceration.
No medication or capsular material is identified. The external
appearance of the small intestine and colon is unremarkable.
The small intestine and colon are opened along their antimesenteric border and no mucosal lesions are present. The
appendix is present. The pancreas occupies a normal position.
The parenchyma is lobular and firm. The pancreatic ducts are
not ectatic. There is no parenchymal calcification.

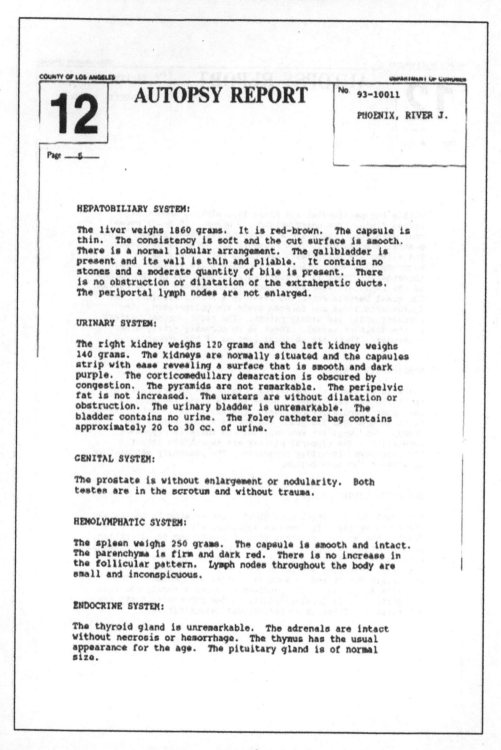

12 AUTOPSY REPORT

No. 93-10011

PHOENIX, RIVER J.

Page ___5___

HEPATOBILIARY SYSTEM:

The liver weighs 1860 grams. It is red-brown. The capsule is thin. The consistency is soft and the cut surface is smooth. There is a normal lobular arrangement. The gallbladder is present and its wall is thin and pliable. It contains no stones and a moderate quantity of bile is present. There is no obstruction or dilatation of the extrahepatic ducts. The periportal lymph nodes are not enlarged.

URINARY SYSTEM:

The right kidney weighs 120 grams and the left kidney weighs 140 grams. The kidneys are normally situated and the capsules strip with ease revealing a surface that is smooth and dark purple. The corticomedullary demarcation is obscured by congestion. The pyramids are not remarkable. The peripelvic fat is not increased. The ureters are without dilatation or obstruction. The urinary bladder is unremarkable. The bladder contains no urine. The Foley catheter bag contains approximately 20 to 30 cc. of urine.

GENITAL SYSTEM:

The prostate is without enlargement or nodularity. Both testes are in the scrotum and without trauma.

HEMOLYMPHATIC SYSTEM:

The spleen weighs 250 grams. The capsule is smooth and intact. The parenchyma is firm and dark red. There is no increase in the follicular pattern. Lymph nodes throughout the body are small and inconspicuous.

ENDOCRINE SYSTEM:

The thyroid gland is unremarkable. The adrenals are intact without necrosis or hemorrhage. The thymus has the usual appearance for the age. The pituitary gland is of normal size.

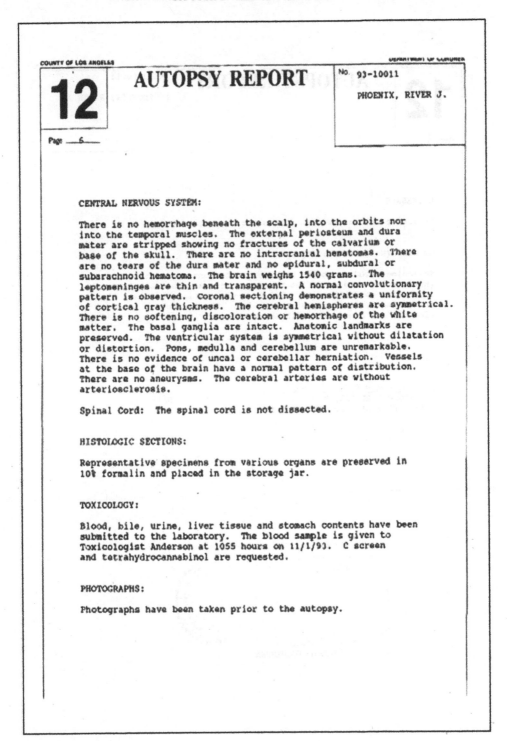

COUNTY OF LOS ANGELES

12

Page 6

AUTOPSY REPORT

DEPARTMENT OF CORONER

No. 93-10011

PHOENIX, RIVER J.

CENTRAL NERVOUS SYSTEM:

There is no hemorrhage beneath the scalp, into the orbits nor into the temporal muscles. The external periosteum and dura mater are stripped showing no fractures of the calvarium or base of the skull. There are no intracranial hematomas. There are no tears of the dura mater and no epidural, subdural or subarachnoid hematoma. The brain weighs 1540 grams. The leptomeninges are thin and transparent. A normal convolutionary pattern is observed. Coronal sectioning demonstrates a uniformity of cortical gray thickness. The cerebral hemispheres are symmetrical. There is no softening, discoloration or hemorrhage of the white matter. The basal ganglia are intact. Anatomic landmarks are preserved. The ventricular system is symmetrical without dilatation or distortion. Pons, medulla and cerebellum are unremarkable. There is no evidence of uncal or cerebellar herniation. Vessels at the base of the brain have a normal pattern of distribution. There are no aneurysms. The cerebral arteries are without arteriosclerosis.

Spinal Cord: The spinal cord is not dissected.

HISTOLOGIC SECTIONS:

Representative specimens from various organs are preserved in 10% formalin and placed in the storage jar.

TOXICOLOGY:

Blood, bile, urine, liver tissue and stomach contents have been submitted to the laboratory. The blood sample is given to Toxicologist Anderson at 1055 hours on 11/1/93. C screen and tetrahydrocannabinol are requested.

PHOTOGRAPHS:

Photographs have been taken prior to the autopsy.

12   AUTOPSY REPORT

No.93-10011

PHOENIX, RIVER J.

Page 7

WITNESSES:

Detective Lee was present during the autopsy.

OPINION (November 12, 1993):

Toxicology studies showed high concentrations of morphine
(heroin) and cocaine in the blood, as well as other substances
in smaller concentrations. Police investigation shows no
indication of foul play at this point. The toxicology
findings are consistent with the history.

Christopher Rogers

CHRISTOPHER ROGERS, M.D.
CHIEF, FORENSIC MEDICINE DIVISION   DATE

CR:rs:c
T-11/2/93

15

AUTOPSY CLASS: ☐ A. ☒ B. ☐ C. ☐ EXAMINATION (D)

Date 11-1-93 Time 1000 Dr Rogers
ADLT NAME

☒ PENDING   ☒ FINAL ON 11-12-93
☒ TOX ☐ NEURO ☐ LAW ENF REPORT
☐ HISTO ☐ MED. HIST. ☐ OTHER _____

APPROX
TIME
INTERVAL
BETWEEN
ONSET
AND
DEATH

93-10011
P. LEVI?, PIVER
L?

22. DEATH WAS CAUSED BY   (ENTER ONLY ONE CAUSE PER LINE FOR A, B, AND C)
IMMEDIATE CAUSE

(A) Acute multiple drug intoxication   ◄

DUE TO, OR AS A CONSEQUENCE OF

(B)   ◄

DUE TO, OR AS A CONSEQUENCE OF

(C)   ◄

Other conditions contributing but not related to the immediate cause of death

☐ NATURAL ☒ ACCIDENT ☐ SUICIDE ☐ HOMICIDE ☐ UNDETERMINED

If other than natural causes
HOW DID INJURY OCCUR?   Intake of drugs

WAS OPERATION PERFORMED FOR ANY CONDITION STATED ABOVE? ☐ Yes ☒ No

TYPE SURGERY_____ DATE_____

☐ PERTINENT COMMENTS: ☐ EVIDENCE RECOVERED AT AUTOPSY
Item Description.

☐ ORGAN PROCUREMENT   ☐ WITNESSES TO AUTOPSY:

Blood samples given to
toxicologist R. Anderson
1055 11-1-93
CR.

This is a true certified copy of record ...
it bears the seal of the ...
Coroner/Inspector ...

Anthony, P. ...

DIRECTOR
DEPARTMENT OF CORONER
LOS ANGELES COUNTY, CALIFORNIA

Christopher Rogers M.D.
DEPUTY MEDICAL EXAMINER

DEATH CERTIFICATE ISSUED

☐ FINAL   DATE ISSUED _____ ISSUED BY_____

REQUEST

☐ Police Report _____
☐ Med History _____
_____
_____
☐ Investigations _____
☐ Criminalistics _____
   ☐ GSR ☐ Other _____

☐ HISTOPATH CUT. ☐ AUTOPSY ☐ LAB
☐ MICROBIOLOGY:
☐ NEUROPATHOLOGY

TOXICOLOGICAL SPECIMENS COLLECTED
☒ YES by _____
   ☒ BLOOD ☒ HEART ☐ (OTHER)
   ☒ BILE ☐ BRAIN
   ☒ LIVER ☐ SPLEEN
   ☒ URINE ☐ KIDNEY
   ☒ STOMACH ☐ VITREOUS
     CONTENTS
     (2) ☐

☐ NO BLOOD
☐ EMBALMED
☐ >24 HR IN HOSPITAL
☐ NOT INDICATED
☐ OTHER_____
       (REASON)

TOXICOLOGICAL ANALYSES ORDERED
SCREEN: ☒ C ☐ H ☐ T
☐ ALCOHOL ONLY
☐ CARBON MONOXIDE
☐ OTHER (SPECIFY DRUG AND TISSUE)
   THC
_____
_____

☐ SUPPLEMENTAL REQUEST (17A)

Typing Blood Taken by CR
☒ HEART ☐ OTHER _____

PRIOR EXAMINATION REVIEW
☒ BODY TAG CR ☒ MED. RECORD CR
☒ CLOTHING CR ☒ AT SCENE PHOTO CR
☐ SPL. PROCESSING ☐ X-RAY
   TAG   ☐ FLUORO

WHITE - FILE COPY
CANARY - FORENSIC LAB COPY

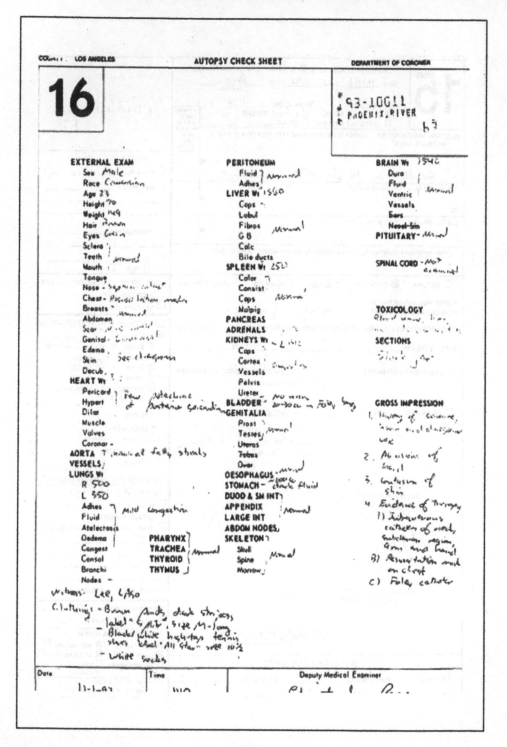

COUNTY LOS ANGELES — AUTOPSY CHECK SHEET — DEPARTMENT OF CORONER

16

93-10011
PHOENIX RIVER

EXTERNAL EXAM
Sex Male
Race Caucasian
Age 23
Height 70
Weight 149
Hair Brown
Eyes Green
Sclera
Teeth normal
Mouth
Tongue
Nose
Chest
Breasts normal
Abdomen normal
Scar
Genital normal
Edema
Skin See diagram
Decub
HEART Wt
Pericard
Hypert
Dilat
Muscle
Valves
Coronar
AORTA normal fatty streak
VESSELS
LUNGS Wt
R 500
L 550
Adhes — Mild congestion
Fluid
Atelectasis
Oedema
Congest
Consol
Bronchi
Nodes

PHARYNX
TRACHEA — normal
THYROID
THYMUS

Witness: Lee, Liho

Clothing - Brown pants, dark stripes,
label - Gap, size M-long
Black white hightop tennis
shoes label All Star - size 10½
- White socks

PERITONEUM
Fluid — normal
Adhes
LIVER Wt 1560
Caps
Lobul
Fibros — normal
GB
Calc
Bile ducts
SPLEEN Wt 252
Color
Consist
Caps — normal
Malpig
PANCREAS
ADRENALS
KIDNEYS Wt
Caps
Cortex
Vessels
Pelvis
Ureter
BLADDER
GENITALIA
Prost
Testes — normal
Uterus
Tubes
Over
OESOPHAGUS — normal
STOMACH — dark fluid
DUOD & SM INT
APPENDIX — normal
LARGE INT
ABDOM NODES
SKELETON
Skull
Spine — normal
Marrow

BRAIN Wt 1540
Dura
Fluid
Ventric
Vessels
Ears
Nasal-Sin
PITUITARY — normal

SPINAL CORD - not examined

TOXICOLOGY

SECTIONS

GROSS IMPRESSION
1. History of cocaine, heroin and diazepam use

2. Abrasion of knee

3. Contusion of skin

4. Evidence of therapy
   1) Intravenous catheter of neck, subclavian region, arm and hand
   B) Resuscitation mark on chest
   C) Foley catheter

Date	Time	Deputy Medical Examiner
11-1-93	1110	

Report of Toxicological Analyses
Department of Coroner
County of Los Angeles

11/15/93   Pending Tox

TO: Christopher Rogers, M.D.
         Chief, Forensic Medicine

FROM: Forensic Toxicology Laboratory
         Forensic Science Laboratories Division

SUBJECT: Coroner's Case Number 93-10011 PHOENIX, RIVER

In accordance with your request, toxicological analyses have been
performed and are now completed on the subject case as tabulated below:

Tissue	Analyses Requested	Drugs Analyzed	Level Found	Assigned Toxicologist	Date Analyzed
Blood	Alcohols	Alcohols	Negative	R. Davol	11/24/93
Blood	Barbiturates		NG	J. Park	11/04/93
Blood	Basic Drugs	Other	Present	J. Anderson	11/04/93
Blood	Narcotics	Free Codeine	0.34 UG/ML	J. Anderson	11/04/93
Blood	Narcotics	Free Morphine	1.79 UG/ML	J. Anderson	11/04/93
Blood	Phencyclidine	Phencyclidine	NG	L. Sidmay	11/04/93
Stomach Contents	Narcotics	CODEINE	0.08 MG	J. Anderson	11/04/93
Stomach Contents	Narcotics	MORPHINE	0.26 MG	J. Anderson	11/04/93
Blood	Cocaine	Benzoylecgonine	4.60 UG/ML	J. Anderson	11/04/93
Blood	Cocaine	Cocaethylene	NO	J. Anderson	11/04/93
Blood	Cocaine	Cocaine	7.90 UG/ML	J. Anderson	11/04/93
Stomach Contents	Cocaine	BENZOYLECGONINE	1.70 MG	J. Anderson	11/04/93
Stomach Contents	Cocaine	COCAETHYLENE	NO	J. Anderson	11/04/93
Stomach Contents	Cocaine	COCAINE	100.89 MG	J. Anderson	11/04/93
Blood		EPHEDRINE	0.57 UG/ML	R. Budd	11/08/93
Blood		MDA	NO	R. Budd	11/08/93
Blood		MDMA	NO	R. Budd	11/08/93
Blood		PSEUDOEPHEDRINE	1.29 UG/ML	R. Budd	11/08/93
Blood	Methamphetamine	Methamphetamine	NO	R. Budd	11/08/93
Urine		EPHEDRINE	Present	R. Budd	11/08/93
Urine		MDA	NO	R. Budd	11/08/93
Urine		MDMA	NO	R. Budd	11/08/93
Urine		PSEUDOEPHEDRINE	Present	R. Budd	11/08/93
Urine	Drug Screen	BENZOYLECGONINE	Present	R. Budd	11/08/93
Urine	Drug Screen	MORPHINE	Present	R. Budd	11/08/93
Blood	Benzodiazepines	DESMETHYLDIAZEPAM	0.05 UG/ML	J. Anderson	11/16/93
Blood	Benzodiazepines	DIAZEPAM	0.19 UG/ML	J. Anderson	11/16/93
Urine		Marijuana Metabolite	Present	L. Chow	11/04/93
Blood	Basic Drugs	Ketamine	NO	J. Anderson	11/15/93
Blood	Basic Drugs	Propoxyphene	NO	J. Anderson	11/15/93

Report of Toxicological Analyses
Department of Coroner
County of Los Angeles

12/06/93   Pending Tox

TO: Christopher Rogers, M.D.
           Chief, Forensic Medicine

FROM: Forensic Toxicology Laboratory
           Forensic Science Laboratories Division

SUBJECT: Coroner's Case Number 93-10011 PHOENIX, RIVER

In accordance with your request, toxicological analyses have been
performed and are now completed on the subject case as tabulated below:

Tissue	Analyses Requested	Drugs Analyzed	Level Found	Assigned Toxicologist	Date Analyzed
Blood	Special Test	Marijuana	Negative	L Mahoney	12/01/93

It is a true certified copy of the record
with the seal of the Department of
Coroner imprinted as shown

(signature)

DIRECTOR
DEPARTMENT OF CORONER
LOS ANGELES COUNTY, CALIFORNIA

LEGEND:
MG/L   = Milligram per Liter   G% = Gram Percent
UG/ML = Micrograms per Milliliter   ND = Not Detected
QNS   = Quanity Not Sufficent   MG = Milligrams
UG/G   = Micrograms per Gram
MG/DL = Milligram per Deciliter
TNP   = Test Not Performed

JOSEPH J. MUTO
CHIEF FORENSIC TOXICOLOGIST

C/2 2-11-94

COUNTY OF LOS ANGELES
Department of Coroner

HOSPITAL AND NURSING
CARE FACILITY REPORT

1104 NORTH MISSION ROAD
LOS ANGELES, CALIF. 90033

18

TO REPORT A DEATH—PHONE (213) 343-0711
COMPLETE ALL LINES. USE INK. IF UNKNOWN OR NOT APPLICABLE, SO STATE

CEDARS-SINAI MEDICAL CENTER
NAME OF FACILITY

001/010954956
RIVER, PHOENIX
/ /
DOS 10/31/93
ER 565717
000/000/000

ADDRESS 8700 Beverly Blvd.   PHONE (213) 855-   2109

NAME OF DECEDENT RIVER, PHOENIX

DATE OF DEATH 10-31-93   TIME 0751   AGE 23 SEX M RACE C

PRONOUNCED BY Dr. Paul Silka   OSP OR LONG.

☒ EMERGENCY ROOM PATIENT
☐ HOSPITAL IN PATIENT

ORGAN/TISSUE DONATION INFORMATION
WAS THE NEXT OF KIN APPROACHED REGARDING ORGAN/TISSUE DONATION?
NO ☐ YES ☐ IF YES WHAT WAS THEIR RESPONSE?

DATE ADMITTED 10-31-93   TIME 0134

TO HOSPITAL BY ☐ POLICE ☐ RELATIVES ☐ FRIENDS ☐ SELF ☒ AMBULANCE (NAME OF R.A. #) 58 8

FROM 8860 SUNSET BLVD. W-H'WOOD CA.
(STATE WHETHER HOME, HOSPITAL OR OTHER) GIVE ADDRESS   (IF HOSPITAL ATTACH THEIR HISTORY)

ADMITTED BY P. Silka   M.D.   ATTENDING PHYSICIAN   M.D.

INJURIES DATE   TIME   PLACE   CAUSE (TRAFFIC, FALL, ETC)

DESCRIBE INJURIES

CLINICAL HISTORY   APPARENT   NARON/COCAINE OVERDOSE - ASYSTOLE

SURGICAL PROCEDURES STATE TYPE, DATE, TIME AND RESULTS OF ANY OPERATION OR AMPUTATION PERFORMED

CENTRAL   LINE

WAS A BULLET OR OTHER FOREIGN OBJECT RECOVERED? SPECIFY

LABORATORY: SPECIFY SPECIMENS TAKEN   DATE & TIME

LABORATORY RESULTS.

OBTAIN LABORATORY SPECIMENS

X-RAY REPORT.   BLOOD/URINA   OVERDOSE TOX

REMARKS: ESPECIALLY SYMPTOMS PRECEDING AND DURING TERMINAL EPISODE

IN MY OPINION, THE IMMEDIATE CAUSE OF DEATH IS:

BY P. Silka   M.D.   OR   OTHER OFFICIAL
SILKA

THE BODY WILL NOT BE REMOVED BY THE CORONER WITHOUT THIS REPORT

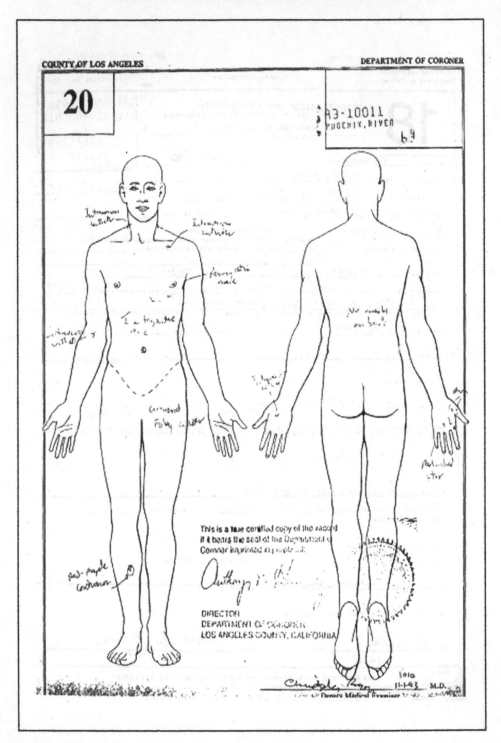

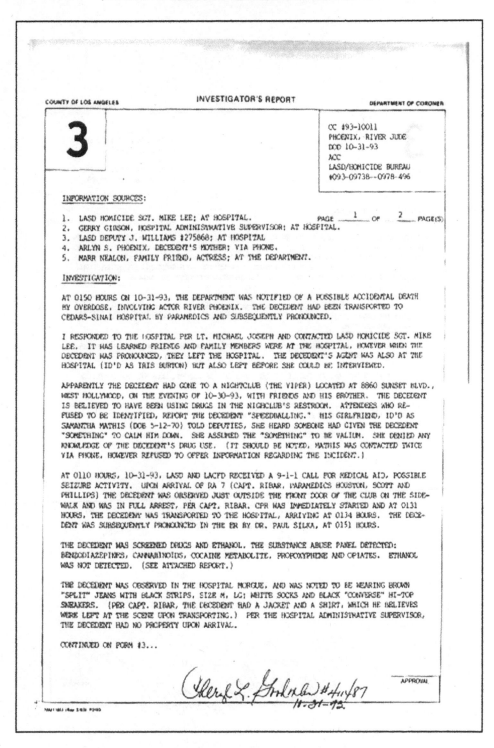

COUNTY OF LOS ANGELES — INVESTIGATOR'S REPORT — DEPARTMENT OF CORONER

3

CC #93-10011
PHOENIX, RIVER JUDE
DOD 10-31-93
ACC
LASD/HOMICIDE BUREAU
#093-09738--0978-496

INFORMATION SOURCES:

PAGE __1__ OF __2__ PAGE(S)

1. LASD HOMICIDE SGT. MIKE LEE; AT HOSPITAL.
2. GERRY GIBSON, HOSPITAL ADMINISTRATIVE SUPERVISOR; AT HOSPITAL.
3. LASD DEPUTY J. WILLIAMS #275868; AT HOSPITAL
4. ARLYN S. PHOENIX, DECEDENT'S MOTHER; VIA PHONE.
5. MARR NEALON, FAMILY FRIEND, ACTRESS; AT THE DEPARTMENT.

INVESTIGATION:

AT 0150 HOURS ON 10-31-93, THE DEPARTMENT WAS NOTIFIED OF A POSSIBLE ACCIDENTAL DEATH
BY OVERDOSE, INVOLVING ACTOR RIVER PHOENIX. THE DECEDENT HAD BEEN TRANSPORTED TO
CEDARS-SINAI HOSPITAL BY PARAMEDICS AND SUBSEQUENTLY PRONOUNCED.

I RESPONDED TO THE HOSPITAL PER LT. MICHAEL JOSEPH AND CONTACTED LASD HOMICIDE SGT. MIKE
LEE. IT WAS LEARNED FRIENDS AND FAMILY MEMBERS WERE AT THE HOSPITAL, HOWEVER WHEN THE
DECEDENT WAS PRONOUNCED, THEY LEFT THE HOSPITAL. THE DECEDENT'S AGENT WAS ALSO AT THE
HOSPITAL (ID'D AS IRIS BURTON) BUT ALSO LEFT BEFORE SHE COULD BE INTERVIEWED.

APPARENTLY THE DECEDENT HAD GONE TO A NIGHTCLUB (THE VIPER) LOCATED AT 8860 SUNSET BLVD.,
WEST HOLLYWOOD, ON THE EVENING OF 10-30-93, WITH FRIENDS AND HIS BROTHER. THE DECEDENT
IS BELIEVED TO HAVE BEEN USING DRUGS IN THE NIGHCLUB'S RESTROOM. ATTENDEES WHO RE-
FUSED TO BE IDENTIFIED, REPORT THE DECEDENT "SPEEDBALLING." HIS GIRLFRIEND, ID'D AS
SAMANTHA MATHIS (DOB 5-12-70) TOLD DEPUTIES, SHE HEARD SOMEONE HAD GIVEN THE DECEDENT
"SOMETHING" TO CALM HIM DOWN. SHE ASSUMED THE "SOMETHING" TO BE VALIUM. SHE DENIED ANY
KNOWLEDGE OF THE DECEDENT'S DRUG USE. (IT SHOULD BE NOTED, MATHIS WAS CONTACTED TWICE
VIA PHONE, HOWEVER REFUSED TO OFFER INFORMATION REGARDING THE INCIDENT.)

AT 0110 HOURS, 10-31-93, LASD AND LACFD RECEIVED A 9-1-1 CALL FOR MEDICAL AID, POSSIBLE
SEIZURE ACTIVITY. UPON ARRIVAL OF RA 7 (CAPT. RIBAR, PARAMEDICS HOUSTON, SCOTT AND
PHILLIPS) THE DECEDENT WAS OBSERVED JUST OUTSIDE THE FRONT DOOR OF THE CLUB ON THE SIDE-
WALK AND WAS IN FULL ARREST. PER CAPT. RIBAR, CPR WAS IMMEDIATELY STARTED AND AT 0131
HOURS, THE DECEDENT WAS TRANSPORTED TO THE HOSPITAL, ARRIVING AT 0134 HOURS. THE DECE-
DENT WAS SUBSEQUENTLY PRONOUNCED IN THE ER BY DR. PAUL SILKA, AT 0151 HOURS.

THE DECEDENT WAS SCREENED DRUGS AND ETHANOL. THE SUBSTANCE ABUSE PANEL DETECTED:
BENZODIAZEPINES, CANNABINOIDS, COCAINE METABOLITE, PROPOXYPHENE AND OPIATES. ETHANOL
WAS NOT DETECTED. (SEE ATTACHED REPORT.)

THE DECEDENT WAS OBSERVED IN THE HOSPITAL MORGUE, AND WAS NOTED TO BE WEARING BROWN
"SPLIT" JEANS WITH BLACK STRIPS, SIZE M, LG; WHITE SOCKS AND BLACK "CONVERSE" HI-TOP
SNEAKERS. (PER CAPT. RIBAR, THE DECEDENT HAD A JACKET AND A SHIRT, WHICH HE BELIEVES
WERE LEFT AT THE SCENE UPON TRANSPORTING.) PER THE HOSPITAL ADMINISTRATIVE SUPERVISOR,
THE DECEDENT HAD NO PROPERTY UPON ARRIVAL.

CONTINUED ON FORM #3...

APPROVAL

Cheryl L. Grolnick #41187
11-31-93

COUNTY OF LOS ANGELES   INVESTIGATOR'S REPORT   DEPARTMENT OF CORONER

3

CC #93-010011
PHOENIX, RIVER JUDE
DOD 10-31-93
ACC
LASD/HOMICIDE BUREAU
#093-09738-0978-496

CONTINUED FROM FORM #3...

PAGE 2 OF 2 PAGE(S)

A BODY EXAMINATION REVEALS FRESH BRUISING TO THE DECEDENT'S LEFT PALM NEAR HIS THUMB, THREE SCABBED OVER ABRASIONS ON THE TOP OF THE RIGHT HAND, ONE FRESH ABRASION ON THE RIGHT INDEX FINGER, FIRST KNUCKLE AND A SCAR ON HIS RIGHT SHIN. ALSO NOTED IS A RED STAR, STAMPED ON THE TOP OF HIS RIGHT HAND. (RECEIVED UPON ENTERING THE NIGHTCLUB.) A LIVER TEMPERATURE WAS TAKEN AT 0337 HOURS SHOWING 99° WITH THE AMBIENT TEMPERATURE AT 68°.

IT SHOULD BE NOTED, THE DECEDENT WAS PRONOUNCED AT 0151 HOURS DAYLIGHT SAVINGS TIME AND WHEN THE LIVER TEMPERATURE WAS TAKEN AT 0337 HOURS, THE TIME THEN CHANGED TO PACIFIC STANDARD TIME.

THE DECEDENT WAS LATER TRANSPORTED FROM THE HOSPITAL TO THE FSC FOR FURTHER EXAMINA- TION. BY J.P. NAVA #412696.

NO OTHER INFORMATION WAS AVAILABLE AT THE TIME OF THE REPORT, HOWEVER THE INVESTIGA- TION BY LASD SGT. LEE AND DET. COMSTOCK IS CONTINUING.

IDENTIFICATION: MADE BY THE DECEDENT'S BROTHER, JOAQIN PHOENIX AT THE SCENE AND BY THE DECEDENT'S AGENT, IRIS BURTON AT THE HOSPITAL.

NOTIFICATION: MADE BY IRIS BURTON AND LATER CONFIRMED BY GOODMAN #411487.

This is a true certified copy of the record
if it bears the seal of the Department of
Coroner imprinted in purple ink.

DIRECTOR
DEPARTMENT OF CORONER
LOS ANGELES COUNTY, CALIFORNIA

#411487
10-31-93

APPROVAL

COUNTY OF LOS ANGELES   **ORDER FOR RELEASE — ORDEN DE ENTEGRA**   **DEPARTMENT OF CORONER**

5

DEPARTMENT OF CORONER   COUNTY OF LOS ANGELES

Please read and answer all questions before signing

WAS THE DECEDENT LEGALLY MARRIED
AT THE TIME OF DEATH? .... no
DOES THE DECEDENT HAVE ANY LIVING CHILDREN? ...... no

Favor de leer y contestar todas las preguntas antes de firmar

¿El Finado tiene hijos vivos? ....
¿El Finado ha sido casado legalmente? ....

Case No.   93-10011
Case Name

PHOENIX, RIVER

Date NOVEMBER 1, 1993

HEALTH AND SAFETY CODE • CHAPTER 3 • CUSTODY AND DUTY OF INTERMENT

7100.   The right to control the disposition of the remains of a deceased person, unless other directions have been given by the decedent, vests in, and the duty of interment and the liability for the reasonable cost of interment of such remains devolves upon the following in the order named: (a) The surviving spouse. (b) The surviving child or children of the decedent. (c) The surviving parent or parents of the decedent. (d) The person or persons respectively in the next degree of kindred in the order named by the laws of California as entitled to succeed to the estate of the decedent. (e) The Public Administrator when the deceased has sufficient assets.

> "WARNING: The person signing this Order for Release is liable for all damages caused by any untruthful statements contained in this document. (Health and Safety Code Section 7100). It is also a criminal offense to knowingly file a false statement with a government agency. (Penal Code Section 115 and 470)" Therefore, please release the body upon completion of your investigation of the death of said deceased on

MORTUARY: Forest Lawn Hollywood Hills

SIGNED X *Arlyn Phoenix*   Relationship mother

Address X 322nd SW 35th Ave. Starneville   State X FL   Zip Code 3468

Telephone No X 904 466-0001   Date Signed November 1, 1993

If not next of kin, sign above and explain why next of kin is not handling. If the executor, attach a copy of the will

Name _____   Relationship _____

Address _____   City _____   State _____   Zip Code _____

CODIGO DE SANIDAD Y SEGURIDAD • CAPITULO 3 • Custodia y Obligacion de Entierro

7100.   El derecho de controlar la disposicion de los restos del finado a menos de que otras instrucciones hayan sido dadas por el finado, dar autoridad, y el deber del entierro y la responsabilidad por el gasto justo de entierro de tales restos para sobre lo siguiente en el orden nombrado, (a) esposo o esposa (b) hijo o hijos del finado (c) padre o padres del finado (d) persona o personas respectivamente en los grados de parentesco es el orden nombrado por las leyes de California como que tiene derecho a suceder al los bienes del finado (e) El Administrador Publico cuando el finado tiene suficientes bienes.

> "AVISO: La persona firmando esta orden para causar es sujeto por todos los perjuicios causados por alguna falsa declaracion contenido en este documento. (Seccion 7100 Del Codigo De Sanidad y Seguridad). Es una ofensa criminal presenta el proposito falsos testimonio con una agencia del gobierno. (Codigo De Pena Section 115 y 470)". Por eso, favor de entregar los restos del finado despues de completar la investigacion a:

FUNERARIA: _____

Firma _____   Parentesco _____

Domicilio _____   Cuidad _____   Estado _____   Zona Postal _____

Telefono _____   Fecha Firmado _____

Si no es el pariente proximo, firme y explique porque el pariente proximo no esta arreglando los tramites en este asunto. Si es el albacea del testamento, incluir una copia del testamento.

Pariente proximo _____   Parentesco _____

Domicilio _____   Cuidad _____   Estado _____   Zona Postal _____

DECEDENT INFORMATION ON REVERSE

COUNTY OF LOS ANGELES — **CASE REPORT** — **DEPARTMENT OF CORONER**

1

APPARENT MODE: NAT **ACC** SUI HOMI

☐ STATE HOSP ☐ O.I.S. ☐ AUTOPSY VIEW/ID ☐ CLOSELY WATCHED ☐ VICTIMS OF CRIME
☐ IN CUSTODY ☐ AT WORK ☐ LAW ENFORCEMENT RELATED

OFFICE CIRCUMSTANCES: COCAINE/HEROIN OVERDOSE

CASE NO: 93-10011

CRPT: 63

LAST, FIRST, MIDDLE / AKA: PHOENIX, RIVER JUDE

ADDRESS: 8916 ASHCROFT AVE CITY: LOS ANGELES STATE: CA 90211

SEX: M RACE: C DOB: 8-23-70 AGE: 23 HGT: 70 WGT: 149 EYES: GRN HAIR: BRN TEETH: OWN IS BODY VIEWABLE: (6) CONDITION: VIEWABLE ☐ EMBALMED

SCARS: RIGHT SHIN TATTOOS AMPUTATIONS DEFORMITIES

ARWN SHARON PHOENIX 8916 ASHCROFT AVE CITY: LA STATE: 90211
RELATIONSHIP: MOTHER PHONE: 310/652-0954 NOTIFIED BY: IRIS BURTON (AGENT) DATE: 10-31-93 TIME:

SSN: 571-61-9058 DL STATE: CA #C8566314 LT MILING EMPT MILITARY C/O: N/A

ID BY (PRINT NAME): JOAQUIN PHOENIX (AT SCENE - TO DEP. E. WILLIAMS #310868) RELATIONSHIP: BROTHER PHONE: DATE: 10-31-93

PLACE OF DEATH: CEDARS-SINAI MEDICAL CENTER ADDRESS OR LOCATION: 8700 BEVERLY BLVD LOS ANGELES 90048

PLACE OF INJURY: NIGHT CLUB AT WORK: 10-31- TIME: 10-31-93 UNK LOCATION OR ADDRESS: 8860 SUNSET BLVD, W. HLYWD

DOD: 10-31-93 PROD: 0151 TIME: PRON. BY: DR. PAUL SILKA

AGENCY & INV. OFFICER: LASO/HOMICIDE SGT. MICHAEL J. LEE #052808 PHONE: 213/974-4341 REPORT NO: #L93-04938-0971 LOCATED: 1/96

DESCRIBE SCENE AND CONTACT MATERIAL TO BODY: HOSPITALIZED CASE WAS BODY EXAM: YES G-NO
TRANSPORTED FROM SCENE TO HOSPITAL.

	TIME	DATE		
AIR 68 ▾	0330	10-31-93	DESCRIBE LIVOR MORTIS: AS POSITIONED ON HOSPITAL TRAY; BLANCHING W/ LT PRESSURE.
LIVER 99 ▾	0337	10-31-93	DESCRIBE RIGOR MORTIS: PRESENT IN WRISTS, ELBOWS AND LOWER EXTREMITIES.
WATER N/A ▾	N/A	N/A	TRANSPORTED BY: JPNAVA #412696 DATE: 10-31-93

PRINTS: ☒ ☐ CLOTHING: ☒ ☐ PA RPT D #69 ☒ NO AUT-SEM FUNERAL CONTAINERS MORTUARY: N/A
MED EV: ☐ ☒ INVEST. PHOTO ③ ☒ ☐ HOSP. RPT: YES ☒ NO ☐
PHYS EV: ☐ ☒ T.S. PHOTO ☐ ☒ HOSP. CHART: YES ☒ NO ☐
SUICIDE NOTE: ☐ ☒ GSR/AB: N/A ROM NO: 117745/116685 PF NO: ER 565717

THE DECEDENT APPARENTLY HAD GONE TO "THE VIPER" NIGHTCLUB LOCATED AT 8860 SUNSET BLVD, WEST HOLLYWOOD, WITH FRIENDS AND A FAMILY MEMBER. WHILE AT THE CLUB, ATTENDEES REPORT THE DECEDENT "SPEEDBALLING" AND THEN TAKING VALIUM. IT'S BELIEVED THE DECEDENT POSSIBLY COLLAPSED WHILE INSIDE THE CLUB, HOWEVER WHEN DEPUTIES AND PARAMEDICS WERE NOTIFIED, DECEDENT WAS TAKEN OUTSIDE. PARAMEDICS WERE NOTIFIED AT 0110 HOURS, TRANSPORTED, ARRIVED AT HOSPITAL AT 0134 HOURS. (SEE FORM #3.)

Cheryl L. Godreau #411487 INVESTIGATOR DATE: 10-31-93 DATE: 11-1-93 TIME: 0411 APPROVAL: DMS

Sharon Tate

Given Name: Sharon Marie Tate
Born: January 24, 1943, Dallas, Texas
Died: August 9, 1969, Los Angeles, California
Cause of Death: Stabbing

Sharon Tate was a Hollywood actress most famous for her Golden Globe–nominated role in *Valley of the Dolls*. She was married to director Roman Polanski and pregnant with a boy when she was brutally stabbed to death in her home along with four other victims. Tate was stabbed by members of the Manson Family cult.

Crypt # _17_

COUNTY OF LOS ANGELES
OFFICE OF CHIEF MEDICAL EXAMINER-CORONER

CASE REPORT

Case No. _69-8796_

REPORTED AS:
- [ ] Natural
- [ ] Accident
- [ ] Suicide
- [x] Homicide
- [ ] Undetermined
- [ ] In Custody
- [ ] Nursing Home
- [ ] At Work

Place of Scene: _____

Taken by _____

gsp stabbing

Post Mortem or _Med. Exam_ _____ Request of _____

NAME _Sharon Tate Polanski_ Occupation _actress_ AGE _25_ Sex _F_ Race _W_

Place of Death _10050 Cielo Dr. - L.A._

Reported by _L. Helder_ Address _Cent. Home_ Phone _____

Due _8-9-69_ Time _1_ A.M./P.M. Pronounced Dead _L.A.P.D. patrol_ Date and Time of Death _8-9-69 9:10 A.M._

Investigating Agency _Cent. Home_

Officer _Henderson_ Due _8-9-69_ Time _2:00_ A.M./P.M. Hospital No. _____

Residence of Deceased _above_ Religion _____

Employer _none_ Name _____ Military No. _____ Vet. _____

Next of Kin _____ Address _out of town_ Phone _____

Relationship _husband_ Notified by _Stanley Tanberg - atty - MA 0266_ at _____ A.M./P.M.

Weight _136_ lbs. Height _66_ in. Hair _blond_ Teeth _white_ Eyes _blue_ Mustache _____

Beard _____ Tattoo or Deformity _stab wounds_ Body Condition _keyed_

Prints [x] Yes [ ] No
Property [x] Yes [ ] No
Clothing [x] Yes [ ] No
Door Sealed [ ] Yes [x] No

Brought in by _Dr. Henry Johnson & Tanberg_ Due _8-9-69 4_ P.M. _place guard on premises_

REMARKS: _Continued -_

OBTAIN appropriate blood at autopsy

_____ Deputy

COUNTY OF LOS ANGELES
OFFICE OF CHIEF MEDICAL EXAMINER—CORONER
MEDICAL REPORT

Name: _Sharon Tate Polanski_   Case No. _69-8796_

Date: _8-9-69_   Dr. _____

CONTINUATION SHEET

apparently entertaining a mixed group of 4 young people at this Cielo Drive excessively artist garde, ranch - estate type home. The party was noticed by neighbors down the street and nearby during mid afternoon into early evening 8-8-69.

At about 12 am 8-9-69 a nearby neighbor reported later he heard a sound of shot echo noise kills. Approximately 9:00 am 8-9-69 house hold maid reported for duty to find a scene of apparent carnage. House doors opened & some lights yet on, windows ajar. An inscription in blood upon front door. One apparently dead body seated in drivers seat of late model Rambler Ambassador parked in parking area at entrance gate (John Doe 85) (69-8792)

Another apparently dead body (69-8793) crumpled to lawn in front of veranda. Body dressed casually for occasion (M/S) The third apparently dead body on lawn about 60 feet south of (69-8793) lying on back and dressed apparently for sleep). This labeled case # 69-8794. (N/C)

Two bodies - a man (69-8795) and woman - decedent were found in living room in front of each fire place at foot of large sofa. Bodies on floor. Man in casual party dress and decedent in bra and briefs (F/S) A long possibly ¾ in nylon cord was looped about each of these persons necks and also looped over a supporting beam of sleeping loft over head. A bath towel apparently placed over head of man prior to looping of rope about neck.

A caretaker - occupying small house at end of large lot and some what away from house had entertained a young man visitor in evening to about 12-5 a.m. 8-9-69 when this young man took leave. The John Doe 85 in auto may possibly have been this same young man. The caretaker being questioned by police appeared unaware of apparent action about the premises at time appeared similar

— Continued —

COUNTY OF LOS ANGELES
OFFICE OF CHIEF MEDICAL EXAMINER—CORONER
MEDICAL REPORT

Name: _Sharon Tate Polanski_   Case No: _69-8796_

Date: _8-9-69_   Dr. _____

CONTINUATION SHEET

Signs of struggle appeared localized in center of living room where decedent and 69-8795 lay upon blood soaked carpeting and amid broken bric-a-brac. Blood on flagstone on front porch covering an area of about 2'x2' and dried. Small amount blood in open garage at parking lot as also a small amount on possible foot smear upon back steps leading to swimming pool at rear of house and adjacent to body (69-8794)

No weapons nor suspects in custody. Central-homicide witnessing autopsy.

Smith

OBTAIN BLOOD AT AUTOPSY

FILE 069-0796
SHARON TATE POLANSKY
AUGUST 10, 1969

2

EXTERNAL FINDINGS:

The unembalmed body is that of a 26 year old, well developed, well nourished Caucasian female, weighing 136 pounds, measuring 66 inches in length. Her hair is blond and eyes are brown.

The examination of the head discloses no evidence of trauma. The forehead, nose, eyelids, right cheek, lips and chin show no ecchymosis or abrasions. Dark red fluid blood is found in the nostrils, but not in the ear canals. Ears are not remarkable. The back of the head is not remarkable. The left side of the face discloses a somewhat linear but slightly curved interrupted slightly irregular abrasion, associated with ecchymosis.

Two abrasions are situated in a horizontal fashion. The upper abrasion measures 2-1/2 inches and the lower 1-1/2 inches. A careful examination of the abrasions reveal interrupted dark red superficial recent loss of epidermis. The upper abrasion extends from the left naris to the lower edge of the zygomatic bone. The abrasion extends slightly upward along the curvature of the posterior aspect of the zygomatic bone. The lower abrasion is on a level of the left side of the maxillary. The left side of the neck shows a faint superficial abrasion, measuring 3 inches in length, extending from the lateral aspect of the upper larynx across the lateral aspect of the neck to the occipital area. This abrasion shows minute irregular skin peeling, suggesting this may be caused by fingernail scraping.

STAB WOUNDS

There are four stab wounds on the chest. Those stab wounds are labeled #1, #2, #3, and #4 for the purpose of identification, and others labeled #5 through #16 are described in a subsequent report.

Stab wound #1 is located in the mid-chest and is located 1-1/2 inches below the nipple line. The stab wound measures 1 inch in length and the edges are sharp. The angulation of the left upper portion shows sharp cutting and the right lower angulation is relatively dull. The dull edge shows a definite tearing appearance, exposing subcutaneous tissue. The sharp angulated area shows slight incisional extension. The probe is inserted through the stab wound in the direction of the stab wound, which is from the front to the back 45° upward and left to right. The probe through the stab wound reaches the left pleural cavity.

Stab wound #2 is located on the left side of the mid-chest and it measures 1-3/4 inches in length. The edges are sharp and the stab wound is located slightly obliquely and sharp angulation is noted in the left upper corner and dull angulation is noted in the right lower portion. The direction of the stab wound is parallel to the direction of stab wound #1.

FILE #69-8796
SHARON TATE POLANSKY
AUGUST 10, 1969

3

Stab wound #3 is located on the left side of the lower chest and is located 3-1/4 inches to the left of the midline, 3-1/2 inches below the nipple line, and 18 inches from the top of the head. The direction of the stab wound is slightly upward, right to left and front to back. A careful examination of this stab wound reveals a sharp edge on the upper portion and a slight dull edge on the lower portion of the stab wound and has a slight rim of abrasion. Stab wound #3 measures 1-1/2 inches in length.

Stab wounds #1, #2 and #3 are located in a close proximity. The distance between #1 and #2 is 1 inch, the distance between #1 and #3 is 1/2 inch, and the distance between #2 and #3 is 2 inches.

Stab wound #4 is located in the upper, outer quadrant of the left breast. It measures 1 inch in length and the stab wound is located in a horizontal fashion. The direction of the stab wound is from left to right in a horizontal fashion. The edges of the stab wound are also sharp.

Authorized personnel present during the autopsy. Sgt. McGuinn of Los Angeles Police Department, Homicide Bureau, and Mr. John Miner, Deputy District Attorney, are present. Autopsy Assistant is Mr. Charles Moore.

Specimens:

1. Sections of vital organs are saved in jars containing formalin solution.
2. Three separate jars are properly labeled and contain elipsical sections of skin showing the stab wounds five (5), seven (7) and eleven (11).
3. Liver, kidney, stomach and other substances are saved.
4. Vaginal smears and smears from the other locations are also made.

Thomas T. Noguchi, M.D.
Chief Medical Examiner-Coroner

TTN:cs

OFFICE OF CHIEF MEDICAL EXAMINER-CORONER

File: #a2736

Date: August 10, 1969 Time: _____

Autopsy begins 11:30 A.M.; completes 2:00 P/M

I performed an autopsy on the body of **SHARON TATE POLANSKY,**

Autopsy Room, County of Los Angeles,
Office of Chief Medical Examiner-Coroner

and from the anatomic findings and pertinent history I ascribe the death to:

Multiple stab wounds of chest and back penetrating heart, lungs, and liver causing massive hemorrhage.

Summary of Wounds:

```
Total stab wounds .............................. 16
        Chest ........................4
        Abdomen ......................1
        Back .........................8
        Right upper arm ..........1
        Left upper arm ...........1
        Right thigh (back of).....1
```

Total incised wounds (left forearm)............... 2

Fatal stab wounds:

Stab wound #1
1. Location - left pericardial area penetrating 4th intercostal space, pericardium, left ventricle of heart covering the descending branch of left coronary artery.
2. Size - 1 1/2 inches long x 4 inches deep sharp cutting edge.
3. Direction - front to back
             left to right
             45° upward

Stab wound #2
1. Location - left side of mid chest penetrating 4th intercostal space, pericardium, heart
2. Size - 1 3/4 inches x 4 inches deep
3. Direction - front to back
             left to right

Stab wound #3
1. Location - left side of lower chest penetrating 6th rib (cartilagenous portion), pericardium, heart
2. Size - 1 1/2 inches x about 4 inches deep

Stab wounds #1, 2 and 3 caused extensive hemorrhage in left pleural cavity and pericardium.

THOMAS T. NOGUCHI, M.D.
CHIEF MEDICAL EXAMINER-CORONER

REPORT OF MICROBIOLOGICAL ANALYSIS
CHIEF MEDICAL EXAMINER-CORONER'S OFFICE
Bacteriology Laboratory
Hall of Justice
Los Angeles, California

File No. 69-8796

Name of Deceased   Sharon Polanski

Date Submitted   8/10/69

Autopsy Surgeon   M.G. Henry, M.D.

Material Submitted   Blood for ABO and Rh typing.

Laboratory Findings:

BLOOD: Group O Rh positive.

Examined By _____   Date 8/25/69

REPORT OF MICROBIOLOGICAL ANALYSIS
CHIEF MEDICAL EXAMINER-CORONER'S OFFICE
Bacteriology Laboratory
Hall of Justice
Los Angeles, California

File No. 09-8796

Name of Deceased___Sharon Polanski

Date Submitted___8/10/69

Autopsy Surgeon___T. Noguchi, M.D.

Material Submitted___Oral and rectal smears for spermatozoa and

acid phosphatase.

Laboratory Findings:

acid phosphatase nonreactive.
Positive control reactive 4+.
Negative control nonreactive.
No spermatozoa found on smears.

Examined By _Roderick H. Baker_ Date_8/11/69

REPORT OF CHEMICAL ANALYSIS
LOS ANGELES COUNTY MEDICAL EXAMINER CORONER
Toxicology Laboratory
Hall of Justice
Los Angeles, California

File No. 69-8796

Name of Deceased ___Sharon Tate Polanski___ Lab No. 8-146-69

Date Submitted ___August 11, 1969___ Time ___8 A.M.___

Autopsy Surgeon ___Thomas T. Noguchi, M.D.___

Material Submitted:
Blood: X   Liver: X   Stomach: X
Brain   Lung   Lavage
Femur   Spleen   Urine
Kidney X   Sternum   Gall bladder
Drugs   Chemicals

Test Desired: Poisons

Laboratory Findings:

1. Blood: Ethanol, Barbiturates, Doriden, Meprobamate,
           Phenacetin, and Soma absent

   Kidney: Amphetamine and Methedrine absent

   Kidney: Methylene dioxy amphetamine absent

2. Kidney: Codeine and Morphine absent

Examined By ___Jack Tillery___ Toxicologist   Date ___August 21, 1969___

___2. L. Park___   Toxicologist   August 21, 1969

COUNTY OF LOS ANGELES
OFFICE OF CHIEF MEDICAL EXAMINER—CORONER
BODY FULL LENGTH ANTERIOR

NAME SHARON TATE POLANSKI Aug 10 1969 File 69-8796

LIVIDITY

STAB WOUND #2

STAB WOUND #1

STAB WOUND #4

STAB WOUND #5

STAB WOUND #3

R

Lo

LIVIDITY

scar

FAINT ecchymosis

small crusted abrasion

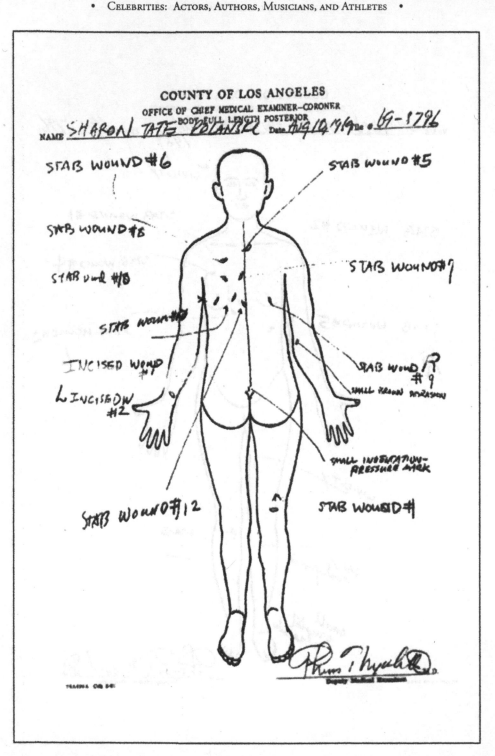

COUNTY OF LOS ANGELES

OFFICE OF CHIEF MEDICAL EXAMINER—CORONER

HEAD - LATERAL LEFT

NAME: SHARON TATE POLANSKI Date Aug 10, 1969 File 69-8296

2-½" Dep
chin

1-½"
long

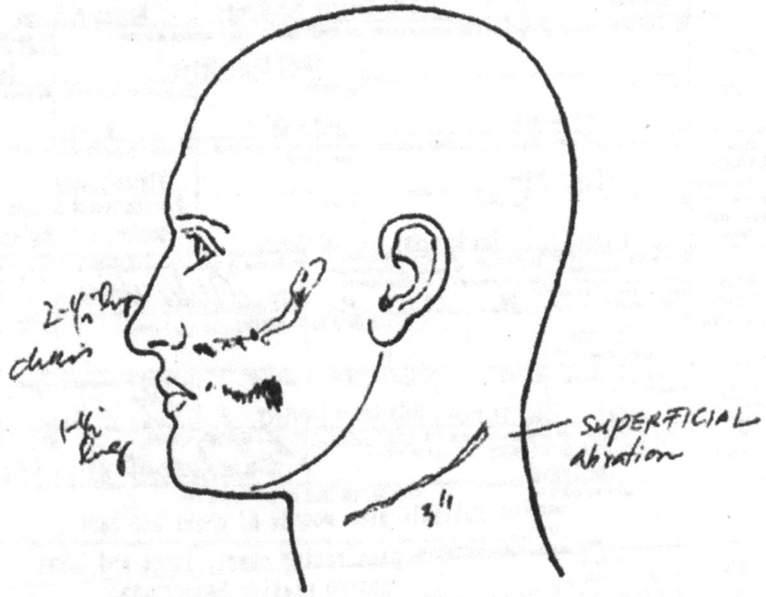

SUPERFICIAL
abration

3"

LEFT

CERTIFICATE OF DEATH

STATE OF CALIFORNIA—DEPARTMENT OF PUBLIC HEALTH

7097-049961

| | Sharon | Tate | Polanski | AUG. 9, 1969 | 9:10 A.M. |
| Female | Caucasian | Texas | January 24, 1943 | 26 | |

DECEDENT PERSONAL DATA

Paul Tate; Texas

Doris Willett, Texas

U.S.A.   452-74-4733   Married   Roman Polanski

Actress   7   20th Century Fox Studio   Motion Pictures

PLACE OF DEATH

10050 Cielo Drive   Yes

Los Angeles   Los Angeles   6   6

USUAL RESIDENCE

10050 Cielo Drive   Yes   Victor Lownes, 1 Connaught Square, London, W. 2, England

Los Angeles   Los Angeles   California

PHYSICIAN'S OR CORONER'S CERTIFICATION

INVESTIGATION

FUNERAL DIRECTOR AND LOCAL REGISTRAR

Burial   Aug. 13, 1969   Holy Cross Cemetery

Cunningham & O'Connor, Hollywood

CAUSE OF DEATH

Multiple stab wounds of chest and back

penetrating heart, lungs and liver causing massive hemorrhage.

BURIAL INFORMATION

STATE REGISTRAR

Billy Mays

Given Name: William Darrell Mays, Jr.
Born: July 20, 1958, McKees Rocks, Pennsylvania
Died: June 28, 2009, Tampa, Florida
Cause of Death: Hypertensive and Atherosclerotic Heart Disease

Billy Mays was most notable for promoting various products like OxiClean, Orange Glo, and Kaboom on America's Home Shopping Network. Mays was found unresponsive in his home in Tampa, Florida, by his wife. The medical examiner concluded that cocaine use had contributed to the development of his heart disease—a claim that was disputed by Mays' family.

HILLSBOROUGH COUNTY, FLORIDA

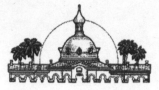

MEDICAL EXAMINER DEPARTMENT
11025 NORTH 46TH STREET
TAMPA, FLORIDA 33617
813-914-4500

Report of Diagnosis and Autopsy
on

William Darrell Mays

File 09-04082

File: 09-04082

2

OPINION

Final Diagnosis:

Atherosclerotic and hypertensive heart disease
    Left ventricular myocardial hypertrophy
    Coronary atherosclerosis
Cocaine use
Narcotic analgesia for avascular necrosis of hip
  (anamnestic)
Intracranial pseudoaneurysm at the optic chiasm
Sigmoid diverticulosis

Cause of Death:

Hypertensive and Atherosclerotic Heart Disease

Contributory Cause of Death:

Cocaine Use

Manner of Death:

Natural

Leszek Chrostowski, M.D.,
Associate Medical Examiner

Date Signed

File: 09-04082

Death: 28 Jun 2009 at 0753 hrs 5823 Bowen Daniel Dr. #1204 *Age:* 50 years	*Autopsy:* 29 Jun 2009 11025 North 46th St, Tampa *Performed by:* Leszek Chrostowski, M.D.

DESCRIPTION OF AUTOPSY FINDINGS

EXTERNAL EXAMINATION: 29 June 2009 at 0850 hours

The body is that of a well developed and nourished adult white man with a large-boned, muscular body habitus, appearing the stated length of 6'0", and compatible with the reported age.

Condition of the Body: The body is cold to touch, with fully developed rigor mortis. Livor mortis is fixed, purple-red, and extends over the anterior surfaces of the body where it is associated with multiple Tardieu spots. On the face, the livor mortis is on the right side. There is also fixed livor mortis on the posterior aspect of the body. The body is neither decomposed, nor embalmed.

Identifying Marks: The body has no tattoos. Scars are described below.

Head and Face: The scalp hair is black with gray roots, straight, and measures 6 centimeters in maximal length. Facial hair consists of approximately 2 centimeters long beard and mustache, also black; there is gray stubble on the neck anteriorly.

Eyes: The irides are brown. The pupils have equal diameter. The corneae are clouded and have mild corneal arches. The conjunctivae are congested due to livor mortis, with rare Tardieu spots in the palpebral portions. The sclerae are white. The upper eyelid of the left eye medially has a small subconjunctival yellow-white nodule measuring 0.3 x 0.2 x 0.1 centimeters.

Nose: The external nares contain a small amount of dried bloody purge. The nasal skeleton is palpably intact.

Mouth: The lips have no injuries. The oral cavity has natural dentition in good repair, and contains a small amount of white foam. The oral mucosa is congested, and has intact frenula, no injuries, and no petechial hemorrhages in the oral vestibule. It is lined with clear mucus.

Ears: The external ears are free of foreign material. The earlobes are not pierced.

Neck: The neck is symmetrical and unremarkable, with no palpable masses or external injuries.

Chest: The thorax is well developed and symmetrical.

Abdomen: The abdomen is somewhat protuberant and soft, and has no palpable masses. The right side of the abdomen in the inguinal region at the right iliac crest has an acrochordon that measures 1.1 x 0.7 x 0.6 centimeters.

External Genitalia: The external genitalia are those of a normal adult uncircumcised man, with no injuries. The testes are descended into the scrotal sac and are unremarkable to palpation.

Lower Extremities: The lower extremities are symmetrical and have no anatomic abnormalities. The right thigh on the anterolateral aspect distally has a red abrasion that measures 0.6 x 0.2 centimeters. The posterolateral aspect of the left thigh proximally, i.e. the left hip area, has an oblique scar that measures 8 centimeters in length and is slightly erythematous.

Upper Extremities: The arms, forearms, wrists, and hands have no anatomic abnormalities. The fingernails are intact.

Back: The back is unremarkable. The anus has no abnormalities.

Therapy: Four electrocardiogram electrodes are adherent to the skin, including one posterolaterally on the left shoulder, one on the right side of the back in the scapular area, and one on each leg on the left lateral aspect.

INTERNAL EXAMINATION: 29 June 2009 at 0910 hours

Head: The galea aponeurotica is unremarkable. The vault and the base of the skull have no fractures. There are no epidural or subdural hemorrhages. The dura mater and falx cerebri are intact. The brain weighs 1,550 grams and has symmetrical cerebral hemispheres. The external surfaces of the brain are not edematous. The arachnoid membranes are thin and delicate, with congested arachnoid vessels, and conceal clear, unremarkable cerebrospinal fluid. The cranial nerves are intact. Just anteriorly to the optic chiasm in the mid sagittal plane is a nodule measuring approximately 1.0 centimeters in diameter; its cut surfaces reveal a cystic globular lesion filled with tan-red mass resembling thrombus.

The cyst does not have any grossly apparent attachment to any nearby blood vessel, and is tightly adherent to the surface of the optic chiasm, which is slightly attenuated. The cyst is also not attached to the infundibulum of the pituitary gland; it is anterior and inferior to the optic chiasm, pushing the chiasm's anterior portion slightly upward. The cerebral arteries have no atherosclerosis. The cut surfaces of the cerebral hemispheres, brainstem, and cerebellum have no structural lesions. The cerebral ventricles are of normal caliber and shape.

Neck: The cervical spine, laryngeal cartilages, and hyoid bone have no fractures or other abnormalities. The strap muscles of the neck have no hemorrhages. The tongue is normal, with no hemorrhages, bite marks, or other lesions. The epiglottic and laryngeal mucosa has no petechiae or edema, and is lined with clear mucus.

Body Cavities: The serosal cavities have no adhesions or abnormal collections of fluid. The pneumothorax test is negative. The organs are congested, in normal anatomic positions, and have no decomposition.

Cardiovascular: The aorta has mild to moderate atherosclerosis, with plaques occupying an estimated 10-15% of the intimal surface in the abdominal portion of the vessel; the plaques are small, but have calcific complications. A 2 x 1.6 centimeter plaque just proximal to the bifurcation of aorta has calcification with ulceration and a small mural thrombus. The venae cavae and their major tributaries return to the heart in the usual distribution and are unremarkable, with no thrombosis. The pulmonary trunk and pulmonary arteries are patent, have no thromboemboli, and have smooth intimal surfaces. The medium size arteries are unremarkable. The large vessels are not distended and contain partially clotted dark red blood.

The heart weighs 580 grams. The weight increase is due to concentric left ventricular myocardial hypertrophy. The epicardial surfaces are smooth and glistening. The coronary arteries arise normally, have patent orifices, and follow a right dominant distribution. The proximal portion of the anterior descending artery has an eccentric, yellow, focally calcified atherosclerotic plaque; it is 1.8 centimeters long and results in a focal stenosis estimated at up to 75%. The remaining coronary arteries have no significant atherosclerosis. The myocardial cut surfaces are firm, brown-red, and have no grossly distinguishable focal lesions. The

parietal and valvular endocardium is smooth, thin and unremarkable. The valvular rings, leaflets and cusps are normal. The atrial and ventricular septa are intact. The chambers of the heart are not dilated. The thickness of myocardium measures 1.7 centimeters at the left ventricular wall, 1.6 centimeter at the interventricular septum, and 0.4 to 0.5 centimeters at the right ventricular wall.

Pulmonary: The upper and lower airways are patent and are lined with clear mucus. The distal bronchial tree contains a small amount of froth. The bronchial mucosal surfaces are yellow-red, smooth, and have no petechiae. The right and left lungs weigh 1,230 and 950 grams, respectively. They have smooth pleural surfaces. The cut surfaces of the pulmonary parenchyma are red, congested and sodden, have no discrete lesions, and exude a large amount of bloody liquid and froth. The pulmonary arteries have smooth intimal surfaces and no thromboemboli.

Hepatobiliary System: The liver weighs 3,380 grams and has a smooth intact capsule. The liver parenchyma is moderately firm, brown-red, congested, and has no lesions except for a few areas of very mild patchy yellow discoloration visible on the cut surfaces. The gallbladder contains a measured 22 milliliters of viscid green bile. Its mucosa is velvety and unremarkable. The extrahepatic biliary tree is patent. The pancreas has tan-brown lobulated parenchyma, clear ducts, and no lesions. It weighs 160 grams.

Hemic and Lymphatic: The spleen weighs 250 grams and has a smooth, intact capsule. The cut surfaces of the splenic parenchyma are dark maroon, very soft, almost liquefied, with inapparent lymphoid follicles. The lymph nodes and tonsils are not enlarged and have unremarkable cut surfaces. The vertebral marrow is red and homogenous, with no gross evidence of abnormalities. The thymus is fat replaced.

Genitourinary: The right kidney weighs 300 grams and the left 310 grams. The kidneys have smooth, thin renal capsules that strip with ease. The cortical surfaces are brown-red and smooth. The cortices are congested, well delineated from the underlying medullary pyramids, and have no lesions. The calyces, pelves, and ureters are not dilated and have unremarkable lining mucosa. There is no significant increase of hilar adipose tissue in the kidneys. The urinary bladder contains a measured 200 milliliters of cloudy yellow urine. Its mucosa is white-tan, smooth, slightly trabecular, and has no lesions. The urethra is unremarkable.

File: 09-04082   7

The prostate gland is of normal size and has monomorphic cut
surfaces. The seminal vesicles, testes and spermatic cords
have unremarkable cut surfaces, with no hemorrhages or other
abnormalities.

Endocrine: The pituitary and adrenal glands have no
abnormalities. The thyroid gland weighs 20 grams, is red,
congested, and has granular cut surfaces with no lesions.

Digestive: The esophagus is lined by smooth gray-white mucosa,
with no lesions. The gastric mucosa has the usual rugal
folds. The stomach lumen contains a measured 600 milliliters
of gray liquid with non-identifiable particulate food. The
duodenum has no lesions. The small and large bowels are
unremarkable except for a few small diverticuli in the
sigmoid colon, with no inflammation. The vermiform appendix
is without note.

Musculoskeletal: The clavicles, sternum, spine, ribs, and pelvis
have no fractures or other abnormalities. The musculature is
normally developed.

LC:kr   06/30/09

MICROSCOPIC DESCRIPTION

Heart: Myocyte hypertrophy. Focal moderate interstitial
fibrosis, mostly perivascular. Moderate hyperplastic
arteriolosclerosis, i.e. hypertensive small vessel disease.
No inflammation or infarction.

Lung: Congestion and edema. Autolytic changes and post mortem
bacterial overgrowth. Scattered deposits of anthracotic
pigment. No inflammation.

Liver: No significant histologic change; a few lymphoid
aggregates in the portal regions.

Cystic lesion from the anterior cranial fossa: Cystic structure filled with
degraded red blood cells, ranging from intact erythrocytes to
amorphous eosinophilic material, partially hyalinized and
with dystrophic calcifications. Its fibrous capsule has
hemosiderin deposits, hemosiderophages, and perivascular
lympho-plasmocytic infiltrates. The structure has a pushing
border; the adjacent nervous tissue is unremarkable. Special
stains reveal no elastic fibers in the cyst wall. Consistent
with pseudoaneurysm.

File: 09-04082   8

HISTOLOGICAL INDEX

Slide 1, 4, 5, 6:   Heart.

Slide 2:   Cystic lesion from anterior cranial fossa.

Slide 3:   Heart, lung, liver.

Slide 7:   Anterior descending coronary artery.

Slide 8, 9:   Lungs.

LC

— End of Autopsy Report; Toxicology Report is Appended —

HILLSBOROUGH COUNTY, FLORIDA

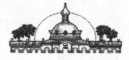

MEDICAL EXAMINER DEPARTMENT
TOXICOLOGY REPORT

July 27, 2009

Name of decedent:	Mays, William Darrell	**Case No:**	09-04082
Medical examiner:	Leszek Chrostowski, MD	**Date of autopsy:**	29 June 2009

The following toxicology procedures were performed:

Procedure	Specimen type
Volatiles by GC/MS	Ocular Fluid
Volatiles by GC/MS	Peripheral Blood
ELISA	Heart Blood
Thin Layer Chromatography	Urine
Opiates by LCMS	Heart Blood
Cocaine and metabolites by LCMS	Peripheral Blood
Cocaine and metabolites by LCMS	Ocular Fluid
Cocaine and metabolites by LCMS	Urine
Cocaine and metabolites by GCMS (via Wuesthoff)	Urine
Benzodiazepines by GCMS (via Wuesthoff)	Peripheral Blood
Benzodiazepines by GCMS (via Wuesthoff)	Urine
Tramadol by GCMS (via Wuesthoff)	Peripheral Blood

The following substances were detected and confirmed:

Substance	Concentration	Specimen type	Method
Ethanol	0.07 g/dL	Ocular Fluid	GCMS
Ethanol	0.05 g/dL	Peripheral Blood	GCMS
Hydrocodone (Free)	<0.02 mg/L	Heart Blood	LCMS
Hydrocodone (Total)	0.03 mg/L	Heart Blood	LCMS
Oxycodone (Free)	0.14 mg/L	Heart Blood	LCMS
Oxycodone (Total)	0.16 mg/L	Heart Blood	LCMS
Tramadol	0.07 mg/L	Peripheral Blood	GCMS
Alprazolam	0.05 mg/L	Peripheral Blood	GCMS

Substance	Concentration	Specimen type	Method
Diazepam	0.12 mg/L	Peripheral Blood	GCMS
Nordiazepam	0.18 mg/L	Peripheral Blood	GCMS
Benzoylecgonine	0.02 mg/L	Peripheral Blood	LCMS
Benzoylecgonine	0.06 mg/L	Ocular Fluid	LCMS
Benzoylecgonine	2.0 mg/L	Urine	LCMS
Benzoylecgonine	1.8 mg/L	Urine	GCMS
Ecgonine Methyl Ester	0.46 mg/L	Urine	GCMS
Alpha-Hydroxyalprazolam	0.41 mg/L	Urine	GCMS
Alprazolam	0.27 mg/L	Urine	GCMS
Nordiazepam	0.16 mg/L	Urine	GCMS
Temazepam	0.35 mg/L	Urine	GCMS

The following volatiles were not detected or confirmed:

Acetone

Isopropanol

Methanol

The following drugs were not detected or confirmed:

6MAM	Fentanyl	Olanzapine
Amphetamines	Fluoxetine	Oxazepam
Barbiturates	Hydromorphone	Oxymorphone
Cannabinoids	Ketamine	Paroxetine
Chlordiazepoxide	Lorazepam	Phencyclidine
Cocaethylene	Meperidine	Propoxyphene
Cocaine	Methadone	Romifidine
Codeine	Methamphetamine	Sertraline
Desalkylflurazepam	Midazolam	Tricyclic Antidepressants
Dextromethorphan	Morphine	

Julia M. Pearson, PhD, DABFT   Date

Chief Forensic Toxicologist

Key to abbreviations	
ELISA	Enzyme-linked immunosorbant assay
GCMS	Gas chromatography mass spectrometry
LCMS	Liquid chromatography mass spectrometry

Anna Nicole Smith

Given Name: Vickie Lynn Hogan
Born: November 28, 1967, Houston, Texas
Died: February 8, 2007, Hollywood, Florida
Cause of Death: Drug Overdose

Anna Nicole Smith was a model, actress, and reality TV star. Most famous for her reality show *The Anna Nicole Show*, she was also a model for *Playboy* and a spokesman for Trimspa diet pills. Smith was the widow of an oil tycoon and the age difference between her and her eighty-nine-year-old husband caused controversy at the time of their wedding. Smith died in her hotel room in Florida. Her death is attributed to an accidental combination of sleeping pills and other prescription drugs.

BROWARD COUNTY MEDICAL EXAMINER
5301 SW 31st AVENUE
FORT LAUDERDALE, FL 33312

NAME: Vickie Lynn Marshall **AUTOPSY NO:** 07-0223
SEX: Female **DATE OF AUTOPSY:** February 9, 2007
RACE: White **TIME OF AUTOPSY:** 10:36 a.m.
AGE: 39 **PROSECTORS:** Gertrude M. Juste, M.D.
DOB: 11/28/1967 Associate Medical Examiner
and
Joshua A. Perper, M.D.
Chief Medical Examiner

FINAL PATHOLOGICAL DIAGNOSES:

I. ACUTE COMBINED DRUG INTOXICATION
A. Toxic/lethal drug:
   Chloral Hydrate (Noctec)
   1. Trichloroethanol (TCE) 75ug/mL (active metabolite)
   2. Trichloroacetic acid (TCA) 85ug/mL (inactive metabolite)
B. Therapeutic drugs :
   1. Diphenhydramine (Bendaryl) 0.11 mg/L
   2. Clonazepam (Klonopin) 0.04 mg/L
   3. Diazepam (Valium) 0.21 mg/L
   4. Nordiazepam (metabolite) 0.38 mg/L
   5. Temazepam (metabolite) 0.09 mg/L
   6. Oxazepam 0.09 mg/L
   7. Lorazepam 22.0 ng/mL
C. Other non-contributory drugs present (atropine, topiramate, ciprofloxacin, acetaminophen)

II. LEFT GLUTEAL PANNICULITIS, WITH ABSCESS FORMATION AND RECENT LINEAR HEMORRHAGE

III. FIBROSIS WITH FAT NECROSIS (CHRONIC REPEATED INJECTIONS OF VARIOUS MEDICATIONS IN BUTTOCKS) OF DERMAL AND SUBCUTANEOUS TISSUES, BILATERAL GLUTEAL REGIONS AND ANTERIOR RIGHT THIGH

IV. GASTROENTERITIS, MILD, OF PROBABLE VIRAL ETIOLOGY

V. DEPRESSION FOLLOWING RECENT DELIVERY OF TERM INFANT AND RECENT DEATH OF ADULT SON (SEPTEMBER 2006)

VI. MODERATE CONGESTIVE HEPATOMEGALY (2550 GRAMS)

VII. FIBROUS PLEURAL ADHESIONS

VIII. CHRONIC THYROIDITIS (HASHIMOTO THYROIDITIS)

IX. WELL HEALED SUPRAPUBIC SCAR (STATUS POST CESAREAN SECTION)

X MINIMAL, INSIGNIFICANT MYOCARDIAL FIBROSIS

XI. STATUS POST MEDICAL INTERVENTION

A. Endotracheal tube placement
B. Right jugular line placement
C. Cardiac Monitoring devices and defibrillator pad placement
D. Bilateral anterior elbow and left anterior wrist venipuncture sites with surrounding ecchymoses

XII. STATUS POST BILATERAL BREAST IMPLANTS WITH SCARRING, LEFT

AREOLA
XIII. MICRO-INFARCT OF BRAIN, LEFT OCCIPITAL WHITE MATTER

XIV. MINOR CONTUSIONS, POSTERIOR SHOULDERS

OPINION:
Vickie Lynn Marshall was a 39-year-old white female who died of acute combined drug intoxication. Abscesses of buttocks, and viral enteritis were contributory causes of death.

The manner of death is determined to be: ACCIDENT

Joshua A. Perper, M.D.,LL.B.,M.Sc. Date
Chief Medical Examiner

Gertrude M. Juste, MD Date
Associate Medical Examiner
GMJ/JAP:jb

OFFICIALS PRESENT AT AUTOPSY:

Joshua A. Perper, M.D.,LL.B.,M.Sc., Chief Medical Examiner; Gertrude M. Juste, M.D., Associate Medical Examiner; Predrag Bulich, M.D., Assistant Medical Examiner; Harold Schueler, Phd., Chief Toxicologist; Stephen J. Cina, M.D., Deputy Chief Medical Examiner; Joseph Anderson, Forensic Photographer; James Fleurimond, Forensic Photographer; Irma Motem, Forensic Technician; Dean Reynolds, Morgue Supervisor; Reinhard W. Motte, M.D., Associate Medical Examiner; Detective Rich Engels of the Broward Sheriff's Office, Crime Scene Unit; Chief Tiger of the Seminole Police Department and Deputy Mike Jacobs of the Seminole Police Department.

CLOTHING:

The body is clad in a light green hospital gown, which is intact, dry and clean. There is no jewelry present.

EXTERNAL EXAMINATION:

The body is that of a well-developed, well-nourished white woman appearing the offered age of 39 years. The body measures 71 inches and weighs 178 pounds.

The unembalmed body is well preserved and cool to touch due to refrigeration. Rigor mortis is fully developed in the major muscle groups. Livor mortis is fixed and purple posteriorly except over pressure points. However, during initial examination in the emergency room, there was no rigor and lividity was at a minimum and unfixed. The skin is intact and shows no evidence of trauma except for medical intervention. The scalp hair is blond and measures up to 5 inches in length in the frontal area and up to 19 inches in length in the back and on top of the head. There are multiple blonde hair extensions including several pink strands attached to the natural hair, which shows light brown roots. The irides are hazel and the pupils are equal, each measuring 0.5 centimeter in diameter. The corneae are clear and the sclerae and conjunctivae are free of petechiae. The nasal bones are intact by palpation. The nares are patent and contain no foreign matter. There is a 3-millimeter raised nodule on the right side of the nose. The natural teeth are in good condition. The frenula are intact. The oral mucosa and tongue are free of injuries. The external ears have no injuries. There are bilateral earlobe piercings; no earring or jewelry were present. There are no earlobe creases.

The neck is symmetrical and shows no masses or injuries. The trachea is in the midline.

The shoulders are symmetrical and are free of scars.

The chest is symmetrical and shows no evidence of injury. There were bilateral breasts with asymmetry of the left breast due to scarring. The flat abdomen has no injuries. There are piercings above and below the umbilicus. The back is symmetrical. The buttocks have inconspicuous small scars, bilaterally. There is a flat, round scar on the lower aspect of the left buttock approximately ½ inch in diameter.

The genitalia are those of a normally developed adult woman. There is no evidence of injury. The anus is unremarkable.

The upper extremities are symmetrical and have no injuries. The fingernails are long and clean. There is a linear ½ inch scar on the anterior right forearm. Two parallel linear scars measuring 1 inch and 2 inches are on the anterior surface of the left forearm.

The lower extremities are symmetrical. The toenails are short and clean. There is no edema of the legs or ankles.

There is no abnormal motion of the neck, the shoulders, the elbows, the wrists, the fingers, the hips and ankles. There is no bony crepitus or cutaneous crepitus present.

EVIDENCE OF INJURY:
A dissection of the posterior neck and upper back show a 2-¼ x 2-¾ inch reddish, recent contusion of the subcutaneous and superficial muscle layer of the left posterior shoulder. A recent, reddish, 1-¾ x 1-½ inch reddish contusion is present on the right posterior shoulder involving the superficial muscular layer.

EVIDENCE OF RECENT MEDICAL TREATMENT:
A properly positioned size 8 endotracheal tube retained by a Thomas clamp is present at the mouth with the marker 22 at the anterior teeth.

Electrocardiogram pads are on the anterior chest in the following order: two on the right anterior shoulder, two on the left anterior shoulder, one on the upper anterior left arm, one each on the anterior side, one each on the anterior leg.

Two defibrillator pads are present: one to the right of the midline, above the right breast, and one to the left of the midline, below the left breast.

There is intravenous line placement at the right anterior neck with hemorrhage into the anterior strap muscles of the neck. One recent needle puncture mark is in the right antecubital fossa and two recent needle puncture marks are at the anterior left elbow with surrounding ecchymoses. There is one recent needle puncture into the medial one-third of the left anterior forearm with surrounding ecchymosis. A recent needle puncture mark is at the left anterior wrist with surrounding reddish ecchymosis, 1 inch in diameter.

OTHER IDENTIFYING FEATURES:

There are multiple scars and tattoos on the body.

SCARS:

A ¾ x ½ inch flat scar is on the upper inner aspect of the right breast quadrant. A ½ x 3/8-inch scar is on the medial aspect of the left nipple. There are circular scars adjacent to both areolae. The right inframammary skin has a linear transverse ¾ inch remote "chest tube" scar. There were bilateral inframammary and transverse linear 3-¾ inch scars compatible with left and right mammoplasty with breast implants. There are circular scars surrounding piercings above and below the umbilicus. A flat 3/8 inch in diameter scar is present on the middle third of the anterior surface of the right thigh. Lateral to this scar is a ½ inch in diameter flat scar. There are several scattered small inconspicuous scars on both buttocks. There is a cluster of multiple, parallel, linear, well-healed scars on the anterior and lateral aspects of the right leg covered by a tattoo.

TATTOOS:

There is a pair of red lips in the right lower abdominal quadrant.

Two red cherries are on the right mid pelvis.

A "Playboy Bunny" is on the left anterior mid pelvis.

The words "Daniel" and "Papas" are on the mid anterior pelvis region.

A mixed tattoo on the right lower leg and ankle represents: Christ's head; Our Lady of Guadalupe; the Holy Bible; the naked torso of a woman; the smiling face of Marilyn Monroe; a cross; a heart and shooting flames.

A mermaid on a flower bed with a pair of lips underneath it laying across the lower back.

INTERNAL EXAMINATION:

The body was opened with the usual Y incision. The breast tissues, when incised, revealed bilateral implants, each containing 700ml of clear fluid. The implants were surrounded by a thick connective tissue capsule with a thick yellow fluid. The content of each capsule was collected for bacteriological cultures.

BODY CAVITIES:

The muscles of the chest and abdominal wall are normal in color and consistency. The lungs are neither hyperinflated nor atelectatic when the pleural cavities are opened. The right lung shows adherence to the parietal pleura and to

the diaphragm interiorly. The ribs, sternum and spine exhibit no fractures. The right and left pleural cavities have no free fluid. There are extensive right pleural fibrous adhesions. The mediastinum is in the midline. The pericardial sac has a normal amount of clear yellow fluid. The diaphragm has no abnormality. The subcutaneous abdominal fat measures 3 centimeters in thickness at the umbilicus. The abdominal cavity is lined with glistening serosa and has no collections of free fluid. The organs are normally situated. The mesentery and omentum are unremarkable.

NECK:

The soft tissues and the strap muscles of the neck, aside from the previously described focal hemorrhages, exhibit no abnormalities. The hyoid bone and the cartilages of the larynx and thyroid are intact and show no evidence of injury. The larynx and trachea are lined by smooth pink-tan mucosa, are patent and contain no foreign matter. There is a focal area of reddish hyperemia at the carina associated with the endotracheal tube. The epiglottis and vocal cords are unremarkable. The cervical vertebral column is intact. The carotid arteries and jugular veins are unremarkable.

CARDIOVASCULAR SYSTEM:

The heart and great vessels contain dark red liquid blood and little postmortem clots. The heart weighs 305 grams. The epicardial surface has a normal amount of glistening, yellow adipose tissue. The coronary arteries are free of atherosclerosis. The cut surfaces of the brown myocardium show no evidence of hemorrhage or necrosis.

The pulmonary trunk and arteries are opened in situ and there is no evidence of thromboemboli. The intimal surface of the aorta is smooth with a few scattered yellow atheromata. The ostia of the major branches are of normal distribution and dimension. The inferior vena cava and tributaries have no antemortem clots (See attached cardiopathology report for additional details).

RESPIRATORY SYSTEM:

The lungs weigh 550 grams and 500 grams, right and left, respectively. There is a small amount of subpleural anthracotic pigment within all the lobes. The pleural surfaces are free of exudates; right-sided pleural adhesions have been described above. The trachea and bronchi have smooth tan epithelium. The cut surfaces of the lungs are red-pink and have mild edema. The lung parenchyma is of the usual

consistency and shows no evidence of neoplasm, consolidation, thromboemboli, fibrosis or calcification.

HEPATOBILIARY SYSTEM:

The liver weighs 2550 grams. The liver edge is somewhat blunted. The capsule is intact. The cut surfaces are red-brown and of normal consistency. There are no focal lesions. The gallbladder contains 15 milliliters of dark green bile. There are no stones. The mucosa is unremarkable. The large bile ducts are patent and non-dilated.

HEMOLYMPHATIC SYSTEM:

The thymus is not identified. The spleen weighs 310 grams. The capsule is shiny, smooth and intact. The cut surfaces are firm and moderately congested. The lymphoid tissue in the spleen is within a normal range. The lymph nodes throughout the body are not enlarged.

GASTROINTESTINAL SYSTEM:

The tongue shows a small focus of submucosal hemorrhage near the tip. The esophagus is empty and the mucosa is unremarkable. The stomach contains an estimated 30 milliliters of thick sanguinous fluid. The gastric mucosa shows no evidence or ulceration. There is a mild flattening of the rugal pattern within the antrum with intense hyperemia. The duodenum contains bile-stained thick tan fluid. The jejunum, ileum, and the colon contain yellowish fluid with a thick, cloudy, particulate matter. There is no major alteration to internal and external inspection and palpation except for a yellowish/white shiny discoloration of the mucosa. The vermiform appendix is identified. The pancreas is tan, lobulated and shows no neoplasia, calcification or hemorrhage.

There are no intraluminal masses or pseudomenbrane.

UROGENITAL SYSTEM:

The kidneys are of similar size and shape and weigh 160 grams and 190 grams, right and left, respectively. The capsules are intact and strip with ease. The cortical surfaces are purplish, congested and mildly granular. The cut surfaces reveal a well-defined corticomedullary junction. There are no structural abnormalities of the medullae, calyces or pelves. The ureters are slender and patent. The urinary bladder has approximately 0.5 milliliters of cloudy yellow urine. The mucosa is unremarkable.

The vagina is normally wrinkled and contains no foreign matter. The uterus shows a reddish endometrial lining with no evidence of intra-uterine pregnancy. The fallopian tubes and ovaries are within normal limits.

ENDOCRINE SYSTEM:

The adrenal glands have a normal configuration with the golden yellow cortices well demarcated from the underlying medullae and there is no evidence of hemorrhage. The thyroid gland is mildly fibrotic and has focally pale gray parenchyma on sectioning. The pituitary gland is within normal limits.

MUSCULOSKELETAL SYSTEM:

Postmortem radiographs of the body show no acute, healed or healing fractures of the head, the neck, the appendicular skeleton or the axial skeleton. The muscles are normally formed.

Dissection of the right anterior thigh in the aforementioned areas of scarring revealed subcutaneous fibrosis and multiple small cysts containing turbid, yellow fluid. The cyst-like structures range in sizes from 0.5 centimeters to 1.2 centimeters in diameter. The cyst associated with the most medial scar is 8 millimeter in diameter and has a calcified wall and the cyst associated with the more lateral scar measures 1 centimeter in diameter.

Dissection of the buttocks reveals diffuse subcutaneous scarring and fat necrosis of the adipose tissue bilaterally with three subcutaneous cystic structures containing light yellow, clear, thick liquid within the left buttock. The right buttock contains similar cysts with similar content, with at least one cyst wall being calcified.

The left and right buttocks have foci of recent, hemorrhagic tracts within the subcutaneous adipose tissue and the superficial and deep muscular layers extending from the skin surface.

There is a deep-seated 3 x 2.5 x 2 centimeter abscess within the musculature of the left buttock with a creamy, yellow-green pus on sectioning. A recent, hemorrhagic, needle tract extends into the abscess

wall from the skin surface.

CENTRAL NERVOUS SYSTEM:

The scalp has no hemorrhage or contusions. The calvarium is intact. There is no epidural, subdural or subarachnoid hemorrhage. The brain has a normal

convolutional pattern and weighs 1300 grams. The meninges are clear. The cortical surfaces of the brain have mild to moderate flattening of the gyri with narrowing of the sulci.

The brain is cut after formalin fixation and a separate neuropathology report is attached.

SPECIAL PROCEDURES:

Layer by layer anterior and posterior neck dissections were conducted. Dissection of the entire back including both gluteal regions was conducted. A biological trace evidence was collected. Multiple hairs were pulled from various parts of the head. The nails of the left hand were cut and preserved. Additional blood and tissue samples for DNA was collected.

Dale Earnhardt

Given Name: Ralph Dale Earnhardt
Born: April 29, 1951, Kannapolis, North Carolina
Died: February 18, 2001, Daytona Beach, Florida
Cause of Death: Car Accident

One of the most famous and well-liked drivers in the sport, Earnhardt is considered one of the most successful drivers in racing history. He won the Sprint Cup seven times and the Daytona 500 once. He was posthumously inducted into the NASCAR Hall of Fame in 2010. Earnhardt died during the 2001 Daytona 500 when he was pushed into a wall on the final lap of the race. The coroner determined his cause of death to be blunt force trauma to the head.

OFFICE OF THE MEDICAL EXAMINER
FLORIDA, DISTRICTS 7 & 24
VOLUSIA & SEMINOLE COUNTIES
1360 INDIAN LAKE ROAD, DAYTONA BEACH, FL 32124-2001
(904) 258-4060

NAME _____ EARNHARDT, RALPH DALE _____ ME # __ 02-0101V

AGE __49__ DOB __APRIL 29, 1951__ RACE __W__ SEX __M__ COUNTY __VOLUSIA__

DATE DEATH (FOUND) __FEBRUARY 18, 2001__ DATE OF EXAM __FEBRUARY 19, 2001__ TIME __0830 HRS.__

GROSS ANATOMIC DIAGNOSES

FINDINGS:
I. Blunt force injuries.
   A. Head and neck.
      1. Ring fracture of base of skull.
         a. Ring includes occipital bone, diastatic fracture of bilateral occipitomastoid sutures, fractures of the clivus behind the dorsum sella and through the body of the sphenoid bone through the lesser wing (with preservation of the hypophysial fossa).
         b. Associated subarachnoid and epidural hemorrhage.
         c. Mild edema of the posterior occipital lobes and posterior temporal lobes bilaterally.
      2. Abrasion, right side of chin.
      3. Contusion of left occipital scalp.
   B. Torso.
      1. Rib fractures.
         a. Left ribs 2 through 8 fractured anteriorly.
         b. Left rib 9 fractured laterally.
      2. Fracture of 3rd sternebra.
      3. Superficial abrasions.
   C. Extremities.
      1. Fracture of left ankle (with fracture of distal fibula).
      2. Superficial abrasions.
II. Cholelithiasis.

FINAL DIAGNOSIS

CAUSE OF DEATH: Blunt Force Injuries of the Head.

DUE TO: Motor Vehicle Accident.

MANNER OF DEATH: Accident.

SPECIAL STUDIES: (See last page of report.)

XC: State Attorney's Office
Daytona Beach Police Department

_____ DATE _____
ASSOCIATE MEDICAL EXAMINER/Thomas A. Parsons, M.D.

THIS DOCUMENT HAS NOT BEEN REVIEWED OR CORRECTED BY THE PHYSICIAN, AND MAY CONTAIN ERRORS AND/OR OMISSIONS WHICH MAY OR MAY NOT AFFECT THE FINAL REPORT.

OFFICE OF THE MEDICAL EXAMINER
DISTRICTS 7 & 24

NAME _____ EARNHARDT, RALPH DALE _____ ME # 91-01017

REPORT OF AUTOPSY

EXTERNAL EXAMINATION

Received is the unembalmed, symmetrically developed, adequately nourished and hydrated, body of an adult white male appearing approximately his reported age of 49 years. The length is 69 inches. The weight is 184 pounds. The body is cool to the touch and has been previously refrigerated. Rigor mortis is fully developed in the muscles of the jaw and extremities. Dorsal livor mortis is spared in areas exposed to pressure, and blanches upon firm pressure. The cranium is symmetrically developed, with brown scalp hair measuring up to 10 cm in length. There is no palpable crepitus over the bridge of the nose. The eyebrows are intact. There is no congestion or petechial hemorrhages within the palpebral or bulbar conjunctivae. The irides are blue. The pupils are round, equal, central and measure 3 mm. The nasal septum is intact and in the approximate midline. Over the upper lip is a well groomed, brown hair mustache. The remaining cheeks, chin, and neck are clean-shaven. The external ears are unremarkable, with no foreign material in the external auditory canals. There is abundant blood in the external auditory canals bilaterally. Dentition is natural and in a good state of repair. There are no oral buccal mucosal injuries. The neck is symmetrically developed, without unusual masses palpable. The trachea is palpated in the midline. The chest is symmetrically developed. The abdomen is soft and without palpable masses or organomegaly. The external genitalia are those of a circumcised adult male with bilaterally descended testes palpable within the scrotum. The anus and perineal region are grossly unremarkable. The lower extremities are symmetrically developed and are without an absence of digits. Attached to the left great toe is a cardboard identification tag which is inscribed with the decedent's identifying information, including the name "Ralph Earnhardt". Encircling the right ankle is a hospital identification bracelet which is inscribed with the name "John Pacific Doe". Attached to the right great toe by a piece of string is a hospital identification disk which has the same name on it. The left ankle has a displaced fracture with contusion, described further subsequently (see EVIDENCE OF INJURY). A white plastic identification bracelet encircles the left wrist with the name "Dale Earnhardt" on it. The upper extremities are symmetrically developed and are without an absence of digits. The fingernails are of medium length, without underlying dirt, debris, hair, or tissue. There are no absent fingernails. There is no tearing of the fingernails on the left hand. There is no acute tearing of the fingernails on the right hand.

EVIDENCE OF THERAPY: A nasogastric tube is present in the right nostril. An endotracheal tube emanates from the right corner of the mouth. An intravenous catheter is secured in the right side of the neck by black suture material. Chest tubes are secured in the chest bilaterally by black suture material. These are inserted cutaneously at approximately the level of the nipples, just anterior to the midaxillary line. An intravenous catheter is secured in the left antecubital fossa. Numerous self-adhesive EKG pads are present over the anterior chest bilaterally, over the left lateral abdomen, and left posterior shoulder. Three needle puncture marks are present over the flexor aspect of the right forearm and antecubital fossa. There are numerous needle puncture marks in the right subclavian area and on the left side of the neck. No other evidence of therapeutic intervention is seen on the surface of the body.

SCARS AND IDENTIFYING MARKS: A nearly vertically oriented, 11 cm scar is present over the left knee, lateral to the patella. A nearly vertically oriented, well healed, curvilinear scar is present over the right knee and measures 12 cm in length. A 3 cm, vertically oriented, well healed, curvilinear scar is present over the distal head of the biceps on the lateral aspect of the left upper arm. There are no other convincing scars, tattoos, or identifying marks observed on the surface of the body.

THIS DOCUMENT HAS NOT BEEN REVIEWED OR CORRECTED BY THE PHYSICIAN, AND MAY CONTAIN ERRORS

OFFICE OF THE MEDICAL EXAMINER
DISTRICTS 7 & 24

NAME _____ MARKHARDT, RALPH DALE _____ ME # 91-0181V

REPORT OF AUTOPSY

EVIDENCE OF INJURY: Over the right side of the chin is a 2.5 x 1.0 cm, superficial abrasion. Over the left clavicular head is a 1.5 x 0.6 cm, superficial abrasion. Over the left hip region is a nearly transversely oriented, 10 x 2 cm area of superficial abrasion. Over the right hip region is a 22 x 5 cm area of faint superficial abrasions. Over the mid abdomen is an area of diffuse purple-red contusion which measures 2.0 x 4.5 cm. Just inferior to the umbilicus in the midline is a 0.5 x 0.4 cm laceration.

Over the inferior left patella is a 0.6 x 0.5 cm, superficial abrasion. Surrounding the palpable dislocation of the left ankle is a purple-blue area of contusion which extends from the medial malleolus inferiorly to the sole of the foot, and from the heel anteriorly to the head of the metatarsals. This continues to the approximate midline. There is palpable fracture of the distal left fibula included in this dislocation and fracture of the left ankle. Over the medial head of the left gastrocnemius is a faint purple contusion measuring 6.5 x 3.5 cm. Over the posterior proximal left forearm is a 2.0 x 0.8 cm, superficial abrasion.

No other evidence of acute injury is seen externally.

DRAFT

INTERNAL EXAMINATION

Through the usual Y-shaped incision, 4.0 cm of yellow subcutaneous adipose tissue and soft, red-brown musculature are revealed. There is generalized congestion of the subcutaneous tissues and musculature. The peritoneal cavity is free of excess fluid. The ends of the chest tubes are present bilaterally within the pleural cavities bilaterally through the 8th intercostal spaces. The omentum and viscera are normally disposed. The appendix vermiformis is intact and grossly unremarkable. The right and left pleural cavities have the associated incisions, without other defects of the pleurae. The remaining pleurae are smooth, glistening, and purple-gray to red-brown with areas of dependent congestion. The pericardial sac is intact and contains a scant amount of pale yellow, clear fluid. The pericardial sac is otherwise unremarkable. The mediastinum is grossly unremarkable. The sternum is transversely fractured at the 3rd sternebra. Left ribs 2 through 9 are fractured anteriorly, with scant hemorrhage surrounding the fractured ends. Left rib 9 is fractured laterally, in approximately the mid axillary line. There are no fractures of the right ribs. There are no unusual odors.

CARDIOVASCULAR SYSTEM: The aorta is of normal course and caliber. There is focal atheromatous streaking with minimal calcification distally. There are no aneurysms identified. The great vessels have their usual anatomical relationships. The pulmonary arteries appear patent and free of thromboemboli. The pulmonary veins are grossly unremarkable. The vena cava is grossly unremarkable. The heart weighs 410 grams. The epicardial surface is smooth, glistening, and red-brown with a moderate amount of yellow subepicardial fat. The coronary ostia are patent and give rise to a normally distributed coronary arterial system which is right dominant. The coronary arteries are thin, elastic, and have focal atheromatous streaking, without significant stenosis. Serial sections through the myocardium are firm and red-brown, with no areas of softening or fibrosis. The cardiac valves and chambers have their usual anatomical relationships. The valve leaflets are thin and delicate, without vegetations. Sections through the area of the conduction system are grossly unremarkable.

THIS DOCUMENT HAS NOT BEEN REVIEWED OR CORRECTED BY THE PHYSICIAN, AND MAY CONTAIN ERRORS AND/OR OMISSIONS WHICH MAY OR MAY NOT AFFECT THE FINAL REPORT.

OFFICE OF THE MEDICAL EXAMINER
DISTRICTS 7 & 24

PAGE 4 OF 6

NAME _____ EARNHARDT, RALPH DALE _____ ME # 01-0101V

REPORT OF AUTOPSY

RESPIRATORY TRACT: The trachea contains an appropriately placed endotracheal tube. A small amount of blood is present over the mucosal surfaces. The mucosal surfaces of the trachea and main stem bronchi are otherwise grossly unremarkable. The right lung weighs 590 grams. The left lung weighs 660 grams. The lungs are moderately collapsed, with a pattern of hemoaspiration beneath the pleural surfaces. The pleural surfaces are otherwise smooth, glistening, and pink-tan to red-brown. Serial sections are pink-tan to red-brown, with areas of dependent congestion and mild hemoaspiration. Mass lesions are not identified. Purulent exudates are not apparent. Emphysematous changes are inconspicuous.

GASTROINTESTINAL TRACT: The esophagus is of normal course and caliber. The surface of the esophagus is grossly unremarkable. The esophagus is free of foreign material. A nasogastric tube is curled above the level of the epiglottis and did not enter into the stomach. The mucosal surface of the esophagus is grossly unremarkable. The serosal surface of the stomach is grossly unremarkable. The stomach contains 50 cc of bloody fluid, a portion of which is retained. No food or medications are identified. The mucosal surface of the stomach is grossly unremarkable. The serosal surface of the small bowel is grossly unremarkable. The small bowel contains a moderate amount of liquid, yellow-green material. Medications are not appreciated. The mucosal surface of the small bowel is grossly unremarkable. The serosal surface of the colon is grossly unremarkable. The colon contains a moderate amount of pasty, greenish brown fecal material. The mucosal surface of the colon is grossly unremarkable.

HEPATOBILIARY TRACT: The liver weighs 1660 grams. The smooth, glistening, red-brown capsular surface is intact. Serial sections are firm and red-brown, with preservation of the normal hepatic lobular architecture. Steatosis is not apparent. Fibrosis is inconspicuous. Mass lesions are not identified. The gallbladder is intact and contains 20 cc of dark green, liquid bile, a portion of which is retained. There are focal, less than 1.0 cm, black-green gallstones. The biliary tract appears free of obstruction.

HEMATOPOIETIC SYSTEM: The spleen weighs 210 grams. ~~DRAFT~~ slate gray connective tissue capsule is intact and slightly wrinkled. Serial sections are soft to gelatinous and red-brown. There are no mass lesions. The lymph nodes and bone marrow are grossly unremarkable.

ENDOCRINE SYSTEM: The right and similar left adrenal glands are of normal size, shape and position. On cut section, the cortices are yellow and the medulla are soft and gray. There are no hemorrhages or mass lesions. The pancreas is of normal size, shape and position. The surface of the pancreas is grossly unremarkable. Serial sections demonstrate preservation of the normal pancreatic lobular architecture. There are no calcifications or hemorrhages. The thyroid gland is of normal size, shape and position. The serosal surface and cut sections are grossly unremarkable. The pituitary is of normal size, shape and position.

GENITOURINARY TRACT: The right and left kidneys weigh 160 grams each. The capsules strip with ease to reveal smooth, dark red-brown cortical surfaces punctuated by occasional fetal lobulations. There are no cortical cysts. On cut section, the cortices and medullae are well demarcated in their respective zones. There are no mass lesions. The renal pyramids are grossly unremarkable. The caliceal systems are grossly unremarkable. Stones are not identified. The ureters are of uniform course and caliber. The serosal surface of the urinary bladder is grossly unremarkable. The bladder contains 300 cc of pale yellow, clear urine, a portion of which is retained. The mucosal surface of the urinary bladder is grossly unremarkable. The prostate gland is of normal size, shape, and position to palpation.

THIS DOCUMENT HAS NOT BEEN REVIEWED OR CORRECTED BY THE PHYSICIAN, AND MAY CONTAIN ERRORS AND/OR OMISSIONS WHICH MAY OR MAY NOT AFFECT THE FINAL REPORT.

OFFICE OF THE MEDICAL EXAMINER
DISTRICTS 7 & 24

NAME _____ EARNHARDT, RALPH DALE _____   ME # __01-0101V__

REPORT OF AUTOPSY

HEAD: Reflecting the scalp demonstrates an 8.0 x 5.5 cm area of contusion on the left side of the occipital scalp. This is included in the area of ring fracture, which extends through the temporal bones and occipital bone. There is hemorrhage beneath the temporalis muscles bilaterally in the area of the fracture. A few other areas of scattered contusion are present over the right side of the scalp and over the vertex. Reflecting the bony calvarium demonstrates epidural and subarachnoid hemorrhage. There is no subdural hemorrhage. Subarachnoid hemorrhage is accentuated in the areas surrounding the fracture and the base of the brain. Epidural hemorrhage is surrounding the fracture sites. Discolorations of the bony calvarium are not apparent. The superior sagittal sinus and all venous dural sinuses appear patent and free of thromboemboli. The brain in the fresh state weighs 1450 grams. From the vertex, the cerebral hemispheres are symmetrical, without significant atrophy. There is flattening of the gyral surfaces and narrowing of the sulci in the posterior occipital and temporal lobes. Anteriorly, there is no evidence of edema. The leptomeninges over the surface of the brain and around the base of the brain are thin and delicate, with the previously described subarachnoid hemorrhage. Purulent exudates are not appreciated. There is no evidence of herniation of the hippocampal unci or cerebellar tonsils. The circle of Willis has its usual anatomical relationships. There are no atheromas or aneurysms present. Serial coronal sections of the cerebral hemispheres demonstrate no gross abnormality of the gray or white matter. Mass lesions are not identified. Serial sagittal sections of the cerebellum demonstrate preservation of the normal cerebellar architecture. There is no gross abnormality of the gray or white matter. Serial transverse sections of the brainstem and midbrain demonstrate preservation of the normal architecture. There is no gross abnormality of the gray or white matter. Mass lesions are not identified. Stripping the dura from the base of the skull demonstrates a ring fracture which extends through the occipital bone to the temporal bone, with diastatic fracture of the occipitomastoid sutures bilaterally and with fracture behind the dorsum sella through the area of the clivus posteriorly and through the lesser wing of the sphenoid anteriorly, to have a preservation of the hypophysial fossa. This ring fracture includes wide separation of the ring anteriorly (through the sphenoid bone and the occipitomastoid sutures) and with minimal to no separation of the fracture through the posterior point of the occipital bone. Although the fracture is seen on both the internal and external tables of the posterior point of the occipital bone, there is no separation of the fractured calvarial plates as there is on the remaining portion of the ring fracture. Examination of the superior cervical spinal canal, upon flexion, extension and rotation of the head, demonstrates no fractures or subluxations.

NECK: The hyoid bone and thyroid cartilage are intact. There are no abnormal collections of extravasated blood over the surface of the hyoid bone or thyroid cartilage. Laminar dissection of the strap muscles of the neck demonstrates no abnormal collections of extravasated blood, except in association with the therapeutic devices and intravenous catheters of the right side of the neck. The cricoid cartilage is intact and grossly unremarkable. The larynx and hypopharynx are free of foreign material. The mucosal surfaces of the larynx are grossly unremarkable. The epiglottis and vocal cords are grossly unremarkable. Posterior dissection of the neck demonstrates no injury to the vertebral arteries or to the ligaments of the posterior cervical spine.

MICROSCOPIC EXAMINATION

(Awaiting slides.)

THIS DOCUMENT HAS NOT BEEN REVIEWED OR CORRECTED BY THE PHYSICIAN, AND MAY CONTAIN ERRORS AND/OR OMISSIONS WHICH MAY OR MAY NOT AFFECT THE FINAL REPORT.

OFFICE OF THE MEDICAL EXAMINER
DISTRICTS 7 & 24

PAGE 6 OF 6

NAME _____ EARNHARDT, RALPH DALE _____ ME # 01-0101V

SPECIAL STUDIES

TOXICOLOGY (Sent to Lab.)

DRAFT

HALIFAX MEDICAL CENTER

PERSONAL EFFECTS INVENTORY

DATE: 62/18/01   TIME: 5⁴⁵ ᵠ M.

John Doe Pacific
Patient's Name

The undersigned hereby certifies that the following personal effects were inventoried as the property of the above patient:

ITEM	REMOVED TO:
1 Pr Black Socks	
Racing suit (. Falls)	
Black Gloves	
1 Helmet & earpiece	Given to wife
Watch	
1 BVD underwear	
1 Black Racing Boots	
1 Yellow colored band @ 4th Finger, left E.H.	

Inventory Witnessed By:

_____
(Signature)

_____
(Signature)

Inventory Taken By:

_____ Dr Daron R. P_____
(Signature)

I hereby acknowledge receipt of the above personal effects (except those removed to Safe).

Mark Marty   DATE: 2-18-01
(Signature)

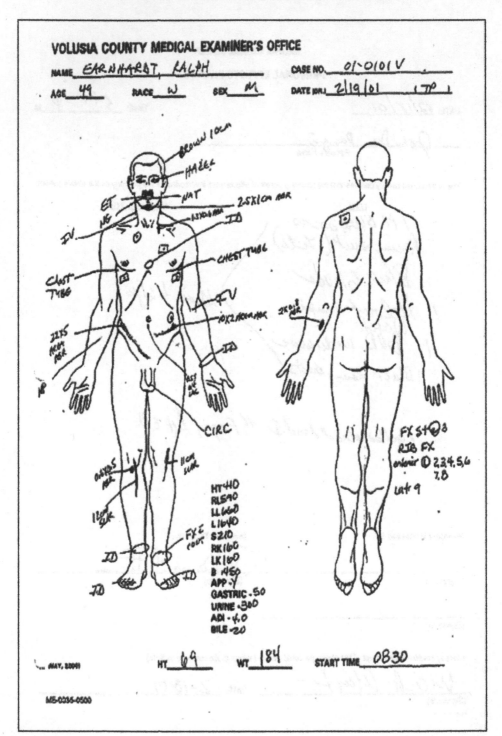

Janis Joplin

Given Name: Janis Lyn Joplin
Born: January 19, 1943, Port Arthur, Texas
Died: October 4, 1970, Hollywood, California
Cause of Death: Heroin Overdose

Janis Joplin was a rock musician during the 1960s. In the course of her career, she had five number one singles including "Me and Bobby McGee" and "Mercedes Benz." Joplin played Woodstock, Madison Square Garden, and the Festival Express. Throughout her career, she struggled with drug addiction, which was the cause of her death. People close to her believe the heroin she overdosed on was overly concentrated.

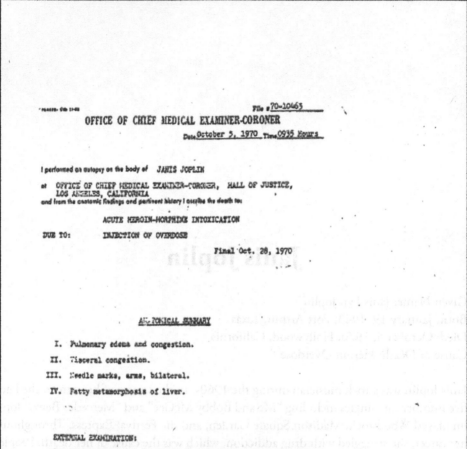

OFFICE OF CHIEF MEDICAL EXAMINER-CORONER

File #70-10463

Date October 5, 1970 Time 0935 Hours

I performed an autopsy on the body of **JANIS JOPLIN**

at OFFICE OF CHIEF MEDICAL EXAMINER-CORONER, HALL OF JUSTICE, LOS ANGELES, CALIFORNIA
and from the anatomic findings and pertinent history I ascribe the death to:

ACUTE HEROIN-MORPHINE INTOXICATION

DUE TO: INJECTION OF OVERDOSE

Final Oct. 28, 1970

AN_TOMICAL SUMMARY

I. Pulmonary edema and congestion.

II. Visceral congestion.

III. Needle marks, arms, bilateral.

IV. Fatty metamorphosis of liver.

EXTERNAL EXAMINATION:

The unembalmed body is that of a Caucasian female, appearing the stated age of 27. A tattoo of a bracelet is present around the left wrist. A small tattoo of a flower is present just behind the lateral malleolus on the right heel. There is also a small heart tattooed over, and medial to, the left breast. Numerous needle marks are present in the arms bilaterally, both in the antecubital fossa and on the left lateral anterior margin of the left arm. On sectioning, there appears to be at least two fresh hemorrhagic areas on the lateral margin of the left arm. The antecubital fossa shows, what appears to be, old needle marks and some are of relatively recent origin. An old surgical scar is present in the right lower quadrant of the abdomen. There is a slight amount of bloody material present in the mouth and on further examination, some disruption of the mucosa is noted. No evidence of major trauma or of violence is present. The hair is of moderate length and shows a varying shade of, from blond to brunette. The eyes are blue and show moderate dilatation of the pupils. The external genitalia is female.. There is some irregular dependent livor with pressure changes chiefly on the left side, suggesting body rest on the left side.

70-10463
JANIS JOPLIN
October 5, 1970

2

INTERNAL EXAMINATION, INCISION:

The usual Y-shaped incision is employed. There is no accumulation of blood or fluid in either abdominal or thoracic spaces. The organs appear in their usual positions.

RESPIRATORY SYSTEM:

The larynx, trachea, and bronchi show moderate congestion of mucosa. A small amount of foamy material is present in the upper portion of the trachea and continues toward the lower portion.. The right lung weighs 550 grams; left 500 grams. The cut surfaces show marked congestion and edema, bilaterally, but no definite recognizable hemorrhage or consolidation. Pulmonary vessels are grossly normal.

CARDIOVASCULAR SYSTEM:

The aorta and its branches show no significant arteriosclerosis. The heart weighs 300 grams, lies within a smooth pericardial sac. The epicardial and endocardial surfaces are smooth. The coronary arteries show no significant arteriosclerosis. The valve appearances and sizes are grossly normal. The cut surfaces of myocardium show no recognizable old, recent, or fresh infarct. Venous system shows no gross abnormalities.

HEMIC AND LYMPHATIC SYSTEM:

The abdominal and mediastinal nodes are not remarkably enlarged. The spleen weighs approximately 290 grams, has a red-purple parenchyma and a smooth capsule.

DIGESTIVE SYSTEM:

The esophagus shows no gross abnormalities. The stomach contains a small amount of fluid and partially digested food particles. The small bowel and colon are grossly normal. The appendix shows no gross abnormality. The pancreas has the usual lobular yellow-tan appearance. The liver weighs 2050 grams and has a smooth capsule. The parenchyma is yellowish-brown and shows some glistening of the surface. There is no significant accentuation of lobules or increase in fibrous components. The gallbladder and biliary tree are grossly normal.

UROGENITAL SYSTEM:

The kidneys weigh: Right 180 grams; left 170 grams. The capsules strip with ease. The cortex is up to 4 or 5 mm. in thickness. The pelves, ureters, and urinary bladder are grossly normal. The uterus contains an intra-uterine contraceptive device, of the serpentine-type. The endometrium is yellow-tan and is somewhat shaggy. The uterine, tubes, and ovaries show no gross abnormalities.

70-10683
JANIS JOPLIN
October 5, 1970

ENDOCRINE SYSTEM:

The adrenals show no recognizable abnormality. The thyroid weighs approximately 78 grams and has the usual glistening pinkish-tan appearance. The pituitary shows no gross abnormality.

SKULL AND CENTRAL NERVOUS SYSTEM:

The scalp, calvarium, and dura are free of abnormality. The brain weighs 1480 grams. The arteries at the base show no significant arteriosclerosis. The leptomeninges are moderately congested. Multiple sections through cerebrum, cerebellum, midbrain and pons show no recognizable hemorrhage, infarct, or neoplasm. The ventricular system is normal in size.

MUSCULOSKELETAL SYSTEM:

No gross deformities of the extremities are noted. The subcutaneous tissues and skin surfaces, bilaterally, show multiple needle marks in the arms. The lower extremities show no gross abnormality. The rib cage show no recognizable fractures. The thoracic and lumbar spine appear grossly normal.

TOXICOLOGY:

Specimen of blood, liver, kidney, stomach contents, gallbladder contents and urine, are submitted for toxicological study. Acetone hold and microscopic sections are also taken.

DAVID M. KATSUYAMA, M.D.
DEPUTY MEDICAL EXAMINER

DMK/jrw/s
10/6/70

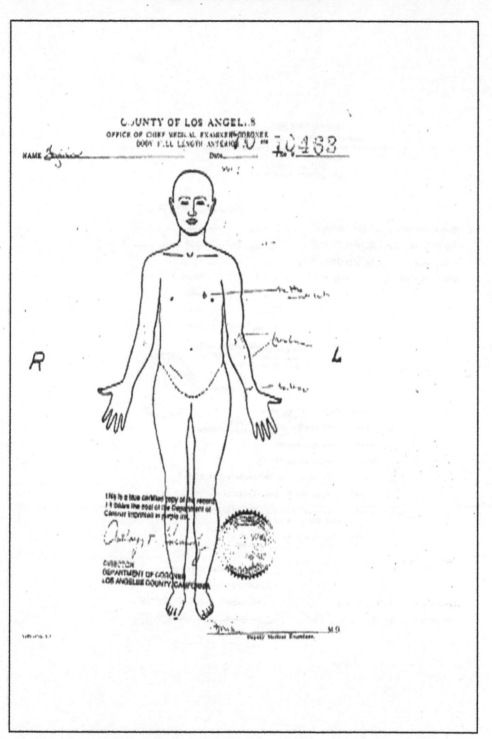

LABORATORY DIVISION
REPORT OF TOXICOLOGICAL ANALYSIS
OFFICE OF THE CHIEF MEDICAL EXAMINER-CORONER
COUNTY OF LOS ANGELES
HALL OF JUSTICE
LOS ANGELES, CALIFORNIA

Coroner's No. 70-10442

Name of Deceased........Janis Joplin

Date Submitted........October 6, 1970........Time........8 A.M.

Autopsy Surgeon........D. Katsuyama, M.D.

Material Submitted:

Blood X	Liver X	Stomach X	
Brain	Lung	Lavage	
Femur	Spleen	Urine X	
Kidney X	Sternum	Bile X	
Drug	Chemical		

This is a true certified copy of the record
it bears the seal of the Department of
Coroner registered in purple ink.

Laboratory Findings:

1. Blood: Ethanol .11 percent
2. Blood: Barbiturates absent
   Urine: Methadone absent
   Urine: Phenothiazine absent
3. Urine: Amphetamine and Methamphetamine absent
   Blood: Librium and Valium absent
4. Blood: Absence of Noludar, Meprobamate, Doriden, Soma and Quaalude
5. Blood: Codeine absent
   Blood: Morphine 0.02 mg. percent
   Bile: Codeine absent
   Bile: Morphine 1.6 mg. percent (Free Morphine)

Analysed by 1........Erik A. Wright........Toxicologist........Date 10-6-70
Analysed by 2........Jack Villaudy........Toxicologist........Date 10-6-70
Analysed by 3........I. Park........Toxicologist........Date 10-6-70

COUNTY OF LOS ANGELES
OFFICE OF CHIEF MEDICAL EXAMINER CORONER

CASE REPORT

This is a true certified copy of the record
if it bears the seal of the Department of
Coroner imprinted in purple ink.

DIRECTOR
DEPARTMENT OF CORONER
LOS ANGELES COUNTY, CALIFORNIA

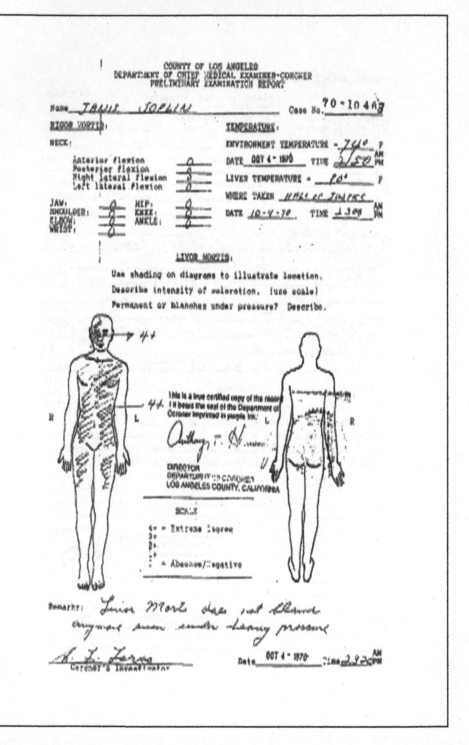

COUNTY OF LOS ANGELES
OFFICE OF CHIEF MEDICAL EXAMINER-CORONER

MEDICAL REPORT
70-10485

Name JANIS JOPLIN   Occupation ENTERTAINER   Case No.

10-5-   9   IN OR Crypt   OUT   MORTUARY M.E. CORONER

INVESTIGATION   AUTOPSY   PENDING   FINAL ON _____

CAUSE OF DEATH:

ACUTE HEROIN-MORPHINE INTOXICATION

INJECTION OF OVERDOSE

DK144
Final Oct. 28, 1970

NATURAL   ACCIDENT   SUICIDE   HOMICIDE   UNDETERMINED

PHYSICAL DESCRIPTION   Age 27   Sex F   Race CAUC   Complexion MED   Ht. 5 ft 5 in.   Wt. 68 lb

Found by: JAMES   License No. 5487   Blood Sample Taken   No — Explain

APARTMENT (ON THE FLOOR)

UNDET (COMB-NARC)

MEDICAL EXAMINER'S COMMENTS:

This is a true certified copy of the record

DIRECTOR
DEPARTMENT OF CORONER
LOS ANGELES COUNTY, CALIFORNIA

COUNTY OF LOS ANGELES
DEPARTMENT OF CHIEF MEDICAL EXAMINER - CORONER
Janis Joplin
MEDICAL REPORT   Case No. 70-10463

10-5-70
                                  Dr.

CONTINUATION SHEET

1100 hrs   - Arrived at decedent's residence (7047 Franklin Avenue,
              Apt. 105) with Dr. Noguchi, Dr. Katsuyama and William
              Lyttrup for further investigation. Public Administrator
              seal broken and apartment entered by above.

1110 hrs   - Gauze noted on decedent's bed; gauze found in waste
              basket in livingroom with apparent dried blood residue.

1120 hrs   - The end of a red balloon or rubber glove was found in
              a waste basket in decedent's kitchen containing a white
              powder. A large disposable towel was found with
              apparent dried blood residue with below evidence.

1140 hrs   - An apparent hype kit consisting of a teaspoon with
              black smudge, a small piece of cotton and dried
              residue; a needle and plastic syringe containing a
              clear liquid and a paper package containing a brownish
              white powder was found in the top right dresser drawer
              in decedent's livingroom. Also found in the drawer
              was a plastic bag containing possible marijuana; and
              a small plastic bag with 4-1/2 small white tablets
              "Lilly 172."

1200 hrs   - All above evidence was impounded and brought in and
              decedent's residence was locked and re-sealed by the
              undersigned.

                                      C. R. Dambacher

                                      C.R.Dambacher

                        This is a true certified copy of the record
                        it bears the seal of the Department of
                        Coroner imprinted in purple ink.

                        DIRECTOR
                        DEPARTMENT OF CORONER
                        LOS ANGELES COUNTY, CALIFORNIA

LOS ANGELES COUNTY, CALIFORNIA — CORONER
MEDICAL REPORT

Name: JANIS JOPLIN   Case No. 70-10409

Age: 27   Dr. _____

CONTINUATION SHEET

Information from Sgt. _____, OIC, and John Cooke, _____ on decedent, Apt. 223 (_____), _____ under contract ō decedent's group.

Decedent was 27-year-old female, and stage singer by occupation. Her group is called "Joplin Full Tilt Boogie" composed of herself and group of musicians — under Fantasity Inc. Licensed to engage in the state of California. On 10-3-70 at about 1400 hrs., decedent was in studio at "Sunset Sound Recorders" located on Sunset. After recording some music, decedent together ō another man (unknown name ō addr.) dropped in at "Barney's Beanery" at 8447 Santa Monica Blvd. and took about two drinks. Decedent was last seen alive by Jack Hagy, mgr. J. Hyssaument (phone nos.) about 0100 hrs., 10-4-70, coming home, alone.

This morning, before 1915 hrs., Mgr. Cooke (phone) saw decedent's car outside of the Barney's. Concerned why the car was parked outside, Cooke called up decedent between 1915 – 1950 hrs. 10-4-70, but no response. He then borrowed key of the manager, entered the room and found decedent lying on the floor between chair and bed, apparently dead. Cooke then called decedent's lawyer ō a Doctor and called police. R.A. #35 at scene 2110 hrs. 10-4-70 and pronounced death at same scene.

Decedent was cold, lying on her left side, clad ē blouse and panties. No rigor mortis noted and lividity marks about ye r. ō small laceration on ye lower lip of decedent noted from ē her fall. Multiple needle ō marks (fresh) noted on ye left antecubital fossa and old marks on ye right. The air-condition at scene was on ō no sign of struggle noted in the room. Balance suspended ō not liable to give pain passing in bed.

No signs of trauma or foul play.

Andy Irons

Given Name: Phillip Andrew Irons
Born: July 24, 1978, Oahu, Hawaii
Died: November 2, 2010, Grapevine, Texas
Cause of Death: Cardiac Arrest

Andy Irons was a professional surfer from Hawaii. He was ranked first in the ASP World Tour three times. He died in his hotel room after being removed from a flight to Honolulu due to illness. The coroner's report states his death was the result of a blockage of the main artery in the heart that resulted from the presence of various drugs in his system.

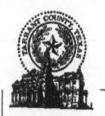

Office of Chief Medical Examiner
Tarrant County Medical Examiner's District
Tarrant County, Texas
200 Feliks Gwiozdz Place, Fort Worth, Texas 76104-4919
(817) 920-5700 FAX (817) 920-5713

AUTOPSY REPORT

Name: Philip Andrew IRONS　　　　　**CASE NO: 1013091**
Approximate Age: 32 years　　　　　**Sex: Male**
Height: 72 inches　　　　　　　　**Weight: 176.6 pounds**

We hereby certify that on the 3rd day of November, 2010, beginning at 1000 hours, we, Shipping Bao, M.D. and Nizam Peerwani, M.D. pursuant to Statute 49.25 of Texas Criminal Code, performed a complete autopsy on the body of PHILIP ANDREW IRONS at the Tarrant County Medical Examiner's District Morgue in Fort Worth, Texas and upon investigation of the essential facts concerning the circumstances of the death and history of the case as known to me, I am of the opinion that the findings, cause and manner of death are as follows:

FINDINGS:

I.　**Investigative Findings:**
　　A. Decedent discovered unresponsive in a hotel room at Dallas-Fort Worth International Airport and pronounced dead at the scene
　　B. Suspected history of dengue fever
　　C. Reported history of drug abuse
　　D. Suicide Profile:
　　　　1.　History of depression: Yes
　　　　2.　Suicide ideations, threatened suicide or previous attempted suicide: None
　　　　3.　Suicide Note at the scene: None

II.　**Postmortem Findings:**
　　A. Atherosclerotic cardiovascular disease with:
　　　　1.　Cardiomegaly (weight = 423 gms)
　　　　2.　Absence of hypertrophy or dilatation
　　　　3.　Severe occlusive coronary atherosclerosis with focal 70-80% stenosis of left anterior descending branch
　　B. Postmortem toxicology:
　　　　1.　Aorta Blood ethanol: Negative
　　　　2.　Femoral vein blood:
　　　　　　a. Alprazolam = 52 ng/mL (lethal > 122 ng/mL)
　　　　　　b. Benzoylecgonine (metabolite of cocaine) = 50 ng/mL

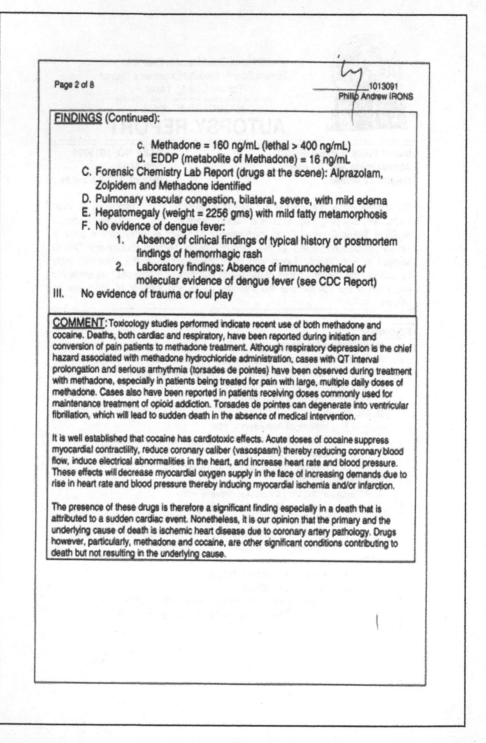

1013091
Philip Andrew IRONS

FINDINGS (Continued):

    c. Methadone = 160 ng/mL (lethal > 400 ng/mL)
    d. EDDP (metabolite of Methadone) = 16 ng/mL
  C. Forensic Chemistry Lab Report (drugs at the scene): Alprazolam, Zolpidem and Methadone identified
  D. Pulmonary vascular congestion, bilateral, severe, with mild edema
  E. Hepatomegaly (weight = 2256 gms) with mild fatty metamorphosis
  F. No evidence of dengue fever:
    1. Absence of clinical findings of typical history or postmortem findings of hemorrhagic rash
    2. Laboratory findings: Absence of immunochemical or molecular evidence of dengue fever (see CDC Report)
III.   No evidence of trauma or foul play

COMMENT: Toxicology studies performed indicate recent use of both methadone and cocaine. Deaths, both cardiac and respiratory, have been reported during initiation and conversion of pain patients to methadone treatment. Although respiratory depression is the chief hazard associated with methadone hydrochloride administration, cases with QT interval prolongation and serious arrhythmia (torsades de pointes) have been observed during treatment with methadone, especially in patients being treated for pain with large, multiple daily doses of methadone. Cases also have been reported in patients receiving doses commonly used for maintenance treatment of opioid addiction. Torsades de pointes can degenerate into ventricular fibrillation, which will lead to sudden death in the absence of medical intervention.

It is well established that cocaine has cardiotoxic effects. Acute doses of cocaine suppress myocardial contractility, reduce coronary caliber (vasospasm) thereby reducing coronary blood flow, induce electrical abnormalities in the heart, and increase heart rate and blood pressure. These effects will decrease myocardial oxygen supply in the face of increasing demands due to rise in heart rate and blood pressure thereby inducing myocardial ischemia and/or infarction.

The presence of these drugs is therefore a significant finding especially in a death that is attributed to a sudden cardiac event. Nonetheless, it is our opinion that the primary and the underlying cause of death is ischemic heart disease due to coronary artery pathology. Drugs however, particularly methadone and cocaine, are other significant conditions contributing to death but not resulting in the underlying cause.

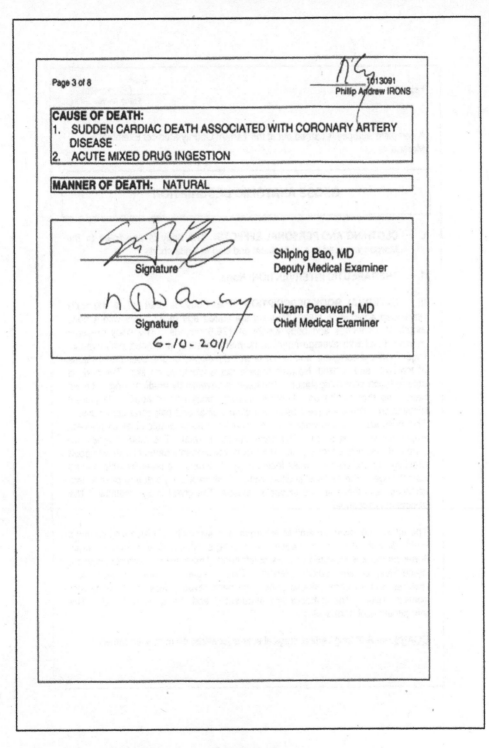

1013091
Phillip Andrew IRONS

CAUSE OF DEATH:
1. SUDDEN CARDIAC DEATH ASSOCIATED WITH CORONARY ARTERY DISEASE
2. ACUTE MIXED DRUG INGESTION

MANNER OF DEATH: NATURAL

Signature

Shiping Bao, MD
Deputy Medical Examiner

Signature

6-10-2011

Nizam Peerwani, MD
Chief Medical Examiner

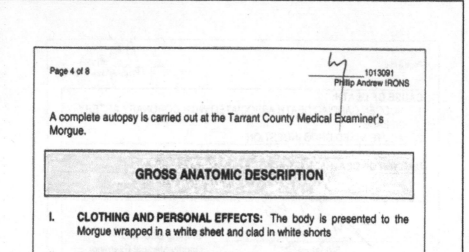

1013091
Phillip Andrew IRONS

A complete autopsy is carried out at the Tarrant County Medical Examiner's Morgue.

GROSS ANATOMIC DESCRIPTION

I.   CLOTHING AND PERSONAL EFFECTS: The body is presented to the Morgue wrapped in a white sheet and clad in white shorts

II. THERAPEUTIC INTERVENTION: None

III. EXTERNAL BODY DESCRIPTION: The body is that of a normally developed adult white male appearing the stated age of 32 years with a body length of 72 inches and body weight of 176.6 pounds. The body presents medium build with average nutrition, normal hydration, and good preservation. Rigor mortis is complete, and lividity is well-developed on the posterior surfaces of the body and is fixed. No rash or petechia is identified on skin. The body is cold to touch post refrigeration. The head is covered by medium length, brown hair. The face is shaven. There is average body hair of adult male pattern distribution. The eyes are closed with clear bulbar and palpebral conjunctivae. The irides are blue with white sclerae. There are no cataracts or arcus present. Pupils are equal at 5 mm. The orbits appear normal. The nasal cavities are unremarkable with intact septum. The oral cavity presents natural teeth with good oral hygiene and contains white foam purge. The ears are unremarkable with no hemorrhage in the external auditory canal. The neck is rigid due to postmortem changes, and there are no palpable masses. The chest is symmetrical. The abdomen is scaphoid.

The upper and lower extremities are equal and symmetrical presenting cyanotic nail beds without clubbing or edema. A ½" long scratch is localized on left wrist. A needle mark is localized on back of left hand. There are no fractures, injuries, deformities, or amputations present. External genitalia present descended testicles and an unremarkable penis. The back reveals dependent lividity with contact pallor. The buttocks are atraumatic, and the anus is intact. The integument is of normal color.

SCARS: An 8.0" long vertical surgical scar is localized on middle abdomen.

_____1013091
Philip Andrew IRONS

<u>TATOOS</u>: None

IV. INTERNAL EXAMINATION

1. INTEGUMENT: A Y-shaped thoracoabdominal incision is made and the organs are examined in-situ and eviscerated in the usual fashion. The subcutaneous fat is normally distributed, moist and bright yellow. The musculature of the chest and abdominal area is of normal color and texture.

2. SEROUS CAVITIES: The chest wall is intact without rib, sternal, or clavicular fractures. The pleura and peritoneum are congested, smooth glistening and essentially dry, devoid of adhesions or effusion. There is no scoliosis, kyphosis, or lordosis present. The left and right diaphragms are in their normal location and appear grossly unremarkable. The pericardial sac is intact, smooth, glistening and contains normal amounts of serous fluid.

3. CARDIOVASCULAR SYSTEM: The heart is slightly enlarged and weighs 423 grams and there is no evidence of chamber hypertrophy or dilatation. The left ventricular wall is 1.5 cm and the right 0.5 cm. The cardiac valves appear unremarkable with normal circumference. The coronary ostia are in the normal anatomical location leading into coronary arteries with atherosclerosis and 70% to 80% stenosis in middle portion of left anterior descending coronary artery. Other major coronary arteries are widely patent. Right dominant circulation is present. The endocardial surface is smooth without thrombi or inflammation. Sectioning of the myocardium presents no gross evidence of ischemic changes either of recent or remote origin. The aortic arch along with the great vessels appears grossly unremarkable.

4. PULMONARY SYSTEM: The neck presents an intact hyoid bone as well as thyroid and cricoid cartilages. The larynx is comprised of unremarkable vocal cords and folds, appearing widely patent without foreign material, and is lined by smooth, glistening membrane. The epiglottis is a characteristic plate-like structure without edema, trauma, or pathological lesions. Both the musculature and the vasculature of the anterior neck are unremarkable. The trachea and spine are in the midline, presenting no traumatic injuries or pathological lesions.

The lungs appear hyperinflated and together weigh 1358 grams. Both the lungs appear severely congested and edematous. There are no gross pneumonic lesions or abnormal masses identified. The tracheobronchial tree contains white foaming liquid. The pulmonary arterial system is intact and grossly unremarkable. The pleural surfaces are pink and smooth with focal mild anthracosis.

1013091
Phillip Andrew IRONS

9. CENTRAL NERVOUS SYSTEM: A scalp incision, craniotomy and evacuation of the brain are carried out in the usual fashion. The scalp is intact without contusions or lacerations. The calvarium is likewise intact without bony abnormalities or fractures.

The brain weighs 1664 grams presenting moderate congestion of the leptomeninges. Overlying dura is intact and unremarkable. Cerebral hemispheres reveal a normal gyral pattern with severe global edema. The brainstem and cerebelli are normal in appearance with no evidence of cerebellar tonsillar notching. The Circle of Willis is patent, presenting no evidence of thrombosis or berry aneurysm. On coronal sectioning of the brain the ventricular system is symmetrical and contains clear cerebrospinal fluid. There are no space occupying lesions present. Spinal cord is not examined.

SPECIMENS AND EVIDENCE COLLECTED

1. 30 mL of aortic blood, 20 mL of femoral blood, 30 ml of urine, 30 ml of gastric content, and 5 mL of vitreous for further examination
2. Representative tissue sections in formalin for further examination
3. Blood card
4. Representative photographs
5. 7 cassettes of tissues
6. Swabs of brain

MICROSCOPY

Sections of the heart reveal normal interdigitating bundles of myocardium with essentially unremarkable interstitium. Individual myocardial fibers are long tapering and without hypertrophy. Well-preserved ovoid nuclei and unremarkable intercalated discs are present. In focal areas, the myocardial fibers appear to be fragmented without accompanying inflammation or fibrosis. Myonecrosis is not identified. Contraction bands are occasionally seen. Mild small vessel disease is noted. Section of middle portion of left anterior descending coronary artery reveals atherosclerosis with 70% to 80% stenosis.

1013091
Phillip Andrew IRONS

9.   CENTRAL NERVOUS SYSTEM: A scalp incision, craniotomy and evacuation of the brain are carried out in the usual fashion. The scalp is intact without contusions or lacerations. The calvarium is likewise intact without bony abnormalities or fractures.

The brain weighs 1664 grams presenting moderate congestion of the leptomeninges. Overlying dura is intact and unremarkable. Cerebral hemispheres reveal a normal gyral pattern with severe global edema. The brainstem and cerebelli are normal in appearance with no evidence of cerebellar tonsillar notching. The Circle of Willis is patent, presenting no evidence of thrombosis or berry aneurysm. On coronal sectioning of the brain the ventricular system is symmetrical and contains clear cerebrospinal fluid.   There are no space occupying lesions present. Spinal cord is not examined.

SPECIMENS AND EVIDENCE COLLECTED

1.   30 mL of aortic blood, 20 mL of femoral blood, 30 ml of urine, 30 ml of gastric content, and 5 mL of vitreous for further examination
2.   Representative tissue sections in formalin for further examination
3.   Blood card
4.   Representative photographs
5.   7 cassettes of tissues
6.   Swabs of brain

MICROSCOPY

Sections of the heart reveal normal interdigitating bundles of myocardium with essentially unremarkable interstitium. Individual myocardial fibers are long tapering and without hypertrophy. Well-preserved ovoid nuclei and unremarkable intercalated discs are present. In focal areas, the myocardial fibers appear to be fragmented without accompanying inflammation or fibrosis. Myonecrosis is not identified. Contraction bands are occasionally seen. Mild small vessel disease is noted. Section of middle portion of left anterior descending coronary artery reveals atherosclerosis with 70% to 80% stenosis.

1013091
Philip Andrew IRONS

Sections of the lung reveal prominent vascular congestion with mild edema. In focal areas, the alveoli appear collapsed. Infrequent lower respiratory tract histiocytes are noted within the alveolar spaces. Inflammation or fibrosis is absent. Bronchi and bronchioles appear unremarkable. Vascular channels likewise appear unremarkable. Pleural lining is intact with minimal anthracosis, focal lymphocytic infiltrate and associated focal patchy fibrosis.

Section of the liver reveals prominent passive congestion with dilated sinusoids. Portal triads appear unremarkable with intact limiting plates. The overall hepatic architecture is preserved and there is no evidence of hepatocellular necrosis or degeneration. Mild fatty metamorphosis is noted of the microvesicular type.

One section of the pancreas reveals autolysis. There is no micropathological lesions present.

Sections of the left and right kidney reveal an intact renal architecture with unremarkable glomeruli, tubular structures and vasculature. Prominent vascular congestion is however noted.

Section of the spleen reveals prominent congestion with enlarged red pulp. The sinuses are however intact and lined by unremarkable elongated flat endothelial cells. Small aggregates of mature lymphocytes and mononuclear cells are present. The white pulp is well-represented with prominent germinal centers. There are no micropathological lesions noted.

One section of the thyroid gland presents a normal lobular architecture with each lobule composed of unremarkable follicles of variable size, filled with pink staining colloid material and lined by lower cuboidal epithelial cells. The interfollicular stroma is sparse and C-cells are difficult to identify. Solid cells nests are not present and there is no evidence of lymphocytic infiltrate.

Sections of the left and right adrenal glands reveal no micropathological lesions noted.

Sections of cerebral cortex, the brainstem and cerebellum are examined. These reveal prominent congestion as well as variable degree of cerebral edema. There is no evidence of neuronal dropout, necrosis or gliosis.

Completed: June 10, 2011
NP/

Toxicology Test Results

Office of Chief Medical Examiner
Toxicology Laboratory Service
200 Feliks Gwozdz Place
Fort Worth, Texas 76104
Name: **Philip Andrew Irons**

Case Number: **1013091**
Toxicology Work Number: **1002235**

Nizam Peerwani, M.D., DABFP
Chief Medical Examiner
Angela Springfield, PH.D., DABFT
Chief Toxicologist
Priority: 0

Service Request Number: 001

Specimen	Drug	Result	Drug Amount	Performed By
AORTA BLOOD	ETHANOL AxSYM	NEGATIVE		B. LANDRY
URINE	CANNABINOIDS AxSYM *	POSITIVE		B. LANDRY
URINE	COCAINE AxSYM	POSITIVE		B. LANDRY
URINE	OPIATES AxSYM	NEGATIVE		B. LANDRY
URINE	AMPHETAMINES AxSYM	NEGATIVE		B. LANDRY
URINE	BENZODIAZEPINES AxSYM	POSITIVE		B. LANDRY
AORTA BLOOD	ACID	NEGATIVE		C. LEWIS
URINE	NAPROXEN	POSITIVE		C. LEWIS
GASTRIC	ACID	NEGATIVE		C. LEWIS
FEMORAL BLOOD	ALPRAZOLAM	POSITIVE	52 NG/ML	C. LEWIS
URINE	ALPRAZOLAM	POSITIVE		C. LEWIS
FEMORAL BLOOD	AMPHETAMINE	NEGATIVE		C. LEWIS
URINE	AMPHETAMINE	POSITIVE		C. LEWIS
FEMORAL BLOOD	METHAMPHETAMINE	NEGATIVE		C. LEWIS
URINE	METHAMPHETAMINE	POSITIVE		C. LEWIS
FEMORAL BLOOD	COCAINE	NEGATIVE		C. LEWIS
URINE	COCAINE	POSITIVE		C. LEWIS
FEMORAL BLOOD	BENZOYLECGONINE	POSITIVE	50 NG/ML	C. LEWIS
URINE	BENZOYLECGONINE	POSITIVE		C. LEWIS
FEMORAL BLOOD	COCAETHYLENE	NEGATIVE		C. LEWIS
URINE	COCAETHYLENE	POSITIVE		C. LEWIS
FEMORAL BLOOD	METHADONE	POSITIVE	160 NG/ML	S. BOTCH
URINE	METHADONE	POSITIVE		S. BOTCH
FEMORAL BLOOD	EDDP	POSITIVE	16 NG/ML	S. BOTCH
URINE	EDDP	POSITIVE		S. BOTCH

*THIS SCREEN IS NOT CONFIRMED

Report Prepared By: _[signature]_

Approved By: _[signature]_

Approved Date: 11/9/10

OFFICE OF CHIEF MEDICAL EXAMINER
AND FORENSIC LABORATORIES
TARRANT COUNTY MEDICAL EXAMINER'S DISTRICT
200 FELIKS GWOZDZ PLACE
FORT WORTH, TEXAS 76104
(817) 920-5700

NIZAM PEERWANI, M.D., DABFP
CHIEF MEDICAL EXAMINER

SUSAN R. HOWE, PH.D., DABFT
INTERIM CHIEF TOXICOLOGIST

FORENSIC CHEMISTRY LABORATORY

NAME: Irons, Philip Andrew
CASE NUMBER: 1013091
OFFENSE DATE: 11-02-10
EVIDENCE REC'D: 11-04-10

AGENCY: Dallas/Fort Worth Airport PD
SERVICE NUMBER: 1003926
REQUESTED BY: Ofc. Herring
ANALYST: John Harris

EVIDENCE RECEIVED:

Tape sealed manila envelope containing

16. plastic prescription bottle holding five blue tablets marked 'GG 258'.
17. plastic prescription bottle holding
    A. twenty six white tablets marked '6469 / V'.
    B. eleven white tablets marked 'M / 57 71' and a visually similar white tablet fragment.
18. white plastic nasal spray bottle with factory label 'Afrin No Drip 12 Hour Pump Mist' containing white liquid.

RESULTS:

16. 0.65 gram of which 0.13 gram (one tablet) was analyzed and found to contain Alprazolam.
17A. 3.33 grams of which 0.12 gram (one tablet) was analyzed and found to contain Zolpidem.
17B. 2.82 grams of which 1.24 grams (five tablets) were analyzed and found to contain Methadone.
18. No controlled substances or dangerous drugs were detected in the liquid.

Analyst: *John Harris*

Administrative Review:
Susan R. Howe / Joyce Ho
Ronald L. Singer

Date: 11/18/10

10 | 3091

Centers for Disease Control and Prevention
National Center for Emerging and Zoonotic Infectious Diseases (NCEZID)
Division of High-Consequence Pathogens & Pathology (DHCPP)
Infectious Diseases Pathology Branch (IDPB)
Pathology Report

IDPB Number:	**2010-1317**
Receipt Date:	11/12/2010
Sign-out Date:	12/17/2010

Patient Name:	**Irons, Andy**
Submitter/Outside #(s):	10-13091
Case Origin:	TX, USA
Specimen(s) Received:	8 unstained slides. 4 blocks rec'd 11/17/10.
Submitted By:	Medical Transcriptionist
	Carol A Lawson,
	Tarrant County
	Office of Chief Medical Examiner
	200 Feliks Gwozdz Place
	Fort Worth, TX 76104 USA
	(817) 920-5700, CALawson@TarrantCounty.com

DASH and other CDC specimen numbers

DASH #	ASTRO #	BT #	Field #	BRRAT #	Outside #'s	Specimen:
2011720074	NBKSHJCK					

Diagnosis:

Liver, kidney, spleen, lung
-- no immunohistochemical or molecular evidence of dengue virus
-- no immunohistochemical evidence of Leptospira spp.

Lung without molecular evidence of influenza A

Comments:

Immunohistochemical (IHC) tests using an indirect immunoalkaline phosphatase technique were performed. The primary antibodies used in the tests included a mixture of 16 reference rabbit polyclonal anti-leptospira antisera (1) and a mouse polyclonal anti-dengue antiserum (2). Appropriate positive and negative controls were run in parallel. No immunohistochemical evidence of dengue virus infection or Leptospira spp. infection was observed.

RNA was extracted from formalin-fixed, paraffin-embedded sections of tissue and tested by using a broad-range, flavivirus-group specific RT-PCR assay, targeting a segment of the NS5 gene. No amplicon was obtained from the assay. House-keeping gene was amplified in all the samples ensuring the presence of amplifiable host nucleic acids.

RNA was extracted from formalin-fixed, paraffin-embedded portions of respiratory tissue and used as template for the CDC Real-time RT-PCR Protocol for Detection and Characterization of novel influenza A H1N1. This assay includes a panel of oligonucleotide primers and dual-labeled hydrolysis (Taqman) probes used in real-time RT-PCR assays for the in vitro qualitative detection and characterization of influenza viruses in respiratory specimens and viral cultures. The influenza A primer and probe set is designed for universal detection of type A influenza viruses. The novel influenza A H1N1 primer and probe set is designed for detection of the novel influenza A H1N1 virus. The samples were negative for influenza A.

CDC, IDPB, 1600 Clifton Road NE, MS: G32, Atlanta, GA 30333   Tel: 404-639-3132   Fax: 404-639-3043   Email: Pathology@cdc.gov

Page 1 of 3

Correlation with clinical history and other laboratory assays is recommended.

1. Zaki Zaki SR, Shieh WJ, et al. Lancet 1996, 347:535-536.
2. This antibody is known to cross-react with all four types of Dengue virus antigens.

Microscopic Examination:

The lungs are congested with mixed inflammation within the submucosa of a single large bronchus. The kidney, liver, and spleen are congested. The appendix shows no significant histopathologic abnormality.

Results:

Specimen	Test	Result
IHC		
Spleen, appendix	Dengue virus and other flaviviruses	Negative
Spleen, appendix	Leptospira spp.	Negative
Kidney	Dengue virus and other flaviviruses	Negative
Kidney	Leptospira spp.	Negative
Liver	Dengue virus and other flaviviruses	Negative
Liver	Leptospira spp.	Negative
Lung	Dengue virus and other flaviviruses	Negative
PCR		
Spleen, appendix	Flavivirus RT-PCR / NS5 / 250 bp	Negative
Kidney	Flavivirus RT-PCR / NS5 / 250 bp	Negative
Liver	Flavivirus RT-PCR / NS5 / 250 bp	Negative
Lung	Flavivirus RT-PCR / NS5 / 250 bp	Negative
Lung	2009 Influenza A H1N1 Real-time RT-PCR	Negative

CDC, IDPB, 1600 Clifton Road NE, MS: G32, Atlanta, GA 30333   Tel: 404-639-3132   Fax: 404-639-3043   Email: Pathology@cdc.gov

Page 2 of 3

• 356 •

David Foster Wallace

Born: February 21, 1962, Ithaca, New York
Died: September 12, 2008, Claremont, California
Cause of Death: Suicide by Hanging

David Foster Wallace was an acclaimed author best known for his short stories and novels. Most widely known for his 1996 novel *Infinite Jest*, his works are regarded as some of the best books of the late twentieth century. Wallace was a MacArthur Fellow and a professor at Pomona College. After struggling with depression for most of his life, he was found dead in his home after a suicide by hanging.

COUNTY OF LOS ANGELES		CASE REPORT		DEPARTMENT OF CORONER

APPARENT MODE	**SUICIDE**	895314	CASE NO. 2008-06413
SPECIAL CIRCUMSTANCES	Celebrity, Media Interest		ON/PT 73

1sv

LAST FIRST MIDDLE	AKA	#
WALLACE, DAVID FOSTER		

ADDRESS	CITY	STATE	ZIP
4205 OAK HOLLOW ROAD	CLAREMONT	CAL	91711

SEX	RACE APPEARS	DOB	AGE	HGT	WGT	EYES	HAIR	TEETH	FACIAL HAIR	O VIEW	CONDITION
MALE	CAUCASIAN	2/21/1962	46	72 in	161 lbs	BROWN	BROWN	ALL NATURAL TEETH	BEARD AND MUSTACHE	Yes	FAIR

MARK TYPE	MARK LOCATION	MARK DESCRIPTION

NOK	ADDRESS	CITY	PHONE

RELATIVE	PHONE	NOTIFIED BY LACO FIRE	DATE 9/12/2008	TIME 21:43

SSN	DL # D5096792	STATE CA	PENDING BY

ID METHOD CALIFORNIA DRIVER'S LICENSE						
LIC #	MAIN #	CII #	FBI #	MILITARY #	POB	

CERTIFIED BY NAME (PRINT)	RELATIONSHIP	PHONE	DATE	TIME
CALPHOTO			9/12/2008	23:45

PLACE OF DEATH / PLACE FOUND	ADDRESS OR LOCATION	CITY	ZIP
RESIDENCE	4205 OAK HOLLOW ROAD	CLAREMONT	91711

PLACE OF INJURY PATIO	AT WORK No	DATE 9/12/2008	TIME	LOCATION OR ADDRESS 4205 OAK HOLLOW ROAD, CLAREMONT, CAL.	ZIP 91711

DOD 9/12/2008	TIME 21:43	FOUND OR PRONOUNCED BY LACOFD ENG 102		

OTHER AGENCY INV. OFFICER CLAREMONT P.D. - OFCR ABARCA	PHONE	REPORT NO 08-3137	NOTIFIED BY	NO

TRANSPORTED BY WITHERS, WENDY	TO LOS ANGELES FSC	DATE 9/13/2008	TIME 01:25

FINGERPRINTS?	No	CLOTHING	Yes	PASPT	No	MORTUARY	
MED EV.	No	INVEST PHOTO #	4	SEAL TYPE	NOT SEALED	HOSP APT	No
PHYS EV.	Yes	EVIDENCE LOG	Yes	PROPERTY?	Yes	HOSP CHART	No
SUICIDE NOTE	Yes	SER NO		ROM NO	233954	FF NO.	

SYNOPSIS
ACCORDING TO POLICE THE DECEDENT WAS FOUND HANGING FROM THE PATIO ROOF RAFTER IN THE REAR YARD. NOTES FOUND. HISTORY OF DEPRESSION.

ALLEN R. MOSES 298382	[signature] INVESTIGATOR	DATE 9/13/2008 TIME 19:40	REVIEWED BY [signature]	DATE TIME

FORM #3 NARRATIVE TO FOLLOW? ☑

County of Los Angeles, Department of Coroner
Investigator's Narrative

Case Number: 2008-06413   Decedent: WALLACE, DAVID FOSTER

Information Sources:

1. Officers Saenz / Abarca – Claremont Police Department

2.

3. On scene investigation

Investigation:

On 09/12/2008 at 2206 hours Officer Saenz reported this case to the Los Angeles County Department of Coroner – reporting desk, receipt by Courtney Morrow. At 2223 hours Kelly Yagerlener assigned this case for investigation. I arrived at the location at 2345 hours and departed at 0100 hours.

Location:

Place of death: 4205 Oak Hollow Road, Claremont, CA 91711

Informant/Witness Statements:

According to information provided by Officer Abarca at the scene, the decedent was found at approximately 2128 hours, hanging in his rear yard by _____ (decedent's wife) who called 911. Los Angeles County Fire Department Squad 101 responded to the location and pronounced death at 2143 hours without medical intervention. The decedent was last seen by his wife at approximately 1730 hours.

While at the scene, I spoke with _____ who stated in essence that she has been married to the decedent for 4 years, she knew him 2 years prior to marriage. The decedent had a history of depression with two prior suicide attempts. The decedent had a mental health expert, Dr. Jodi Rawles (714) _____ who the decedent last saw two weeks ago. The decedent had been issued Nardol, Clonopin, and Restoril. The decedent was also status post ECT treatments x 12.

Scene Description:

The location was a single story, family style residence with a large outdoor yard on the south side of the residence. Attached to the residence structure was a wood patio cover, the decedent had used a black leather belt as a ligature and nailed it to a 2 x 6 support. There was a lawn chair that was knocked over on its side next to the decedent which measured 1'4" from the seat to the ground. The top of the support beam to the concrete patio measured 8'10 ½".

Evidence:

One black belt ligature was collected at the scene and brought back to the Forensic Science Center as physical evidence. Duct tape around both wrists were left in place pending the examination by the DME.

County of Los Angeles, Department of Coroner
Investigator's Narrative

Case Number: 2008-08413   Decedent: WALLACE, DAVID FOSTER

Body Examination:

The decedent is a male, Caucasian, who appears to be the reported 46 years of age. He was wearing gray shorts, blue t-shirt, brown underwear, white socks and white gym shoes. The ambient temperature – unregulated was 69.2 degrees at 2355 hours. The liver temperature was 91.7 degrees at 0005 hours. Livor mortis blanched to light pressure and was consistent with the position found. Rigor mortis was 3 throughout. The decedent has a ligature mark about the front of the neck. The decedent also has duct tape about both wrists.

Identification:

CALPHOTO.

Next of Kin Notification:

» present at the scene.

Tissue Donation:

One legacy handling.

Autopsy Notification:

No law enforcement request.

ALLEN R. MOSES   KELLY YAGERLENER

09/13/2008

Date of Report

COUNTY OF LOS ANGELES

DEPARTMENT OF CORONER

AUTOPSY REPORT

12

Page __2__

No

2008-06413

WALLACE, DAVID

INJURY DATE: Unknown.

HOSPITAL DATE: None.

CIRCUMSTANCES:

Please see the Investigator's reports and Forms 1, 3 and 6, copy of evidence log (two), copy of suicide note, copy of paperwork from decedent, and a material from the internet about the life of the decedent. The decedent was found in the backyard of his residence on the evening of September 12, 2008. He was found hanging by a belt noose from the ceiling rafter on the patio in the backyard of his home. The decedent was pronounced dead at the scene on September 12, 2008 at 2123 hours.

There had been a history of prior depression with multiple suicide attempts and history of electroconvulsive therapy treatment.

EXTERNAL EXAMINATION:

The body is identified by toe tags and is that of an unembalmed, refrigerated adult White male with the stated age of 46 years. The decedent weighs 161 pounds and measures 76 inches in height. The decedent appears thin.

There is a furrow/impression present around the neck. The furrow is present around the anterior neck at the level of and above the thyroid cartilage. It measures approximately 2.5 cm in maximal width and up to 10 mm in depth. It slants slightly upward on both sides laterally. No noose is present.

No other trauma is present.

There is a tattoo on the right upper arm laterally with word "Karen" and a symbol of the heart.

The head is normocephalic and is covered by brown hair of medium to long length. The hair is straight. Frontal balding is present. A mustache and beard are present. Examination of the eyes reveals that the irides are brown. No petechiae are noted. There are no petechial hemorrhages of the lids or sclerae. The oronasal passages appear unobstructed.

76A79BP—Rev 2-91

Ludwig van Beethoven

Given Name: Ludwig van Beethoven
Baptized: December 17, 1770, Bonn, Germany
Died: March 26, 1827, Vienna, Austria
Cause of Death: Apparent Liver Failure

One of the most famous and successful musicians of all time, Beethoven was a German classical composer. He lost his hearing at the age of twenty-six and was unable to hear most of the music he created. In the course of his career, Beethoven composed nine symphonies, eleven concertos, thirty-two piano sonatas, and sixteen string quartets. His autopsy was performed by Dr. Johann Wagner and compiled in Latin. It was only recently translated to English.

General appearance

The body of the deceased was emaciated, and the skin was dotted with black petechiae especially at the extremities; the abdomen was swollen and the skin was stretched because of fluid in the abdominal cavity.

The external ear

The aural cartilage appeared large and was of irregular shape; the fossae of the helix (scapha) and the concha were larger and deeper than usual by about one half. The crura and notches were more prominent than usual. Shiny scales of skin lined the external auditory canal, especially around the tympanic membrane, which they concealed.

The middle and internal ear

The Eustachian tube was thickened, and its mucus membrane was swollen, but it became shrunken near its bony section. The mastoid process was sectioned and a vascular membrane lined the cellular structures within. Similarly, the petrous bone was covered by many blood vessels, especially towards the cochlea. The membranous part of the spiral lamina of the cochlea appeared redder than usual.

Both facial nerves were thickened. On the other [sic] and, the two auditory nerves were wrinkled and lacked a central core. The auricular arteries encircled the auditory nerves, and were larger in size than a crow's feather. They also were cartilaginous. The left auditory nerve was much thinner than the right nerve, and had three dull white streaks on its surface; the right auditory nerve had a thick white streak of a substance having a dense consistency. It was vascularized as it curved around the floor of the fourth ventricle.

Brain and cranium

The convolutions of the brain were softer and moister, and appeared to be deeper and more numerous than usual. In general, the bones of the cranium showed increased density and were almost one half inch thick.

The thorax

The thoracic cavity, and the organs it contained, appeared normal.

The abdomen

The abdominal cavity was filled with four quarts ['measures'] of a reddish, cloudy fluid. The liver was half of its usual size. It was compact and leathery in consistency, blue-green in color, and its surface was covered by nodules the size of a

bean. Its vessels were very narrow and thickened and there was no blood in them. The gall bladder contained a dark colored fluid, and much gravel-like sediment. The spleen appeared twice its usual size, and was compact and black in color. The pancreas also appeared larger and more compact, and the end of the pancreatic duct was the width of a goose feather. The stomach and the intestines were both distended with air.

Both kidneys were pale red and soft in consistency. They were covered by cellular tissue about one inch in thickness, and this tissue was filled with a dark cloudy fluid. In each calyx there was a calcareous concretion approximately the size of half a pea.

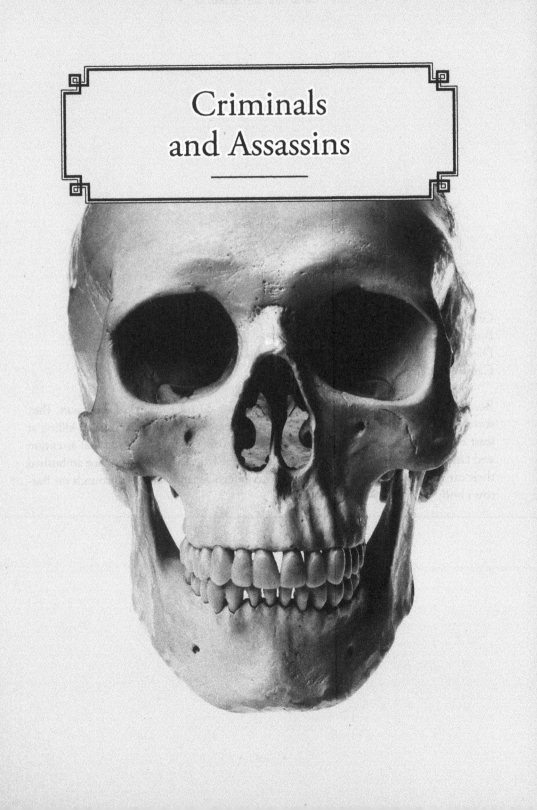

Criminals
and Assassins

Bonnie Parker

Given Name: Bonnie Elizabeth Parker
Born: October 1, 1910, Rowena, Texas
Died: May 23, 1934, Bienville Parish, Louisiana
Cause of Death: Shooting

Bonnie Parker was part of the famous Barrow Gang during the Great Depression. They traveled through the central United States robbing up to a dozen banks and killing at least nine police officers. The exploits of the Barrow Gang gained national attention and fame. Parker was killed along with her lover Clyde Barrow after police ambushed their car in Louisiana. The autopsy listed seventeen separate gunshot wounds on Barrow's body and twenty-six on Parker's.

Bonnie Parker

One gold wedding ring on third finger of left hand. Small watch on left arm. A three acorn brooch on dress, in front. One small catholic cross under dress. Red dress and red shoes. Tattoo of two hearts with arrow, above the right knee, names Roy on right side, and Bonnie on the left side. Gunshot wound around edge of hair, 1 1/2" above the left ear. Another through the mouth on left side, exiting at top of jaw. Another at middle, just below left jaw. Another above clavicle, left side, going into the neck. Another entering chest 2" below the inner side of left shoulder. Two shots entered about 2" below left shoulder, fracturing the bone. Another wound on elbow of left arm. Another entering left chest above the heart, breaking ribs. Six shots entering 3" on back region left side. Five pellet wounds about the middle of left side. Cut places on left leg. Cut glass on the left ankle. Cut on top of left foot, apparently from glass. Cut on center of right thigh. Cut 6" in length, about 3 1/2" center of right leg. Eight metal fragments centering across the front of face. Exit wounds 6" on the inner side of right leg. Flesh wound underside of right knee. Gunshot wound entering fleshy portion of left thigh. Eight bullet wounds striking almost in parallel line on left side. Three parallel lines of bullets striking right side of back from base of neck to angular right capular to middle of back bone, one striking midway of back, breaking backbone.

Office of the Coroner of Bienville Parish
Arcadia, Louisiana

Report of Death of _Bonnie Parker_

Age _23_ Color _White_ Sex _Female_ Marital State _Married_

Notified by _Curtis Oakley (Deputy Sheriff)_

Place Where Injury Occurred (street, city or parish, etc.) _Bienville Parish_
on highway between Sailes & Mt. Lebo

Place of Death _Bienville Parish_

Time of Death (day and hour) _May 23, 1934 about 9:15 a.m._

Witnesses: Name _A. P. Alcorn_ Address _Dallas Texas_

Remarks: _Was found dead in car_
V8 Desoto sand color 4 door
Sedan on Sailes highway
about 8 miles out of Gibsland

Conclusion or Recommendation:

I hereby certify that on the _23_ day of _May_ 193_4_

I made an _inquest_ on the body of _Bonnie Parker_
and upon investigation of the essential facts concerning the circumstances of the death and history of the
case, I am of the opinion that the cause of death was _Gun shot wounds in_
the hands of Texas Rangers and Sheriffs
Jordan and Curtis Oakley

J. L. Wade m.d.
Coroner of Bienville Parish.

*somewhat round entering
fleshy portion left thigh.
8 bullet wounds entering
almost in parallel line
left side. 2 parallel
striking right side,
back of neck bore of neck
to angular right scapula
to side both bone
one striking midway back
breaking both bone*

Dr. F. L. Wade
Coroner

DR. J. L. WADE
CORONER
BIENVILLE PARISH
ARCADIA, LOUISIANA

We the undersigned coroners
jury after diligent inquiry
and through investigation
find that Bonnie Parker
came to her death from
gun shot wounds fired
from rifles pistols and
shot guns in the hands
of officers.

M. N. Parker
G. R. Taylor
J. M. Prudhomme Jr.
EB Perry
J. R. Goff

Clyde Barrow

Given name: Clyde Chestnut Barrow
Born: March 24, 1909, Ellis County, Texas
Died: May 23, 1934, Bienville Parish, Louisiana

Clyde Barrow was a criminal and bank robber during the 1930s. Barrow and Parker grew to national prominence as the bank robbing, gun wielding couple that was wildly in love. He was gunned down by police while speeding down the highway in a stolen Ford V-8.

Clyde C. Barrow

On the right arm, tattoo picture of girl under which is written Grace. on the inner side, an anchor and shield USN. On left side, a tattoo through forearm dagger through heart with "E.B.W." On left shoulder, a tattoo rose and leaves. Gunshot wound in head, center front of left ear, exiting about 2" above right ear. One entering edge of brain above left eye. Several shots entering left shoulder joint. Small glass cut at joint, first finger of right hand. Seven small bullet wounds around middle of right knee. A number of glass cuts. Bullet wound right leg, about middle of outer left knee. Bullet wound on exterior ankle. Wound 2" above back, a great hole. Gunshot wound, back of first finger. Another wound, middle finger at bone, severing the member.

We the undersigned concur fully after diligent inquiry and through investigation, find that Bonnie Parker came to her death from gun shot wounds fired from rifles, pistols, and short range in the head and of affrience.

We the undersigned concur fully after diligent inquiry and through investigation, find that Clyde Chestnut Barrow met his death from gun shot rounds fired from affrience.

Office of the Coroner of Bienville Parish
Arcadia, Louisiana

Report of Death of *Clyde Champion Barrow*

Age *26*　　　Color *W.*　　　Sex *Male*　　　Marital State *Single*

Notified by *Puntis Oakley Depty Sheriff*

Place Where Injury Occurred (street, city or parish, etc.) *Bienville Parish between Mt. Lebanon + Sailes.*

Place of Death *Bienville Parish Highway between Sailes + Mt. Lebanon*

Time of Death (day and hour) *May 23. 1934 about 9:15 am*

Witnesses:　Name *R. F. Alcorn*　　　Address *Dallas Texas*

Remarks: *Was found dead in car V8 Desent sand color 4 door Sedan on Sailes highway about 8 miles out of Gibsland*

Conclusion or Recommendation:

I hereby certify that on the *23* day of *May* 193*4*

I made an *Inquest* on the body of *Clyde Champion Barrow* and upon investigation of the essential facts concerning the circumstances of the death and history of the case, I am of the opinion that the cause of death was *Gun shot wounds in the hands of Texas Rangers and Henderson Jordan and Puntis Oakley*

J. L. Wade M.D.
Coroner of Bienville Parish.

Clyde C Barrow.

On right arm tattooed Picture of girl on top which is written Grace on inner side a tattoo anchor and shield U. S. N.

On left arm a tattoo on forearm dagger through heart and E. B. W.

On left shoulder a tattoo Rose and leaves.

Gun shot wound in head entering front of left ear left about 2 inches above right ear, and at edge hair above left eye

Gun shot wound entering left shoulder joint.

Small place cut at first joint right hand.

7 small bullet inside of right knee.

a bullet gone into

Bullet wound right leg about
mid way ankle & knee,
another B wound at again
ankle, came up past about
2 in above bone chest tate
gun shot wound bone of right
finger small middle finger at bone
bearing the member

Dr. J. L. Wade
coroner

DR. J. L. WADE
CORONER
BIENVILLE PARISH
ARCADIA, LOUISIANA

We the undersigned coroner jury after diligent inquiry and thorough investigation find that Clyde Champion Barrow met his death from gun shot wounds fired by officers.

M. N. Barber
G. C. Taylor
J. W. Pentecost Jr.

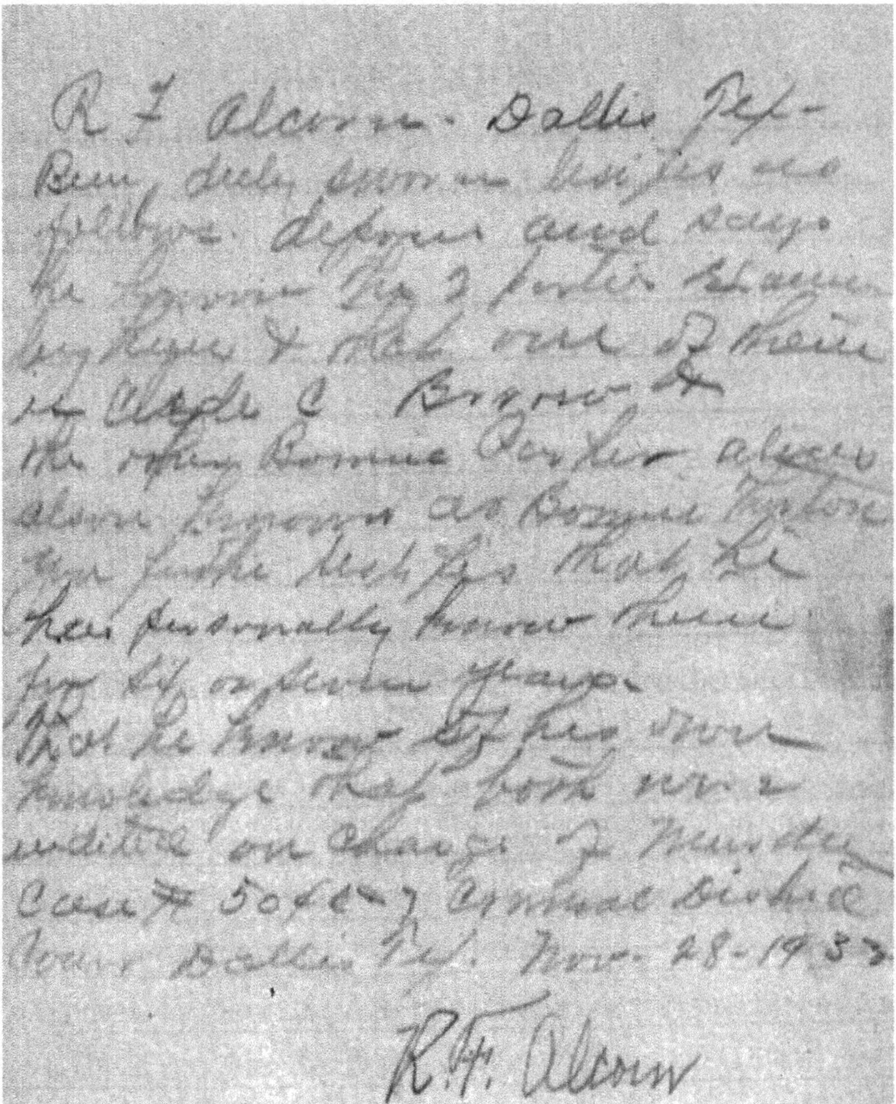

Jack Ruby

Given Name: Jacob Leon Rubenstein
Born : March 25, 1911, Chicago, Illinois
Died: January 3, 1967, Dallas, Texas
Cause of Death: Pulmonary Embolism

On November 22, 1963, Lee Harvey Oswald was arrested for the assassination of John F. Kennedy. Two days later, Dallas nightclub owner Jack Ruby shot Oswald while he was being moved from the basement of police headquarters to the local jail. Ruby was convicted of murder and he died while appealing his conviction. His last words were reported to be "There is nothing to hide . . . There was no one else."

February 1, 1967

Honorable W. E. Richburg
Justice of the Peace
410 South Beckley
Dallas, Texas

Re: Jack Ruby
Our ML 67-007

Dear Judge Richburg:

The autopsy studies on the above named deceased have been completed. The protocol is closed to show the cause of death as follows: Pulmonary emboli as immediate cause of death secondary to bronchiolar carcinoma of the lungs.

With kindest personal regards,

Very sincerely yours,

Earl F. Rose, M. D.

EFR:bh

cc: Hon. Henry Wade
    Capt. J. W. Fritz
    Dr. J. M. Pickard
    Mrs. Maurine Loan
    Sheriff Decker

Charles Whitman

Full name: Charles Joseph Whitman
Born: June 24, 1941, Lake Worth, Florida
Died: August 1, 1966, Austin, Texas
Cause of Death: Shooting

Known as the Texas Sniper, Charles Whitman was a former marine who killed fourteen people and wounded thirty-two others while firing from the top of the clock tower at the University of Texas. After murdering his mother and wife the previous day, Whitman purchased additional guns and ammo and made his way to the Austin campus. After approximately an hour and a half after he fired his first shot, Whitman was killed by Austin police. His autopsy revealed that Whitman had a highly aggressive and invariably fatal brain tumor, but the tumor was not believed to have caused psychosis although this finding was later disputed. The mass shooting is claimed to have resulted in the formation of America's first SWAT teams.

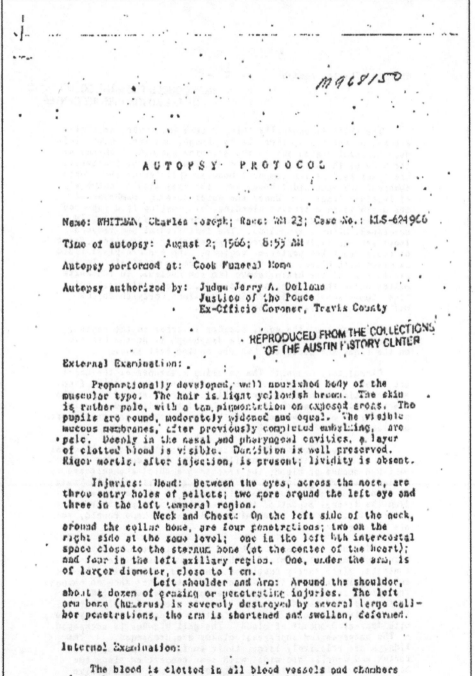

M968150

A U T O P S Y · P R O T O C O L

Name: WHITMAN, Charles Joseph; Race: WM 23; Case No.: MLS-624966

Time of autopsy: August 2, 1966; 8:55 AM

Autopsy performed at: Cook Funeral Home

Autopsy authorized by: Judge Jerry A. Dellana
                       Justice of the Peace
                       Ex-Officio Coroner, Travis County

External Examination:

Proportionally developed, well nourished body of the
muscular type. The hair is light yellowish brown. The skin
is rather pale, with a tan pigmentation on exposed areas. The
pupils are round, moderately widened and equal. The visible
mucous membranes, after previously completed embalming, are
pale. Deeply in the nasal and pharyngeal cavities, a layer
of clotted blood is visible. Dentition is well preserved.
Rigor mortis, after injection, is present; lividity is absent.

Injuries: Head: Between the eyes, across the nose, are
three entry holes of pellets; two more around the left eye and
three in the left temporal region.
Neck and Chest: On the left side of the neck,
around the collar bone, are four penetrations; two on the
right side at the same level; one in the left 4th intercostal
space close to the sternum bone (at the center of the heart);
and four in the left axillary region. One, under the arm, is
of larger diameter, close to 1 cm.
Left shoulder and Arm: Around the shoulder,
about a dozen of grazing or penetrating injuries. The left
arm bone (humerus) is severely destroyed by several large caliber penetrations, the arm is shortened and swollen, deformed.

Internal Examination:

The blood is clotted in all blood vessels and chambers
of the heart, after the complete injection.

WHITMAN, Charles Joseph   - 2 -

The skull is unusually thin, 2 to 4 mm. Over the hemispheres of the brain, there is no change, however, on the left deep temporal region and in the anterior and median thirds of the base of the skull, there are numerous lines of fractures. The lower half of the temporal bone is splintered; the frontal, temporal and sphenoidal bones over the eyes show a 'network' of fracture lines. - Under the outer covering membrane of the brain is an extensive bleeding, originating from ruptured venous sinuses and arteries. - The brain is symmetrically developed, without anomalies. The left frontal and temporal lobes are partially destroyed by penetrating bone pieces, some of these reach the posterior regions. The cerebrospinal fluid is mixed with blood. The ventricles are symmetrical. In the middle part of the brain, above the red nucleus, in the white matter below the gray center thalamus, is a fairly well outlined tumor about 2x1.5x1 cm in dimensions, grayish-yellow, with peripheral areas of red as blood.

The organs of the neck, besides injuries in the region, are unchanged. The level of the diaphragm is at the 6th rib on the right and above the 4th rib on the left side.

Circulatory Organs: The covering membranes of the heart are smooth, the cavity is filled with blood, originating from a penetrating wound into the right ventricle, around which the heart muscle is hemorrhagic. The heart is collapsed, its inner membrane and valves are smooth, the coronary arteries, aorta and large arteries are unchanged.

Respiratory Organs: The lining membrane of the right chest cavity is smooth, there is no fluid. The lung contains a diminished amount of blood; the tracheo-bronchial channels are filled with frothy blood. The left chest cavity contains some 50 ml of blood and a considerable amount of air, originating from the lateral aspect of the lobes which were penetrated by projectiles. Several areas of both lobes are hemorrhagic, so are all the air channels.

Abdomen: The lining membrane is smooth, the cavity contains embalming fluid mixed with blood and gastrointestinal contents, after cavity embalming. Besides perforations by the embalming instrument, the stomach and intestines show no change. The spleen is of average size, the capsule is corrugated, due to some loss of blood. - The liver is proportionally large, its capsule is smooth, its inner matter is pale brownish-yellow, with decreased amount of blood. The gall bladder is unchanged. - The pancreas and suprarenal glands are unchanged. - The kidneys are relatively large, their surface is smooth, both cortex and medulla are wide, with some congestion along the borderline of the two layers. The bladder and reproductive organs show no pathological change.

WHITMAN, Charles Joseph   - 3 -

    Histological Findings: The tumor of the brain is composed
of elements of the connective tissue of the brain (glia) and
of blood vessels of enlarged calibers. Some of these blood
vessels have thick walls, others thin ones, with defective con-
struction of the layers and microscopically small bleedings
into the surrounding intercellular spaces, however, only a dozen
or less red blood cells enters those spaces around. The cells
are rather small, round or elongated, with a small amount of
cytoplasm and mostly well staining nucleus. The chromatin substance of the nucleus is well organized, round or somewhat elongated
and in some places, vesicular. Cell divisions occur only very
exceptionally, indicating a minimal level of activity, just on
the borderline to malignant formations. There are areas of cell
death (necrosis), surrounded by a fence-like arrangement (pali-
sade formation) of elongated cells.

    Diagnosis: Fatal injuries to the head and to the heart.
            Additional finding: a small brain tumor in the
white matter above the brain stem, composed of connective
tissue elements of the brain, mixed with numerous enlarged
blood vessels; no evidence of malignantly fast growth, but
that of partial tissue death, necrosis. (Astrocytoma). No
correlation to psychosis or permanent pains.

                                    C. de Chenar, M.D.
                                    Pathologist
                                    Neuropathologist

Eric Harris and Dylan Klebold

Full Name: Eric David Harris
Born: April 9, 1981, Wichita, Kansas
Died: April 20, 1999, Columbine, Colorado
Cause of Death: Suicide

Full Name: Dylan Bennett Klebold
Born: September 11, 1981, Lakewood, Colorado
Died: April 20, 1999, Columbine, Colorado
Cause of Death: Suicide

Eric Harris and Dylan Klebold were the two shooters who planned and executed the Columbine High School Massacre. The two youths armed themselves with an array of guns and two propane bombs and entered the school. The propane bombs did not go off, but Harris and Klebold killed twelve students and one teacher while injuring another twenty-four students. After they finished their massacre, they headed to the library and shot at police before killing themselves in unison.

HARRIS, Eric   Dr. Galloway

FINAL ANATOMIC DIAGNOSES:

1. Through and through high energy contact gunshot wound
    involving the roof of the mouth associated with:

    A. Extensive lacerations of the scalp and soft tissues of
        the face
    B. Massive fracturing of the skull
    C. Evacuation of the brain - cerebral cortex and brain
        stem
    D. Extensive fracturing of the facial bones

COMMENT: The autopsy findings in this case reveal that the cause
of death is due to massive head injury secondary to a high energy
gunshot wound involving the roof of the mouth, consistent with a
shotgun. This wound is consistent with self-infliction.

Ben Galloway MD
Ben Galloway, M.D.
Forensic Pathologist

This autopsy is performed in the Jefferson County Coroner's Office in Golden, Colorado on 04/22/99 at 2:00 p.m. The autopsy is done at the request of Dr. Nancy Bodelson, the Coroner of Jefferson County. Identification is by fingerprints. The position identification for this individual is #12. Members of the Jefferson County Sheriff's Department attended the autopsy. I am assisted in the autopsy by Mr. Rob Kulbacki.

HISTORY: This is the case of an 18-year-old, white male who was the alleged victim of a self-inflicted gunshot wound to the head that occurred in the Columbine High School library on 04/20/99. No other history is available at the time of autopsy.

EXTERNAL EXAMINATION: The body is clothed in a blood stained white T-shirt with the inscription "Natural Selection" on the front; green plaid jockey shorts; black combat boots; white socks; and a black glove on the right hand with the fingers cut away. This is the unembalmed, well-developed, well-nourished, extensively traumatized body of a white male appearing consistent with the stated age of 18. Height is measured at 5'8-1/2"; weight is estimated at 135-140 pounds. Rigor is present in the lower extremities only. Faint reddish-purple livor is present over the dorsal aspects of the body with appropriate blanching of the pressure points.

HEAD: The scalp is covered by short, blood stained, black hair. The normal contour of the head is prominently distorted by extensive laceration of the scalp and associated massive fracturing of the cranium. Present in the mid-aspect of the lower forehead and extending downward to involve the bridge of the nose; the distal portion of the right side of the nose; and the medial aspects of both orbits; is an oblong configured blow-out type of laceration measuring 3" in length by 2" in width, associated with underlying multiple fracture fragments which extend outward from the wound. Present on the right lower forehead, extending upwards and across the lateral aspect of the right side of the head; extending up over the apex of the head; and then extending downward to involve the posterior aspect of the scalp to the level of the horizontal plane of the ears; is a large gaping laceration which measures 8" in length by 3" in width. Ears - both ears are intact. There is blood in both external auditory canals. There is blood staining of the earlobes. Present anterior to both of the ears are vertical lacerations. The one on the right measures 1-1/2" in length; the one on the left measures 3/4" in length; and these are consistent with blow-out injuries from a gunshot wound involving the mouth. Eyes - the eyebrows are brown. The orbits are distorted by fracturing of the underlying skeleton. The sclera on the right is bluish-gray; the sclera on the left is white. The right iris is gray; the left iris is hazel. The pupils are round, measure 8 mm, and are directed anteriorly. The conjunctivae are minimally congested. No petechiae are observed. A reddish-purple periorbital contusion involves the left orbit. Nose - there is, as previously described, injury to the external surface of the

nose with extensive underlying fractures. Present adjacent to the right lateral margin of the nose are two vertical lacerations, each measuring 1/4". Present on both sides of the face are multiple linear, curvilinear, punctate lacerations and cuts, more dense on the right. Palpating the face reveals massive fracturing of the facial bones. Mouth - there are several lacerations involving the corners of both sides of the mouth, the largest of which is on the right side, measuring 1/2" in length. There are multiple mucosal lacerations involving the mid-aspect of the lower lip. Slightly downward from the right side of the mouth is a laterally diagonal laceration measuring 1/2" in length. There is extensive laceration of the buccal mucosa. The tongue is intact, reddish-purple, with some black staining consistent with powder. There are central fractures of the upper and lower alveolar ridges. The teeth are intact with the exception that the lateral lower incisor on the right side of the jaw is absent. There is dense powder (soot) staining the mucosal surface of the hard palate. There is a large cavitary defect involving the roof of the mouth, including the hard palate, the soft palate, extending upwards involving the nasal pharynx and nasal passages, communicating directly into the base of the skull. This represents a contact entrance high energy gunshot wound. Present on the lateral surface of both sides of the face are brown whiskers.

NECK: The external surface of the neck reveals no evidence of trauma. The neck organs are in the midline without palpable masses.

CHEST: The chest demonstrates a mild pectus excavatum with some central decrease in the anterior-posterior diameter. Present in this area is a curvilinear, horizontally oriented scar. No external trauma involves the chest. The breasts are normal male. Palpating the chest reveals no instability. The axillae are negative to observation and palpation.

ABDOMEN: The abdomen is flat. No external trauma is present. There is no evidence of previous surgical exploration. There is green discoloration of the lower abdomen. On deep palpation, no organomegaly or masses are noted grossly.

GENITALIA: A normal appearing male, black, genital hair pattern is present. The penis is of normal size, shape, and position; circumcised. Both testicles are bilaterally descended in their respective scrotal sacs without palpable masses. There is a pigmented nevus in the right groin.

BACK: Present on the right upper back is a horizontal area of soft tissue indentation with postmortem drying artifact. There is a small pigmented nevus on the right lower quadrant of the back. The anus is intact without any unusual dilatation or trauma.

EXTREMITIES: The upper extremities are intact. The nails are

intact, short and slightly dirty. The lateral surfaces of the
hands are unremarkable. The forearms are unremarkable. The
antecubital fossae reveal no evidence of recent needle puncture
marks or scars. Present on the lateral aspect of the left upper
arm is a small cluster of punctate lacerations and cuts. Present
on the lateral aspect of the right upper arm is a reddish-brown
abrasion associated with purple contusion measuring 3/8" in size.
Arm spans: the right arm from the right shoulder to the tip of
the right index finger is 30-1/2"; the left arm from the left
shoulder to the tip of the left index finger is 31". The lower
extremities are intact without evidence of congenital abnormality
or trauma. There is a small reddish-brown abrasion on the
lateral aspect of the right foot.

INTERNAL EXAMINATION: Through the usual Y-shaped incision, a
thin layer of yellow subcutaneous adipose tissue and reddish-
brown musculature are revealed. The diaphragms are intact and
arch to the level of the 5th left intercostal space and the 4th
right intercostal space. The peritoneal cavity contains no
unusual accumulation of fluid. The lining is smooth, gray and
glistening. The viscera and omentum are normally disposed.

PLEURAL SPACES: The pleural spaces are without any unusual
accumulation of fluid. The parietal pleurae are smooth, gray and
glistening. The ribs of the chest are intact and unremarkable
grossly. There is a mild pectus excavatum deformity of the
sternum. The clavicles are intact. The pericardial sac is
intact. The lumen contains 8 cc of clear fluid. The pericardium
is smooth, gray and glistening.

THYMUS: Five (5) grams of pink, lobular, firm, thymic tissue is
present in the anterior-superior mediastinal space.

NECK: The lumen of the upper esophagus and pharynx is patent.
The mucosal surface is tan and wrinkled. The lumen of the upper
respiratory tract is patent. The mucosal surface is tan and
smooth. The hyoid bone and cricothyroid cartilages are intact.
There are contusions involving the mucosal surface of the
piriform sinus consistent with the blast impact of the contact
gunshot wound to the roof of the mouth.

THYROID: The thyroid is of normal size, shape, and position, and
has a reddish-brown, lobular, firm, gross appearance. The
cervical vertebrae are intact. There is no obstruction to the
posterior nasopharynx or the posterior aspect of the oral cavity.
I can palpate a large defect of the nasopharynx associated with
multiple fracture fragments. The major vessels of the neck are
intact and unremarkable grossly. There is no soft tissue
hemorrhage in the neck.

HEART: The heart is intact and weighs 290 grams. The epicardial
surface is reddish-brown, smooth, and glistening. Very little
epicardial yellow fat is present. The myocardium is reddish-
brown and firm without gross evidence of fibrosis or softening.

The ventricular walls are of normal thickness. The endocardial surface is reddish-brown, smooth, and glistening. The cardiac valves are intact. The valve leaflets are thin and fully pliable. The valve circumferences are normal for this size heart. The chordae tendineae are tan and delicate. The papillary muscles are intact. The foramen ovale is closed. The atrial septum is intact. The coronary sinus is patent. The ventricular septum is intact. The coronary ostia are in a normal anatomic position and widely patent. The coronary arteries demonstrate a normal anatomic distribution with normal gross features.

AORTA: The aorta is intact and of normal course and calibre throughout. The intimal surface is tan and smooth. The wall is thin and elastic. The main abdominal tributaries are intact.

RESPIRATORY SYSTEM: The lumen of the lower respiratory tract contains a small amount of hemorrhagic fluid on the right side. The mucosal surface is hyperemic and smooth. The lungs are moderately well aerated. The pleural surfaces are pink, smooth and glistening. The lungs together weigh 600 grams. Serial sections reveal moderately well aerated, soft, spongy, lung tissue. The pulmonary arteries are intact without evidence of thromboembolic disease. The pulmonary veins empty into the left atrium in a normal fashion.

GASTROINTESTINAL SYSTEM: The esophagus is of normal course and calibre throughout. The lumen is patent. The mucosal surface is tan with longitudinal furrowing. The wall is thin. The stomach is in a normal anatomic position. The lumen contains 250 cc of brown, liquid, gastric contents. The gastric mucosa is tan with intact rugae. No peptic ulcer disease or tumor are noted grossly. The small bowel demonstrates a normal anatomic distribution with normal gross features. The appendix is present and unremarkable grossly. The large bowel demonstrates a normal anatomic distribution with normal gross features.

SPLEEN: The spleen is intact and weighs 160 grams. The external surface is purple and smooth. Serial sections reveal a firm, reddish-purple, splenic parenchyma.

LIVER: The liver is intact and weighs 1250 grams. The external surface is reddish-brown, smooth, and glistening. Serial sections reveal a soft, reddish-brown, lobular, normal appearing, liver tissue.

GALLBLADDER: The gallbladder is intact. The lumen contains 10 cc of liquid, yellowish-brown bile. The mucosal surface is smooth and bile stained. The cystic duct and common bile duct are intact and patent throughout. The portal vein, splenic vein, and superior mesenteric vein are intact and patent.

PANCREAS: The pancreas is of normal size, shape, and position, and has a tan, lobular, soft, partially autolyzed, gross

appearance.

ADRENALS: Both adrenals are identified. Serial sections reveal a thin yellow cortex and gray medulla.

KIDNEYS: Both kidneys are identified. The capsules strip easily. The left kidney weighs 120 grams; the right kidney weighs 110 grams. The cortical surfaces are reddish-brown and smooth. Bivalving of each kidney reveals a well-demarcated, reddish-brown cortex and medulla. The renal papillae are normal. There is no calyceal scarring. There is no unusual pelvic dilatation. Both ureters are present, patent, and uniform in diameter throughout.

BLADDER: The bladder is intact. The lumen contains 2 cc of cloudy yellow urine. The bladder mucosa is tan and wrinkled. The prostate, seminal vesicles and testicles are intact and unremarkable grossly.

MUSCULOSKELETAL SYSTEM: Other than the injuries to be described under the observation of the head, no other injuries are observed.

LYMPHATICS: There are reactive lower respiratory tract lymph nodes. A biopsy is taken.

VENOUS SYSTEM: There is no evidence of hepatic vein, renal vein, or portal vein thrombosis. The superior and inferior vena cavae are intact.

CENTRAL NERVOUS SYSTEM: As previously described, the scalp is massively lacerated. The external cranium is markedly distorted with a large area in the right lateral and posterior aspects of the head absent, having been blown away. The cranium is a mass of fracture fragments. The cerebral cortex and brain stem have been evacuated. All that remains is a small portion of medulla oblongata. Several large fragments of brain are submitted separately consisting of portions of cerebral cortex; examined and there is no evidence of any underlying disease. There is massive fracturing of the base of the skull, and there is a large cavitary defect involving the base of the skull, including the posterior aspect of the orbital plates, the temporal fossae, portion of the posterior fossae, and the sphenoid bone and clivus. This is the area that represents entry of the gunshot wound into the skull. C1 and C2 are intact. The odontoid ligament and odontoid processes are intact.

TOXICOLOGY:

Blood: I obtained two gray-stoppered test tubes of blood from the heart.

Urine: I obtained one gray-stoppered test tube of urine.

Bile: I obtained one gray-stoppered test tube of bile.

Gastric Contents: I obtained one gray-stoppered test tube and one red-stoppered test tube of gastric contents.

Vitreous Humor: I obtained one gray-stoppered test tube of vitreous humor.

I also obtained approximately 100 grams of liver and 100 grams of kidney which will be retained and frozen.

TRACE EVIDENCE:

1. Hair samples: I obtained random scalp and pubic hair.
2. I obtained left and right nail scrapings.
3. I obtained one yellow-stoppered test tube of blood, one purple-stoppered test tube of blood, and one red-stoppered test tube of blood.

The hair samples and nail scrapings are given to the Jefferson County Sheriff's Officers in attendance at the autopsy.

We will keep the blood samples with the toxicology specimens for a year for any possible evidentiary need.

X-RAY EXAMINATION: Revealed no evidence of retained bullets.

WOUND SUMMARY: The wound of entrance is a high energy gunshot wound to the roof of the mouth consistent with shotgun. The major force of the wound extended upward, backwards, and slightly to the right, causing large cavitary defects in the base of the skull and the right lateral posterior aspect of the skull. The characteristics of the wound are consistent with self-infliction.

04/29/99 ADDENDUM:

Additional material obtained from the scene is submitted for examination includes:

A. Skull fragments with one tooth.
B. Decomposed brain tissue - 600 grams

IMPRESSIONS:

1. Decomposing cerebral cortex and cerebellar cortex - containing bone fragments - one circular shotgun wad - one tiny piece of what appears to be metal

    A. Wad and metal given to Sheriff's Office.

2. Skull fragments demonstrating circular perforations with outward beveling

3. Separated dried blood for any future DNA testing - frozen

5. Other specimens frozen separately - i.e. bone from decomposing brain tissue

HARRIS, Eric   Dr. Galloway

MICROSCOPICS:

Thymus: Normal histologic features.

Adrenal: Normal histologic features.

Brain Fragments: Sections reveal early autolysis and small foci of intraparenchymal hemorrhage involving the medulla.

Liver: Sections reveal moderate autolysis.

Kidney: Sections reveal moderate autolysis.

Lymph Node: Sections reveal benign reactive lymphoid hyperplasia.

Stomach: Sections reveal early autolysis involving the gastric mucosa.

Heart: Normal histologic features.

Spleen: Normal histologic features.

Thyroid: Normal histologic features.

Lung: Sections reveal patchy atelectasis.

TOXICOLOGY:

Blood Alcohol   Negative

Blood Drug Screen - Gas Chromatography/Mass Spectroscopy
        Only drug detected is Fluvoxamine - 390 ng/ml
        (therapeutic levels 50-900 ng/ml)

Urine Drug Screen   Negative

KLEBOLD, Dylan   Dr. Galloway

FINAL ANATOMIC DIAGNOSES:

1. Through and through close contact large calibre gunshot
    wound involving the left side of the head (region of the
    left temple) associated with:

    A.   Brain injuries - lacerations and contusions
    B.   Skull fractures
    C.   Subdural hemorrhage

2   Aspiration blood lower airway and lungs

COMMENT: The autopsy findings in this case reveal that the cause
of death is due to brain injuries secondary to a close contact,
large calibre, through and through gunshot wound involving the
left side of the head. This gunshot wound is consistent with
self-infliction.

Ben Galloway, M.D.
Forensic Pathologist

This autopsy is performed in the Jefferson County Coroner's
Office in Golden, Colorado on 04/22/99 at 10:30 a.m. This
autopsy is done at the request of Dr. Nancy Bodelson, the Coroner
of Jefferson County. The identification was made by
fingerprints. Concerning location, this body is identified as
#11. Members of the Jefferson County Sheriff's Department
attended the autopsy. I am assisted in the autopsy by Mr. Rob
Kulbacki.

HISTORY: This is the case of a 17-year-old, white male who is
allegedly a victim of a self-inflicted gunshot wound to the head.
The decedent was found dead in the library at Columbine High
School, and the death occurred on 04/20/99. No other history is
available at the time of autopsy.

EXTERNAL EXAMINATION: The body is clothed in a black T-shirt
with the inscription "Wrath" across the front; a black glove on
the left hand with the fingers cut away; blue-green plaid boxer
shorts; black pants with a black belt which have been partially
cut away; white socks; and black boots. A large calibre, copper-
jacketed bullet is present in the right boot. This is given to
the Sheriff's Officer along with the clothing. Present on the
left boot was a red star medallion containing a sickle and a
hammer. Black suspenders were in close proximity of the body.
This is the unembalmed, well-developed, well-nourished,
traumatized body of a white male appearing consistent with the
stated age of 17. Height is measured at 74-1/2"; weight is 143
pounds. Rigor is minimal in the neck and the right lower
extremity; absent in the other areas of the body. Paint reddish-
purple livor is set over the dorsal aspects of the body with
appropriate blanching of the pressure points.

HEAD: The scalp is covered by long, thick, blood-stained, brown
hair which measures 6" in length at the apex. Present on the
left side of the head, in the region of the temple, 1/4" above
and 3/4" anterior to the left ear, is a circular, large calibre,
entrance type of gunshot wound. The wound is surrounded by
marginal abrasion, and what appears to be powder, although there
is extensive drying artifact which makes this determination
difficult. There are small irregular tears in the wound margins.
The perforated area of the wound measures 3/4" in diameter; the
marginal abrasion 1-1/4" in diameter. There is no powder
stippling associated with the wound. For identification
purposes, this wound will be referred to as "A". Present on the
right lateral surface of the head, 1/2" anterior to the midportion of the right ear, is a generally circular exit type of
gunshot wound showing irregular tearing of the margins. This
wound measures 1/2" in diameter. No marginal abrasion or powder
residue are observed. For identification purposes, this wound
will be referred to as "B". Ears - the ears are intact. Both
ears are blood stained. Eyes - the eyebrows are brown. The
sclerae are white. The irides are bluish-gray. The pupils are
round, measure 7 mm, and are directed anteriorly. The
conjunctivae are pale. Bilateral periorbital reddish-purple

contusions are present. Nose - the nose is externally
unremarkable. The nasal passages contain bloody fluid. The
septum is in the midline. Mouth - the lips are reddish-purple
with some drying artifact. There is a blond mustache on the
upper lip. The oral mucous membranes are tan and moist. The
tongue is reddish-brown and finely granular without evidence of
lacerations or contusions. The teeth are in a good state of
dental repair. There is a small amount of hemorrhagic fluid in
the oral cavity. Chin - a blond beard, fashioned in a goatee,
involves the chin. Dried blood smears the forehead; there are
dried blood flow patterns extending across both sides of the face
in a predominantly horizontal plane.

NECK: The external surface of the neck reveals no evidence of
injury. The neck organs are in the midline without palpable
masses.

CHEST: The chest demonstrates a normal anterior-posterior
diameter. No external trauma is present. The breasts are normal
male. Palpating the chest reveals no instability. The axillae
are negative to observation and palpation. A moderate amount of
brown hair is present in both axillae.

ABDOMEN: The abdomen is flat. No external trauma is present.
There is some green discoloration of the lower abdomen due to
early decomposition. Present in the right upper quadrant of the
abdomen, is a linear, horizontal scar which measures 3" in
length. Palpating the abdomen reveals no organomegaly or masses.

GENITALIA: A normal appearing male, brown, genital hair pattern
is present. The penis is of normal size, shape, and position;
circumcised. Both testicles are bilaterally descended in their
respective scrotal sacs without palpable masses. There is
postmortem drying artifact on the anterior surface of the
scrotum.

BACK: The external surface of the back reveals no evidence of
trauma. The anus is intact without any unusual dilatation or
trauma.

EXTREMITIES: The upper extremities are intact. The nails are
intact, short and clean. A silver-colored ring with a black
stone is present on the ring finger of the left hand. There is
accentuated dark purple livor involving the portions of the
fingers external to the glove on the left hand. Present on the
lateral aspect of the left hand involving the thumb and middle
finger are several small reddish-brown abrasions, measuring 1/8"
in diameter. Present overlying the proximal knuckle of the index
finger of the right hand is a purple contusion which also
involves a portion of the hand, and measures 1-1/4" in size. The
forearms are unremarkable. The antecubital fossae reveal no
evidence of recent needle puncture marks or scars. The upper
arms are intact and unremarkable grossly. The lower extremities
are intact. Present on the anterior aspect of the proximal

portion of the right lower extremity are several tiny healing
reddish-brown abrasions. There is a cluster of three yellow-
brown contusions on the anterior-lateral aspect of the right
lower leg, varying in size from 1/4" to 1". Present on the
lateral aspect of the left knee is a cluster of three yellow-
brown contusions, varying in size from 1/4" to 5/8". The soles
of the feet are intact and unremarkable grossly.

Also present in close proximity to the body, in the body bag,
were the following personal effects: a pierced earring, a
silver-colored pocket watch, and a beaded cloth necklace.

INTERNAL EXAMINATION: Through the usual Y-shaped incision, a
thin layer of yellow subcutaneous adipose tissue and reddish-
brown musculature are revealed. The diaphragms are intact and
arch to the level of the 5th left intercostal space and the 4th
right intercostal space. The peritoneal cavity contains no
unusual accumulation of fluid. The lining is smooth, gray and
glistening. The viscera and omentum are normally disposed.

PLEURAL SPACES: The pleural spaces are without any unusual
accumulation of fluid. The parietal pleurae are smooth, gray and
glistening. The bony structures of the chest are intact and
unremarkable grossly. The clavicles are intact. There is no
soft tissue injury involving the chest wall. The pericardial sac
is intact. The lumen contains 10 cc of clear fluid. The
pericardium is smooth, gray and glistening.

THYMUS: Eight (8) grams of pink, lobular, firm, thymic tissue is
present in the anterior-superior mediastinal space.

NECK: The lumen of the upper esophagus and pharynx is patent.
The mucosal surface is tan and wrinkled. The lumen of the upper
respiratory tract contains blood. The mucosal surface is tan and
smooth. The hyoid bone and cricothyroid cartilages, are intact.

THYROID: The thyroid is of normal size, shape, and position, and
has a reddish-brown, lobular, firm, gross appearance. The
cervical vertebrae are intact. There is no obstruction to the
posterior nasopharynx or the posterior aspect of the oral cavity.
The major vessels of the neck are intact and unremarkable
grossly. There is no soft tissue hemorrhage in the neck.

HEART: The heart is intact and weighs 300 grams. The epicardial
surface is reddish-brown, smooth, and glistening. Minimal
amounts of epicardial yellow fat are present. The myocardium is
reddish-brown and firm without gross evidence of fibrosis or
softening. The ventricular walls are of normal thickness. The
endocardial surface is reddish-brown, smooth, and glistening.
Early subendocardial flame type hemorrhages are present in the
left ventricle. The cardiac valves are intact. The valve
leaflets are thin and fully pliable. The valve circumferences
are normal for this size heart. The chordae tendineae are tan
and delicate. The papillary muscles are intact. The foramen

ovale is closed. The atrial septum is intact. The ventricular septum is intact. The coronary ostia are in a normal anatomic position and widely patent. The coronary arteries demonstrate a normal anatomic distribution with normal gross features.

AORTA: The aorta is intact and of normal course and calibre throughout. The intimal surface is tan and smooth. The wall is thin and elastic. The main abdominal tributaries are intact.

RESPIRATORY SYSTEM: The lumen of the lower respiratory tract contains blood. The mucosal surface is tan, smooth and blood stained. The lungs are mildly hyperaerated. The pleural surfaces are pink, reddish-purple, smooth and glistening. The lungs together weigh 850 grams. Serial sections reveal soft, spongy, mildly hyperaerated lung tissue showing evidence of vascular congestion, early pulmonary edema, and aspirated blood. The pulmonary arteries are intact without evidence of thromboembolic disease. The pulmonary veins empty into the left atrium in a normal fashion.

GASTROINTESTINAL SYSTEM: The esophagus is of normal course and calibre throughout. The lumen is patent. The mucosal surface is tan with longitudinal furrowing. The wall is thin. The stomach is in a normal anatomic position. The lumen contains 160 cc of yellow-orange, liquid, gastric contents containing fragments of what appears to be potato skins. The mucosal surface is tan with intact rugae. No peptic ulcer disease or tumor are noted grossly. The small bowel demonstrates a normal anatomic distribution with normal gross features. The appendix is present and unremarkable grossly. The large bowel demonstrates a normal anatomic distribution with normal gross features.

SPLEEN: The spleen is intact and weighs 180 grams. The external surface is purple and smooth. Serial sections reveal a firm, reddish-purple, splenic parenchyma.

LIVER: The liver is intact and weighs 1300 grams. The external surface is reddish-brown, smooth, and glistening. Serial sections reveal a firm, reddish-brown, lobular, normal appearing, liver tissue.

GALLBLADDER: The gallbladder is intact. The lumen contains 12 cc of cloudy yellow-brown, liquid bile. The mucosal surface is smooth and bile stained. The cystic duct and common bile duct are intact and patent throughout. The portal vein, splenic vein, and superior mesenteric vein are intact and patent.

PANCREAS: The pancreas is of normal size, shape, and position, and has a tan, lobular, soft, partially autolyzed, gross appearance.

ADRENALS: Both adrenals are identified. Serial sections reveal a thin yellow cortex and gray medulla.

KIDNEYS: Both kidneys are identified. The capsules strip easily. The left kidney weighs 160 grams; the right kidney weighs 150 grams. The cortical surfaces are reddish-brown and smooth. Bivalving of each kidney reveals a well-demarcated, reddish-brown cortex and medulla. The renal papillae are normal. There is no calyceal scarring. There is no unusual pelvic dilatation. Both ureters are present, patent, and uniform in diameter throughout.

BLADDER: The bladder is intact. The lumen contains 20 cc of clear yellow urine. The bladder mucosa is tan and wrinkled. The prostate, seminal vesicles and testicles are intact and unremarkable grossly.

MUSCULOSKELETAL SYSTEM: Other than the injuries to be described under the head, no other significant injuries are observed.

LYMPHATICS: No gross abnormality.

VENOUS SYSTEM: There is no evidence of hepatic vein, renal vein, or portal vein thrombosis. The superior and inferior vena cavae are intact.

CENTRAL NERVOUS SYSTEM: Reflection of the scalp reveals wound tracts in the soft tissues involving both the left and right side of the head in the temporal areas. There appears to be some powder staining of the soft tissues comprising the margin of the wound tract on the left side of the head. There is also a contusion measuring 1-1/2" on the apex of the scalp. There is a circular perforation which is beveled inward involving the left temporal bone. There is a circular perforation which is beveled outward involving the right temporal bone. Numerous fractures radiate from the circular perforations. Removal of a portion of the calvarium reveals no epidural hemorrhage. 40 cc of subdural hemorrhage overlies the right cerebral hemisphere and on the undersurface of this hemisphere. There is no subarachnoid hemorrhage. There are contusions on the undersurface of both temporal lobes. There is a wound tract across the undersurface of the brain, involving both cerebral hemispheres in the temporal and frontal areas. The brain demonstrates laceration and some pulverization of brain tissue involving the previously mentioned areas. The brain weighs 1500 grams. Serial sectioning the cerebral cortex, the midbrain, the pons, the medulla, the spinal cord, the cerebellum and the pituitary reveals internal injury to the brain involving the anterior aspects of both cerebral hemispheres involving the frontal and temporal areas; and there is injury to the midbrain with predominantly contusion. There is no evidence of any underlying disease of the brain. Examination of the base of the skull reveals a transverse basal skull fracture that involves both temporal fossa and interconnects across the sphenoid bone in the region of the sella turcica. C1 and C2 are intact. The odontoid ligament and odontoid processes are intact. Removal of the dura on the left side of the head reveals powder staining (soot) in the margins of the dura

adjacent to the perforated area of skull.

TOXICOLOGY:

Blood: I obtained two gray-stoppered test tubes of blood from the heart.

Urine: I obtained two gray-stoppered test tubes of urine.

Gastric Contents: I obtained two gray-stoppered test tubes and one red-stoppered test tube of gastric contents.

Vitreous Humor: I obtained one gray-stoppered test tube of vitreous humor.

Bile: I obtained one gray-stoppered test tube of bile.

Approximately 100 grams of liver and kidney were also obtained and will be frozen.

TRACE EVIDENCE:

Hair: I obtained random samples of scalp hair and pubic hair. I obtained scalp hair adjacent to the wounds involving the right and left sides of the head.

Nail Scrapings: I obtained nails scrapings of both hands.

Blood: I obtained one yellow, one purple and one red-stoppered test tube of blood from the heart.

All of the trace evidence, with the exception of the blood samples, are given to the Jefferson County Sheriff's Officers upon completion of the autopsy. The blood samples for any evidentiary need are going to be stored along with the toxicology specimens for up to a year.

X-RAY EXAMINATION: Revealed no evidence of retained bullets.

WOUND SUMMARY:

The wound of entrance is designated wound "A" in the region of the left temple. The projectile penetrated the cranium through the left temporal bone; extended across the undersurface of both cerebral hemispheres; exiting the head through the right temporal bone. The perforated area on the left side is beveled inward; the perforated area on the right side is beveled outward. Powder is associated with the wound on the left side of the head. The projectile traveled left to right slightly front to back and slightly downward. The characteristics of the wound are consistent with a large calibre weapon; with a close contact range of fire; consistent with self-infliction.

The wound is consistent with 9 mm ammunition.

KLEBOLD, Dylan   Dr. Galloway

MICROSCOPICS:

Heart: Normal histologic features.

Lung: Sections reveal intra-alveolar edema.

Liver: Sections reveal moderate autolysis.

Kidney: Sections reveal moderate autolysis.

Spleen: Normal histologic features.

Adrenal: Normal histologic features.

Thymus: Normal histologic features.

Thyroid: Normal histologic features.

Stomach: Sections reveal early autolysis involving the gastric mucosa.

Brain: Sections reveal fragmentation and intraparenchymal hemorrhage.

Entrance Wound A: Sections are of skin revealing a central deeply penetrating wound associated with a few scattered fragments of powder residue in the deeper margins of the wound.

Dura: Sections reveal scattered foci of powder residue adhering to one side of the dural surface.

TOXICOLOGY:

Blood Alcohol   Negative

Blood Drug Screen - Gas Chromatography/Mass Spectroscopy
    Acid Neutral Extract   No drugs detected
    Basic Extract   No drugs detected

Urine Drug Screen   Negative

John Wilkes Booth

Born: May 10, 1838, Bel Air, Maryland
Died: April 26, 1865, Port Royal, Virginia
Cause of Death: Shooting

John Wilkes Booth, the assassin of Abraham Lincoln, was killed after he was surrounded by US soldiers but refused to surrender. Before his assassination plot, he was an actor at Ford's Theatre. He killed Lincoln with the intent of bringing down the American government. He had two co-conspirators who had agreed to attack the Vice President and the Sectary of State, but the men were unable to carry out the task. The autopsy of Booth was performed by Dr. Woodward—the same doctor that performed Lincoln's autopsy.

Case JWB: Was killed April 26, 1865, by a conoidal pistol ball, fired at the distance of a few yards, from a cavalry revolver. The missile perforated the base of the right lamina of the 4th cervical vertebra, fracturing it longitudinally and separating it by a fissure from the spinous process, at the same time fracturing the 5th vertebra through its pedicle, and involving that transverse process. The projectile then transversed the spinal canal almost horizontally but with a slight inclination downward and backward, perforating the cord which was found much torn and discolored with blood (see Specimen 4087 Sect. I AMM). The ball then shattered the bases of the left 4th and 5th laminae, driving bony fragments among the muscles, and made its exit at the left side of the neck, nearly opposite the point of entrance. It avoided the 2nd and 3rd cervical nerves. These facts were determined at autopsy which was made on April 28. Immediately after the reception of the injury, there was very general paralysis. The phrenic nerves performed their function, but the respiration was diaphragmatic, of course, labored and slow. Deglutition was impracticable, and one or two attempts at articulation were unintelligible. Death, from asphyxia, took place about two hours after the reception of the injury.

-Dr. Woodward

Sir,

I have the honor to report that in compliance with your orders, assisted by Dr. Woodward, USA, I made at 2 PM this day, a postmortem examination of the body of J. Wilkes Booth, lying on board the Monitor Montauk off the Navy Yard.

The left leg and foot were encased in an appliance of splints and bandages, upon the removal of which, a fracture of the fibula (small bone of the leg) 3 inches above the ankle joint, accompanied by considerable ecchymosis, was discovered.

The cause of death was a gun shot wound in the neck - the ball entering just behind the sterno-cleido muscle - 2 1/2 inches above the clavicle - passing through the bony bridge of fourth and fifth cervical vertebrae - severing the spinal chord (sic) and passing out through the body of the sterno-cleido of right side, 3 inches above the clavicle.

Paralysis of the entire body was immediate, and all the horrors of consciousness of suffering and death must have been present to the assassin during the two hours he lingered.

-Surgeon General Barnes

Jim Jones

Full Name: James Warren Jones
Born : May 13, 1931, Randolph County, Indiana
Died: November 18, 1978, Jonestown, Guyana
Cause of Death: Suicide

Jim Jones was the leader of the People's Temple, a communist community and religion. He moved the temple throughout the United States before settling on a location in Guyana. He called the community Jonestown and it was a safe haven for communist ideals. Many of his followers were American citizens who were not allowed to leave the compound. When an American delegation came to assess any human rights violations in Jonestown, members of the armed guard opened fire, killing a US Congressman and several members of the news community. Jones then told his people that the only course of action was to drink cyanide-laced Flavor Aid or they would be tortured and forced into fascism. Jones died from a self inflicted gunshot wound to the head. Though it was not the cause of death, Jones's autopsy revealed that he had ingested enough drugs to die of an overdose.

Standard Form 503
Burau of the Budget
Canale A-32 Rev. 1

CLINICAL RECORD | AUTOPSY PROTOCOL

DATE AND HOUR DIED | DATE AND HOUR AUTOPSY PERFORMED | CHECK ONE
18 November 1978 P.M. | 15 December 1978 P.M. | FULL AUTOPSY | HEAD ONLY | TORSO ONLY
PROSECTOR | ASSISTANT |
Kenneth H. Mueller, LTCOL, USAF | Robert L. Thompson, CAPT, MC, USN | X

CLINICAL DIAGNOSES (Indicate operation)

This body (later identified as James Warren Jones) was one of a large number of bodies discovered at Jonestown, Guyana on or about 19 November 1978 by members of the Guyanese Defense Force. The scene, as reported in various news media and by government officials of Guyana, was said to be grotesque in the extreme. A few witnesses, again reported in various news media, said that most of these people, some willingly and others unwillingly, had ingested poison(s) which fairly quickly led to their deaths.

After inquiries into the cause and manner of death by Guyanese officials, including Dr. Leslie Mootoo, forensic pathologist to the government of Guyana, the bodies, which were rapidly putrefying in the hot and humid tropical climate of Guyana, were released by the government of Guyana and transported by the United States Air Force from Jonestown, Guyana to Dover AFB, Delaware between 23 and 26 November 1978. Efforts to identify the bodies and add to the store of reliable information about the causes and manners of their deaths were carried on at Dover AFB from 27 November 1978 onward.

PATHOLOGICAL DIAGNOSES

1. Gunshot wound, head, hard contact, perforating, with extensive skull fractures.
   a) Entrance wound: left temple area.
   b) Wound track: left to right, anterior to posterior, and slightly inferior to superior.
   c) Exit wound: right temple area.

2. Postmortem decomposition.

3. Embalming artifacts.

Cause of Death: Gunshot wound of head.

Manner of Death: Undetermined.

APPROVED—SIGNATURE |
KENNETH H. MUELLER, LTCOL, USAF, MC | ROBERT L. THOMPSON, CAPT, MC, USN
MILITARY ORGANIZATION (If not military) | AGE | SEX | RACE | IDENTIFICATION NO. | AUTOPSY NO.
 | 47 | Male | Caucasian | |

PATIENT'S IDENTIFICATION | REGISTER NO. | WARD NO.
JONES, JAMES WARREN | | AUTOPSY PROTOCOL
AFIP #1680342 | | Standard Form 503

AUTOPSY REPORT - (B013)   AFIP #1680342

Name: JAMES WARREN JONES
Age: 47 years
Date of Birth: 13 May 1931
Sex: Male
Race: Caucasian
Date of Death: 18 November 1978
Date of Autopsy: 15 December 1978
Prosector: Kenneth M. Mueller, Lt.Col, USAF, MC
Witnesses: Robert L. Thompson, CAPT, MC, USN
                   Joseph M. Ballo, LTC, MC, USA
                   Douglas S. Dixon, MAJ, MC, USA
                   Rudiger Breitenecker, M.D., Baltimore, Maryland

This is one of the bodies (B013) transported by the USAF from Jonestown,
Guyana to Dover Air Force Base, Delaware.

Body Identification:

The body is identified as James Warren Jones on the basis of the comparison
of antemortem and postmortem fingerprint and dental records. No medical
records are available.

Description of Clothing:

The body is clothed in a red shirt with the label "Fruit of Loom, Extra
Large", tan trousers labeled "Sears Permapress, 36 X 30", no belt, brief
type underwear with the label "3H Fruit of Loom" and the name "Steve"
initialed into the waist band, black socks and black lace shoes with the
label "84550, Cont, 305Z".

External Description:

The body is that of a Caucasian male with moderate to severe decomposition
changes. There is a tag attached to the toe with the name Reverend James W.
Jones and the number 138 is also attached to the body. The body is well
nourished, well developed and measures 68 inches in length. The age is
estimated to be 45-60 and the weight 175 lbs. The color of the hair is
black. The body has been previously embalmed and is covered with a white-
tan powder. The examination of the teeth reveal them to be in good repair
and a few of the anterior lower teeth have a pink coloration. The eyes are
sunken. The face has been incised at each corner of the mouth for previous
examination of the teeth. In the anterior midline of the body there is a
26 inch sutured incision which begins in the area of the left sterno-clavicular
junction and ends in the supra-pubic area. There are coils of intestine protruding through the sutured incision. Examination of the external genitalia
reveals the penis to be circumcised. No scars or tattoos are identified.

AUTOPSY REPORT - (B013)   AFIP #1680342

Evidence of Embalming:

Trocar stab wounds are identified in the following areas: beneath the chin, in the cheek areas bilaterally, the right forearm near the antecubital fossa, the left anterior shoulder area, the right side of the anterior abdominal wall at the level of the umbilicus, the supra-pubic area slightly to the right, the right anterior upper thigh area, the area of the right medial thigh near the knee, the left lower leg anterior near the knee.

Evidence of Injury:

The entrance of a gunshot wound is located in the left temple area 3+7/8 inches below the top of the head, 1/2 inch anterior to the external auditory canal and 5 inches to the left of the midline of the face. The entrance wound is triangular shaped and measures 3/4 by 2+1/2 inches. No powder residue or muzzle imprint is identified around the wound.

The track of the wound perforates the underlying tempo-parietal skull with internal beveling. The wound track within the brain is not identified because of severe postmortem decomposition. The wound then perforates the right temporal bone with external beveling.

The exit gunshot wound is located in the right temple area superior to the right ear. The wound measures 3/8 by 1/4 inch, and is 3+1/2 inches below the top of the head, 1/2 inch posterior to the external auditory canal and 6 inches to the right of the midline of the face.

The path of the wound is directed from left to right, anterior to posterior and slightly inferior to superior.

Internal Examination:

The thorax and abdomen are opened by extending, in the usual Y shape, the previously described incision. The original incision on the chest is seen to have extended through the skin and subcutaneous tissue, but not the rib cage. The abdominal segment of this incision extends into the abdominal cavity. The usual intermastoid coronal scalp incision is employed for examination of the cranial cavity.

Cranial Cavity: The examination of the skull reveals multiple comminuted fractures in the areas of the frontal bone, parietal bone, occipital bone and base of the skull. There is a fracture of the base of the skull in the area of the ethmoid bone. The brain is severely decomposed and is in a semi-liquid state. No grossly identifiable structures are noted within the brain. Except for fractures, the sella turcica shows no abnormality and the pituitary gland is not enlarged. The gunshot wound of the head has previously been described.

-2-

AUTOPSY REPORT - (8013)   AFIP #1680342

Neck: The examination of the neck structures reveals no hemorrhage and no fractures of the hyoid bone or laryngeal cartilages. Examination of the interior of the larynx reveals no evidence of obstruction.

Body Cavities: Each chest cavity has approximately 150 cc's of reddish-brown, foul smelling fluid. The abdominal cavity contains a small amount of yellowish-brown fluid.

Cardiovascular System: The heart is of normal size and shape. Examination of the coronary arteries reveals no thickening and they are of normal size and distribution. Examination of the chambers of the heart reveals all valves to be normal and the myocardium shows no abnormalities except for the changes of decomposition. The examination of the aorta reveals a few small atheromatous plaques at the ostia of the coronary arteries.

Respiratory Tract: The lungs have an extensive honey-combed appearance due to decomposition, but they are of normal size and shape. Examination of the bronchi reveals a small amount of brownish material within the lumens.

Biliary Tract: The liver is of normal size and shape and there is no abnormality except for decomposition changes on the cut surfaces. The gall-bladder is empty.

Spleen: The spleen is of normal size and shape and there is no abnormality except for decomposition changes on the cut surface.

Pancreas: The pancreas is extensively decomposed, but no abnormality is noted.

Genitourinary System: The kidneys are of normal size and shape and examination of the cut surface reveals an extensive honey-combed appearance due to decomposition on the cut surfaces. There is no abnormality of the ureters. The bladder is empty, and the mucosa of the bladder shows no abnormality. The prostate gland is small and no nodules are noted on the cut surface.

Alimentary Tract: Examination of the pharynx reveals no obstruction. The esophagus is empty. The stomach is empty and no identifiable food or drugs are identified. Examination of the small and large intestine reveals no external abnormality.

Endocrine System: Examination of the area of the pituitary gland reveals extensive fractures of the bone in this area. The pituitary gland is extensively decomposed, but no gross abnormality is noted. Examination of the thyroid gland and adrenal gland reveals no abnormality except for changes of decomposition.

-2-

AUTOPSY REPORT - (8013)   AFIP #1680342

Musculoskeletal System: The extensive fractures of the skull have been
previously described. Examination of other areas of the musculoskeletal
system reveals no gross abnormality.

Toxicology: The following tissues are submitted for toxicological examination: the stomach and stomach contents, spleen, liver, kidney, lung.

X-Ray Examination: Total body X-rays reveal the only obvious trauma to be
confined to the head. The calvarium is fractured in a massive, comminuted
fashion. Within the head are scattered small metallic densities, consistent
with a bullet track, but no large fragments are seen. There is no obvious
evidence of sella turcica or pituitary problems, but the sella is not ideally
evaluated on the available films.

Microscopic Description

All of the tissues show moderate to severe changes of postmortem decomposition:

   Skin: Sections from the entrance and exit wounds are examined. No
          definite powder residue is identified. The changes of decom-
          position preclude further evaluation.

   Coronary arteries: Sections of coronary artery show slight to moderate
                       intimal thickening.

   Lung: Sections of lung show focal intra-alveolar hemorrhage.

Sections of liver, kidney, thyroid, myocardium, and prostate show no changes
except decomposition.

After fungus and bacterial stains were prepared, the microscopic stains were
evaluated by the Department of Infectious Diseases. It is the opinion of
this Department that fungi and bacteria seen in the sections are postmortem
contaminants, and no changes to indicate antemortem infectious disease are
noted.

-4-

AUTOPSY REPORT - (B013)   AFIP #1680342

Summary:

This is the case of a 47 year old Caucasian male who was found dead in
Jonestown, Guyana. The cause of death is a gunshot wound of the head.
The caliber of the gun was large enough to produce the typical stellate
tearing of the skin surrounding the wound. The hands were not swabbed
for powder residue because the embalming and extensive handling of the
body after death would have led to the high probability of either false
positive or false negative results.

The tissue levels of pentobarbital are within the toxic range, and in
some cases of drug overdose have been sufficient to cause death. The
liver and kidney pentobarbital levels are within the generally accepted
lethal range. The drug level within the brain is not within the generally
accepted lethal range, and brain levels are the most important as far as
vital functions are concerned. The cause of death is not thought to be
pentobarbital intoxication because: (1) the brain level is low, as
stated above (2) tolerance can be developed to barbiturates over a period
of time and (3) the lethal level of a drug varies from individual to individual. The level of chloroquine within the liver is within the therapeutic
range.

. No anatomic evidence of antemortem disease is found.

The manner of death is consistent with suicide because of the finding of
a hard contact gunshot wound of the head. The possibility of homicide
cannot be entirely ruled out because of the lack of specific and reliable
information.

KENNETH H. MUELLER
LTCOL, USAF, MC
Division of Forensic Pathology

ROBERT L. THOMPSON, M.D.
Captain, MC, USN
Chairman, Department of
    Forensic Sciences

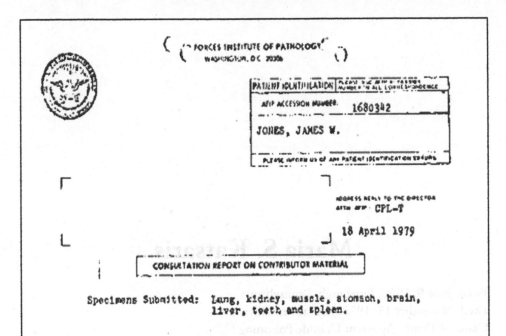

(FORCES INSTITUTE OF PATHOLOGY
WASHINGTON, DC 20306)

PATIENT IDENTIFICATION	PLEASE USE ABOVE ACCESSION NUMBER IN ALL CORRESPONDENCE
AFIP ACCESSION NUMBER	1680342
JONES, JAMES W.	
PLEASE INFORM US OF ANY PATIENT IDENTIFICATION ERRORS	

ADDRESS REPLY TO THE DIRECTOR
ATTN AFIP CPL-T

18 April 1979

CONSULTATION REPORT ON CONTRIBUTOR MATERIAL

Specimens Submitted: Lung, kidney, muscle, stomach, brain,
liver, teeth and spleen.

AFIP DIAGNOSIS:

REPORT OF TOXICOLOGIC EXAMINATION

1. All tissues submitted were putrefied; the body was embalmed
prior to autopsy.

2. Neutral drugs - LIVER - None Found.

3. The following drugs were identified and quantitated by
gas chromatography and uv spectrophotometry and verified by
mass spectrometry. Amounts reported are in milligrams per
100 grams tissue.

	LUNG	STOMACH	BRAIN	KIDNEY	MUSCLE	LIVER	SPLEEN
Pentobarbital	0.5	37.3	0.3	8.4	0.03	5.7	19.3
Chloroquine	NR	NR	NR	NR	NR	8.3	NR

WILLIAM W. MANDERS
LTCOL, USAF, BSC
Chief, Division of Toxicology

AFIP FL 61 (1 May 78)

Maria S. Katsaris

Born: June 9, 1953, Pittsburgh, Pennsylvania
Died: November 18, 1978, Jonestown, Guyana
Cause of Death: Apparent Cyanide Poisoning

On November 18, 1978, 909 members of the People's Temple were massacred. They were given cyanide-laced juice and told that if they didn't drink it, people would come to torture them and their loved ones. The leaders of the temple called this action revolutionary suicide. The people, convinced by their leader they were doing the right thing, calmly took the poison despite the screams they heard from the others. One of the members of the group, Maria Katsaris, was twenty-five years old at the time. When her autopsy was performed, coroners could not determine the exact cause of death. This was attributed to the nature of cyanide and the low level of toxins in Katsaris' and many of the others' systems.

Standard Form 503
Revised August 1954
Bureau of the Budget
Circular A-51 (Rev.)

CLINICAL RECORD		AUTOPSY PROTOCOL				
DATE AND HOUR DIED	A. M.	DATE AND HOUR AUTOPSY PERFORMED	A. M.	CHECK ONE		
18 November 1978	P. M.	15 December 1978	P. M.	FULL AUTOPSY	HEAD ONLY	TRUNK ONLY
PROSECTOR		ASSISTANT		X		
Robert L. Thompson, CAPT, MC, USN		Kenneth H. Mueller, LTCOL, USAF				

CLINICAL DIAGNOSIS (Autopsy Narrative)

This body (later identified as Maria Katsaris) was one of a large number of bodies discovered at Jonestown, Guyana on or about 19 November 1978 by members of the Guyanese Defense Force. The scene, as reported in various news media and by government officials of Guyana, was said to be grotesque in the extreme. A few witnesses, again reported in various news media, said that most of these people, some willingly and others unwillingly, had ingested poison(s) which fairly quickly led to their deaths.

After inquiries into the cause and manner of death by Guyanese officials, including Dr. Leslie Mootoo, forensic pathologist to the government of Guyana, the bodies, which were rapidly putrefying in the hot and humid tropical climate of Guyana, were released by the government of Guyana and transported by the United States Air Force from Jonestown, Guyana to Dover AFB, Delaware between 23 and 26 November 1978. Efforts to identify the bodies and add to the store of reliable information about the causes and manners of their deaths were carried on at Dover AFB from 27 November 1978 onward.

PATHOLOGICAL DIAGNOSES

1. Cause of Death: Probable cyanide poisoning.

2. Young adult Caucasian female (embalmed) in advanced stages of postmortem decomposition with maggot infestation.

3. Manner of Death: Undetermined.

Robert L. Thompson   *K H Mueller*

APPROVED SIGNATURE

ROBERT L. THOMPSON, CAPT, MC, USN   KENNETH H. MUELLER, LTCOL, USAF, MC

MILITARY ORGANIZATION (Item record)	AGE	SEX	RACE	IDENTIFICATION NO.	AUTOPSY NO.
	25	Female	Caucasian		

PATIENT'S IDENTIFICATION

KATSARIS, MARIA
AFIP #1683272

AUTOPSY PROTOCOL
Standard Form 503
503-101

AUTOPSY REPORT - (A006)   AFIP # 1680273

Name: MARIA KATSARIS
Age: 25 years
DOB: September 16, 1953
Sex: Female
Race: Caucasian
Date of Death: November 18, 1978
Date of Autopsy: December 15, 1978
Prosector: Robert L. Thompson, Capt, MC, USN
Witnesses: Kenneth H. Mueller, LtCol, USAF, MC
           Joseph M. Ballo, LTC, MC, USA
           Douglas S. Dixon, Major, MC, USA
           Rudiger Breitenecker, M.D.

This is one of the bodies (6A) transported by the USAF from Jonestown,
Guyana to Dover Air Force Base, Delaware.

Body Identification:

The body is identified as MARIA KATSARIS by fingerprints taken by the
Federal Bureau of Investigation and by comparing post-mortem dental observations
with ante-mortem dental records by Colonels Hooker and Morlang, USAF, DC.
Physical characteristics are also consistent.

Description of Clothing and Personal Effects:

When first seen during the week of 27 November through 2 December 1978, the
body is clothed in a green checked shirt, tan trousers with a brass belt
buckle, white socks, blue sneakers, and white panties and bra. Gold-colored
earrings are held in place by pierced ears.

External Description:

When first seen sometime during the week of 27 November through 2 December
1978, the body is received clothed (see above) and in a body bag. Post-mortem
decomposition is advanced. Maggots are present. The height is measured at
70 inches and weight is measured at 118 pounds. No scars, tattoos, or moles
are noted. The scalp hair is brown to black, straight, and drawn up in a
pony-tail. The race is judged to be Caucasian. The sex is female. The age
is estimated to be somewhere between 25 and 40 years. Upper and lower teeth
are present, in good repair, and pink-stained.

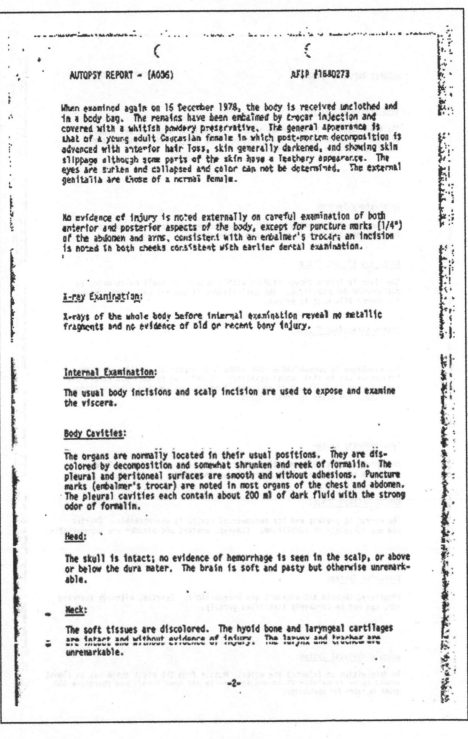

AUTOPSY REPORT - (A036)   AFIP #1680273

When examined again on 15 December 1978, the body is received unclothed and in a body bag. The remains have been embalmed by trocar injection and covered with a whitish powdery preservative. The general appearance is that of a young adult Caucasian female in which post-mortem decomposition is advanced with anterior hair loss, skin generally darkened, and showing skin slippage although some parts of the skin have a leathery appearance. The eyes are sunken and collapsed and color can not be determined. The external genitalia are those of a normal female.

No evidence of injury is noted externally on careful examination of both anterior and posterior aspects of the body, except for puncture marks (1/4") of the abdomen and arms, consistent with an embalmer's trocar; an incision is noted in both cheeks consistent with earlier dental examination.

X-ray Examination:

X-rays of the whole body before internal examination reveal no metallic fragments and no evidence of old or recent bony injury.

Internal Examination:

The usual body incisions and scalp incision are used to expose and examine the viscera.

Body Cavities:

The organs are normally located in their usual positions. They are discolored by decomposition and somewhat shrunken and reek of formalin. The pleural and peritoneal surfaces are smooth and without adhesions. Puncture marks (embalmer's trocar) are noted in most organs of the chest and abdomen. The pleural cavities each contain about 200 ml of dark fluid with the strong odor of formalin.

Head:

The skull is intact; no evidence of hemorrhage is seen in the scalp, or above or below the dura mater. The brain is soft and pasty but otherwise unremarkable.

Neck:

The soft tissues are discolored. The hyoid bone and laryngeal cartilages are intact and without evidence of injury. The larynx and trachea are unremarkable.

-2-

AUTOPSY REPORT - (A006)   AFIP #1680273

Cardiovascular System:

The heart appears to be normal sized; the coronary arteries are widely patent; the valves are normally shaped. The great vessels pursue their normal courses to and from the heart.

Respiratory System:

The lungs appear normally shaped; no parenchymal lesions are seen; the tracheobronchial tree is patent and unremarkable.

Liver and Biliary Tract:

The liver is intact though studded with a network of small holes owing to post-mortem decomposition. The gall-bladder is present and green-stained; the common bile duct is patent.

Gastro-intestinal Tract:

The esophagus is unremarkable; the stomach is empty; the small and large intestines are in their usual positions and deflated by multiple punctures; the pancreas is difficult to recognize owing to post-mortem decomposition: no lesions are noted in these organs.

Hematopoietic System:

The spleen weighs 80 grams; it is soft, mushy and reddish-brown; lymph nodes are not enlarged; bone marrow is unremarkable.

Genito-urinary Tract:

The uterus is present and its endometrial cavity is unremarkable. Ovaries can not certainly be identified. Kidneys, ureters and bladder are unremarkable.

Endocrine System:

Pituitary, thyroid and adrenals are unremarkable. Ovaries, although searched for, can not be certainly identified grossly.

Musculo-skeletal System:

No deformities or injuries are noted. Muscle from the right thigh has an almost normal color (embalming fluid had apparently not penetrated) and therefore 350 grams is taken for toxicology.

AUTOPSY REPORT - (A006)   AFIP #1680273

Specimens for Toxicology:

Brain, stomach, liver, kidney, spleen, and thigh muscle.

Microscopy:

Representative sections from all organs except brain are examined: they
all reveal advanced post-mortem degeneration.

Summary and Opinion:

Postmortem examination of the body of Maria Katsaris demonstrated advanced
putrefaction and evidence of embalming. These findings are consistent
with the circumstances at and after her death as reported or known to us.
Morphological alterations sufficient to account for death were not seen.
Toxicological examination (the specimens being taken about one month after
death and about 2 weeks after embalming) revealed a mixture of an anti-

histamine, an anti-malarial, and a phenothiazine--all of these at tissue
levels not ordinarily thought to be lethal--and a level of cyanide in the
brain of 0.08 mg%, an amount that could be significant.

In view of the above mentioned observations, the reports of seemingly
reliable witnesses, the presence of cyanide in the stomach contents of at
least some of the bodies studied at the scene by Dr. Mootoo, and the presence
of apparently significant amounts of cyanide in other bodies studied at Dover
AFB (as reported by the Toxicology Division of the AFIP), it seems reasonable
to say that, in our opinion, the death of Maria Katsaris was probably caused
by cyanide poisoning. The manner of death, in our opinion, remains undetermined owing to the lack of reliable and specific information about her own
intent and the possibility of coercion by others.

Robert L. Thompson
ROBERT L. THOMPSON, M.D.
Captain, MC, USN
Chairman, Department of
        Forensic Sciences

K H Mueller
KENNETH H. MUELLER
LtCol, USAF, MC
Division of Forensic Pathology

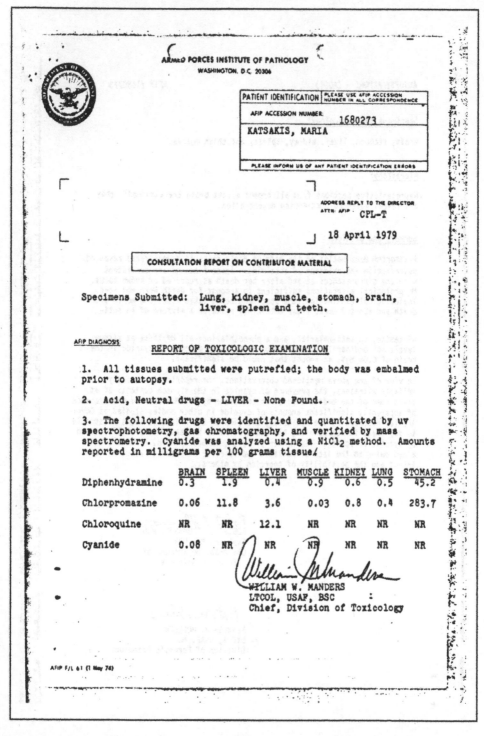

ARMED FORCES INSTITUTE OF PATHOLOGY
WASHINGTON, D.C. 20306

PATIENT IDENTIFICATION	PLEASE USE AFIP ACCESSION NUMBER IN ALL CORRESPONDENCE

AFIP ACCESSION NUMBER: 1680273

KATSAKIS, MARIA

PLEASE INFORM US OF ANY PATIENT IDENTIFICATION ERRORS

ADDRESS REPLY TO THE DIRECTOR
ATTN: AFIP · CPL-T

18 April 1979

CONSULTATION REPORT ON CONTRIBUTOR MATERIAL

Specimens Submitted: Lung, kidney, muscle, stomach, brain, liver, spleen and teeth.

AFIP DIAGNOSIS:

REPORT OF TOXICOLOGIC EXAMINATION

1. All tissues submitted were putrefied; the body was embalmed prior to autopsy.

2. Acid, Neutral drugs – LIVER – None Found.

3. The following drugs were identified and quantitated by uv spectrophotometry, gas chromatography, and verified by mass spectrometry. Cyanide was analyzed using a $NiCl_2$ method. Amounts reported in milligrams per 100 grams tissue:

	BRAIN	SPLEEN	LIVER	MUSCLE	KIDNEY	LUNG	STOMACH
Diphenhydramine	0.3	1.9	0.4	0.9	0.6	0.5	45.2
Chlorpromazine	0.06	11.8	3.6	0.03	0.8	0.4	283.7
Chloroquine	NR	NR	12.1	NR	NR	NR	NR
Cyanide	0.08	NR	NR	NR	NR	NR	NR

WILLIAM W. MANDERS
LTCOL, USAF, BSC
Chief, Division of Toxicology

AFIP F/L 61 (1 May 74)

Lee Harvey Oswald

Born: October 18, 1939, New Orleans, Louisiana
Died: November 24, 1963, Dallas, Texas
Cause of Death: Shooting

On November 22, 1963, Lee Harvey Oswald set up in the Dallas book depository building and assassinated John F. Kennedy—although whether or not he acted alone continues to be a source of controversy. Oswald was a former marine who defected to the Soviet Union. He was originally arrested for killing Dallas police officer J. D. Tippet and on suspicion of shooting the President. He denied both charges telling reporters, "I'm just a patsy!" Oswald was unable to stand trial as he was killed by Jack Ruby while being transferred by police on November 24.

OFFICE OF THE

COUNTY MEDICAL EXAMINER

5201 HARRY HINES BLVD.

DALLAS, TEXAS 75235

Autopsy Number: M63-356

Name: OSWALD, Lee Harvey   Age: 24   Race: White Sex: Male

Autopsy date: 11-24-63, 2:45 P.M.   Coroner: Judge Pierce McBride

Autopsy by: Earl F. Rose, M.D.
Assistant: Sidney C. Stewart, M.D.

EXTERNAL EXAMINATION:

External examination reveals a 5 foot, 9 inch white male, the estimated weight
is 150 pounds. Rigor is not present, slight cooling of the body. There is faint
posterior mottling lividity.

Identification bands on the left wrist, the right wrist, the left great toe.
The head is examined. The hair is brown, slightly wavy. Small amount of dried
blood is the hair which has run from the hairline to the right and backward.
Slight frontal balding. To the right of the midline over the forehead is a
1/2 x 1/16 inch crusted superficial abrasion. The hairline, left temporal region,
is a 1/16 inch very superficial abraded area. There is a left periorbital hematoma which is purple in the central portion, fading at the margins to a faint
lemon-yellow. Total diameter of this is 1 3/4 x 1½ inch. The irides are grey-blue,
the pupils are equal at 8 mm. The sclera and conjunctiva are not remarkable.
Poorly defined scar on the dorsum of the nose which measures ¼ x ¼ inch. There
is black material in the nares. Midline, upper lip, terminating at the vermillion
margin is a ¼ inch pale scar. To the left of the midline, the upper lip, is a
1/16 inch abrasion. The buccal cavity is otherwise not remarkable. Oral hygiene
is fair with some fillings. The tongue is not remarkable. The beard measures
between 1 to 2 mm. Examination of the neck is made. At the upper end of the
right sternocleidomastoid over the skin is a transverse very superficial 3/4 inch
scratch with some reddish antiseptic type of paint surrounding this. Hair distribution is normal. The pubic hair has been shaved. The penis is circumcised.
The testes are descended. The abdomen is flat.

Over the left pectoral region, 14 inches from the top of the head and 2 3/4 inches
to the left of the midline there is a 1½ inch wound. The edges of this are sharp.
Over the left chest is an oblique wound which originates 17 inches from the top of
the head and runs forward, downward toward the midline anteriorly measuring 7½ inches
and closed by 12 running black sutures. This wound goes inferior to the left nipple.
Over the lateral aspect of the left arm, 16 inches from the top of the head is a
3/4 x 3/8 inch wound. It goes into the subcutaneous tissue. 18 inches from the
top of the head over the lateral aspect anteriorly of the right arm there is a
1 x ½ inch wound which goes into the subcutaneous tissue. 21½ inches from the top
of the head originating slightly below the xiphoid running in the midline to above
the pubis is a 10½ inch anterior midline wound closed by 5 wire sutures. Above

M63-356

the medial malleolus on the right side there is a 1 3/4 inch transverse cut-down incision. Cephalad to this is a transverse 1 3/4 inch superficial transverse incised wound. Above the left medial malleolus there is a 1½ inch cut-down type of incised wound. To the left of the midline region of the second thoracic vertebra there is a very faint 3/8 inch bluish discolored area. In the right antecubital fossa is a very tiny needle puncture type of wound surrounded by bluish discoloration. In the left antecubital fossa there are three small needle puncture type of wounds surrounded by bluish discoloration. The nails are examined. They are somewhat dirty although quite well cared for. No evidence of injury is noted. On the midportion dorsum of the left hand, there is a poorly defined pale white oblique ½ inch scar. Over the volar aspect of the right wrist there is a transverse superficial ¼ inch abrasion. Volar aspect of the left wrist there is a transverse 1 3/4 inch slightly raised white scar. Medial aspect of the right knee reddish very poorly defined 7/8 x 1/4 inch reddish discoloration. Over the left arm, below the deltoid there is a transverse 5/8 x 3/4 inch somewhat puckered and irregular scar. A few striae along the lateral aspect of the thighs. Some of the hair of the chest has been shaved. In addition, to the left of the midline there is a round poorly defined round impression on the skin, the diameter of which is 2 inches. Over the medial aspect mid-distal third of the left arm there is a 1½ inch vertical scar with cross hatching.

23 inches from the top of the head and 3 3/8 inches to the left of the midline anteriorly and 10 3/4 inches to the left of the midline posteriorly, over the lower aspect of the left chest there is an entrance type of wound which measures 1/4 x 5/16 inch in diameter. This is surrounded by a contusion ring, the total diameters of the contusion ring are 3/8 of an inch.

22 inches from the top of the head and 9 3/4 inches to the right of the midline anteriorly and 8½ inches to the right of the midline of the back there is a vertical 2 x 1 inch gaping wound. Posterior to this by ½ inch there is a 3/4 x 3/8 inch irregular contused area.

INCISIONS: The standard "Y" thoracoabdominal and intermastoid incisions are utilized. Reflecting the skin there is found to be a wound between the fourth and fifth rib which extends through the soft tissue and measures 6 inches in length. This conforms to the wound on the left chest. The incision is continued through the abdominal wound as well as the thoracotomy wound to the left of the midline of the chest.

SEROUS CAVITIES: Examination of the serous cavities is made. In the left pleural space approximately 175 cc. of blood. In the right pleural space there is in excess of 600 cc. of blood. In the peritoneal cavity there is in excess of 1000 cc. of blood with clot formation. In addition, there is massive retroperitoneal hemorrhage. The omentum adjacent to the transverse colon and stomach is hemorrhagic and irregularly torn.

The abdominal panniculus measures 1 3/4 inches.

THE COURSE OF THE WOUND IS FOLLOWED. It is found to notch the undersurface of the seventh rib at the costochondral junction, this is surrounded by hemorrhage. In its course it notches the diaphragmatic attachment in this region, however, the left lung is not penetrated. The course is found to go from left to right and backward. In its course it is found to strike the anterior edge of the spleen and there is a cruciate laceration of the spleen measuring approximately 1.5 x 2 cm.

M63-356

The missile is found to penetrate the stomach along the greater curvature of the body of the stomach, the penetration measuring 9 cm. It exits from the stomach along the posterior wall, lesser curvature, 2 cm. distal to the cardioesophageal junction. The penetration measures 8 cm. It pursues a course backwards and to the right slightly cauded to the celiac axis and there is extensive hemorrhage in this area. The anterior and right anterio-lateral aspect of the aorta is torn with the superior mesenteric artery being severed. The right renal artery shows destruction and hemorrhage along the cephalad portion. The right renal vein is torn and the tear involves the inferior vena cava, the dorsal surface. It courses through the upper pole of the right kidney along the anterior surface causing a jagged and irregular laceration covering a distance of 5 x 2 cm. with penetration into the calyces. It becomes peritonealised in the hepatorenal pouch and there is a jagged and irregular laceration of the liver covering a distance of 9.5 x 2 x 2 cm. From the liver it penetrates the diaphragm posteriorly on the right side. It then passes adjacent to the lung in the pleural space and the right lung is not penetrated. The eleventh rib to the right of the midline is irregularly fractured and an exit type of wound in this region and in the soft tissue along the posterior axillary line right side there is an incised wound and fragmentation of the rib.

NECK ORGANS: The neck organs are examined. They are not remarkable. The hyoid is intact. No evidence of injury is noted. The thyroid gland is not remarkable grossly.

LUNGS: The trachea and bronchi are not remarkable. The right lung is quite well aerated. The left lung is atelectatic. The peribronchial tissue is not remarkable, however, there is hemorrhage in the posterior mediastinum.

HEART: Examination of the right atrium as well as the right ventricle and a pulmonary artery shows frothing bubbles. The epicardium is markedly congested with petechial hemorrhages, more marked over the left ventricular portion. The heart weighs 330 gm. There are a few subendocardial petechial hemorrhages. Along the anterior right ventricular surface there is a single suture. This is in the epicardial fat. The right ventricle measures 2 to 3 cm., the left 1.2 to 1.3 cm. The valvular circumferences are as follows: aortic valve - 7 cm., mitral valve - 10.5 cm., tricuspid valve - 11.5 cm., and pulmonic valve - 7 cm. The coronary ostia are in the normal location. The coronary arteries are examined in situ, found to be thin, delicate, of normal distribution and free of occlusions. There are left ventricular myocardial hemorrhages.

LIVER: The liver weighs 1260 gm. The penetration of the liver has previously been described.

GALLBLADDER & BILIARY TREE: Not remarkable.

PORTACAVAL SYSTEM: Examination of the portacaval system is made. There is frothing blood in the portacaval system. Extensive hemorrhage is noted to surround this, particularly in the region of the pancreas.

PANCREAS: The pancreas is surrounded by hemorrhage. The parenchyma of the pancreas is not penetrated and the ductal system is not remarkable.

SPLEEN: The spleen weighs 300 gm. The penetration of the spleen has previously been described.

DIAPHRAGM: The penetrations of the diaphragm have previously been described.

N63-356

RETROPERITONEAL TISSUE: There is massive hemorrhage.

GREAT VESSELS: The penetration of the aorta has previously been described. The aorta is otherwise smooth and elastic. There is extensive periaortic hemorrhage which extends above the diaphragm in the posterior mediastinal tissue.

KIDNEYS: The kidneys weigh 450 gm. The destruction to the right kidney has previously been described. The capsule strips with slight difficulty. The cortical surfaces are smooth and pale. The corticomedullary junction is indistinct. The cortices measure 5 to 7 mm. There is hemorrhage into the parenchyma with destruction of the right kidney as previously described. The penetration of the calyces has also been described. About the pelvis of the right kidney there is extensive hemorrhage. The pelvis and ureters are otherwise not remarkable. The bladder contains bloody urine. The prostate is grossly not remarkable.

ADRENALS: The adrenals are both surrounded by hemorrhage, however, both are intact.

INTESTINAL TRACT: The small and large bowel are examined. They are free of penetrations. The appendix is identified. The large bowel contains some formed stool. The penetrations of the stomach have previously been described and there is blood in the stomach. The rugal pattern is not remarkable. The duodenum is not remarkable.

THYMUS: The thymus weighs approximately 15 gm., is quite fibrotic.

SCALP, SKULL, CRANIAL CAVITY & DURA: Not remarkable No evidence of injury is noted

BRAIN: The brain weighs 1450 gm. The brain is symmetrical. The external surface of the brain is not remarkable Configuration is normal. Multiple sections through the brain are taken and fail to reveal any abnormalities. The ventricular system is symmetrical. No abnormalities are encountered. The vascular system is not remarkable and the vessels are thin and delicate. The calvarium is not remarkable. The cervical vertebra and odontoid are not remarkable

M63-356

MICROSCOPIC:

Aorta: There is disruption with fresh hemorrhage. No inflammation or organisation.

Heart: There are hemorrhages in the epicardial fat, mild interstitial edema and
        focal fragmentation of the muscle fibers.

Lung: Areas of atelectasis and focal alveolar hemorrhagic extravasations.

Liver: Disruption with fresh hemorrhages, otherwise non-contributory.

Bowel: There are disruptions of the stomach with hemorrhages adjacent.
        The remainder of the bowel sections are non-contributory.

Spleen: There is disruption along one margin, otherwise non-contributory.

Thyroid: Non-contributory.

Pancreas: Non-contributory.

Gallbladder: Non-contributory.

Prostate: Non-contributory.

Lymph Nodes: Non-contributory.

Adrenals: There is extensive fresh hemorrhage adjacent, otherwise non-contributory.

Skin: Section through the entrance wound shows disruption with fresh hemorrhages.
       There is no organisation or inflammation. Some amorphous debris and fibers
       in the depths of the wound.

Kidney: Sections show disruption of the right kidney with hemorrhages which are
         marked in the pelvic fat and perirenal tissue.

Central Nervous System: Multiple sections are examined and they are non-contributory.

M63-356

FINDINGS:

Chest, left, gunshot wound.
    Penetration of the spleen, stomach, aorta, kidney, liver and diaphragm.
    Massive retroperitoneal hemorrhage.
    Massive peritoneal hemorrhage.
    Right and left hemothorax.
    Heart, left ventricular epicardial and myocardial hemorrhages.
    Atrium, right; ventricle, right; pulmonary artery, - air.
    Lung, left, atelectasis.
Chest, left, thoracotomy.
Abdomen, laparotomy incision.
Arm, left; arm, right; ankle, right; ankle, left - cut-down incisions.
Chest, right, incised wound.
Eye, left, periorbital hematoma.
Forehead and lip, abrasion.
Left wrist and left arm, scars.

CAUSE OF DEATH:

Hemorrhage, secondary to gunshot wound of the chest.

_____
Earl F. Rose, M D.

DALLAS CITY-COUNTY CRIMINAL INVESTIGATION LABORATORY
(Parkland Memorial Hospital
Dallas, Texas
BLOOD and BOX TEST

Case of **M-63-356**   Referred by **Medical Staff**

Blood drawn by _____   At   **Parkland Hospital**
            M.

Date _____ Time _____ .M. Antiseptic used _____

Officers, identification, etc.: _____

_____

Specimen received from:

☐ Dallas P.D. Lock Box at _____ .M. Date _____ By _____

☐ P.D. Lab. Lock Box at **1:15** .M. Date **11/25/63** By **M. Patterson**

☒ Other (Describe): **Morgue ice box.**

_____

Specimen transferred to **M. R. Ray** _____ (Analyst).

Time **1:30** .M. Date **11/25/63** By **M. Patterson**

Specimen container: **One test tube stoppered with rubber stopper.**

_____

Information from _____

Analytical

    Specimen: Date and time of analysis **11/25/63**   **2:20**   .M.

    ☒ Whole Blood

    ☐ Plasma or serum   Analyst: **M. R. Ray**

Data (Micro-Greenberg Method):

U1 = 2.82	U1 = 2.78		Calculation:		
2 = 2.82	2 = 2.78				
av. = 2.82	av. = 2.78		**Negative for alcohol.**		
B1 = 2.86	B1 = 0.19				
B2 = 2.86	B2 = 0.19				
B av. = 2.86					

Gas chromatogram   ☐ Yes   ☒ No

Result: Alcohol content **Negative** %

[signature]

Dallas City-County Criminal
Investigation Laboratory

DALLAS COUNTY HOSPITAL DISTRICT
(Parkland Memorial Hospital)

Date __11/24/63__

TOXICOLOGICAL REPORT

Case of __Lee Harvey Oswald__ ____ Autopsy No. __M163-356__

Autopsy by Dr. __Rose__ ____ On __11/24/63__

Examined for __Alcohol and barbiturate.__

Organs submitted __Blood (see also report on skin, below).__

RESULT OF ANALYSIS:

Poisonous Gases _____ •

Volatile Poisons _____ __Negative.__

Acid-Ether soluble poisons _____ __Negative.__

Alkaline-Ether soluble poisons _____ •

Ammonia-Ether or Amn.-Chloroform soluble poisons _____ •

Metallic Poisons _____ •

Mineral acids and alkalies _____ •

Halogens and their salts _____ •

Salts of Oxy-acids _____ •

Poisons isolated by special methods _____ •

REMARKS: __Blood type = "A"__

__No nitrates were detected around the bullet hole in the
specimen of skin and specimen of ligament submitted.__

(signature)

Toxicologist, Dallas County Hospital
District

John Dillinger

Full Name: John Herbert Dillinger, Jr.
Born: June 22, 1903, Indianapolis, Indiana
Died: July 22, 1934, Chicago, Illinois
Cause of Death: Shooting

John Dillinger was an American bank robber during the Depression. He robbed two dozen banks throughout the Midwest, escaped from jail twice, and was charged but not convicted of killing a police officer. When he needed supplies, he and his gang took police officers hostage and robbed the supply rooms of the stations. At the height of his criminal career, he was declared "Public Enemy Number One" by the US government. Some people believe it was Dillinger's status as a nationally wanted man that sparked the FBI to organize into the powerful law enforcement agency we know today. He was shot by FBI agents while visiting his ailing father in Chicago.

Form 12

CORONER'S PROTOCOL
FRANK J. WALSH—CORONER—COOK COUNTY, ILL. #116 of July

NAME ....JOHN DILLINGER............................ DATE OF DEATH ..7/22/34.....

ADDRESS ....Unknown.................................. AUT. ..Yes.... CERT. ..No.. INQ. Yes

DATE OF EXAM.........7/23/34...................... COR. PHY. ..J. J. Kearns....

SEX ..Male.......... AGE ..33........ LENGTH ..5'7"..... WEIGHT ..#160...

RACE ..White........... NAT'LTY ..American..... EXAM. AT ..Cook County Morgue....

AUTOPSY PERFORMED BY...........J. J. Kearns, M.D.,...........

SIGNATURE OF IDENTIFIER............Cook County Morgue Records.............

HISTORY OF CAUSE OF DEATH:

Gunshot. Removed from sidewalk at 2600 Lincoln Ave. 37th District Police.

ANATOMIC DIAGNOSIS:

1. Multiple (4) (3 superficial: two of the face and one of the chest) and (1) thru and thru of the face, causing laceration of the soft tissues of the neck, comminuted fractures of the lateral processes of the 3rd, 2nd and 1st cervical vertebrae and body of the 2nd cervical vertebra, laceration of the vertebral artery and veins, lower portion of the medulla oblongata and spinal cord to the level of the 5th cervical segment.
2. Anemia and edema of the brain and lungs.
3. Hemorrhagic softening of the myocardium, liver, kidneys and spleen.
4. Multiple healed scars of the face, chin and volar surface distal phalanges of the fingers of both hands.
5. Healed thru and thru bullet wound of the left thigh. ✔
6. Healed scars in the left thigh and leg.
7. Rheumatic mitral (partly stenosing) verrucous endocarditis.
8. Eccentric hypertrophy of the myocardium. ✔

The following order of description will be followed on this and succeeding pages:

1. External findings (in detail)	7. Blood Vessels	13. Spleen	19. Skull
2. Thoracic Cavity	8. Upper Digestive Tract	14. Lymph Glands	20. Meninges
3. Abdominal Cavity	9. Stomach	15. Adrenals	21. Brain
4. Upper Respiratory Tract	10. Intestines	16. Kidneys	22. Miscellaneous
5. Lungs	11. Liver—Gall Bladder	17. Pelvic Organs	23. Chemical Microscopic
6. Heart Aorta	12. Pancreas	18. Testicle—Ovary	24. Bacteriologic

EXTERNAL EXAMINATION (Inspection)

Development of skeleton { Slender / Medium •• / Powerful / Deformed

Musculature....well-developed........ Panniculus adiposus (subcutaneous)....2 cm.

Skin—Color...white....   Edema........none......

Pigmentation...none...........   Bed Sores.......none......

SIGNS OF DEATH

Body Heat.......absent.......   Lividity....dorsal....   Rigor-mortis....present..

Cornea { Turbid / Cloudy } { Smooth / Dry }.....cloudy.........   Putrefaction....none...

Color of hair.........brown scalp hair and mustache (dyed black)....

Size of pupils.............dilated.......Color of Iris......brown...Color of Sclera....gray..

Size and shape of neck { Long / Short / Slender } { Slender / Medium / Thick }.....medium....

Size and shape of thorax { Deformities / Symmetric / Asymmetric } { Massena / Vertebral / Column }....symmetric.....

Abdomen { Flat / Normal / Distended / Retracted }.......flat...

Evidences of External Injury, with description:

There were two superficial "gutter-like" abrasions of the skin, such as a bullet would make: #1—adjacent to the outer angle of the left eye: #2—in the cheek over the zygoma, on the left side.

#3—Bullet wound of entrance at the level of the 6th cervical vertebra 5 cm. to the right of the midline. This bullet passed upward in the neck causing laceration of the soft tissues, comminuted fractures of the lateral processes of the 3rd, 2nd and 1st cervical vertebrae, comminuted fracture of the body of the 2nd cervical vertebra, laceration of the vertebral artery and vein, laceration of the meninges of the spinal cord, posterior, lateral and anterior tracts from the level of the 4th thru the medulla oblongata on the right side, from here the bullet passed upward along the postero-lateral pharynx causing hemorrhage around the internal jugular and internal carotid arteries, leaving thru an open' in the lower lid of the right eye at its outer angle. There was an extensive sub-periosteal hemorrhage from the level of the jugular foramen to the 6th cervical vertebra, in the spinal canal. The spinal canal contained clotted an fluid blood.

#4—Bullet wound of entrance in the mid-clavicular line over the 7th costal interspace. This bullet passed superficially leaving thru an opening in the mid-axillary line over the 8th rib on the left side.

There were superficial abrasions of the skin of the nose and face. There were healed scars in the chin, oblique in direction, 2 cm. on either side of the midline. There were healed verticle scars over the temporo-mandibular joint, 3 cm. long, on either side. There was a purple-red area in the skin, 2½ cm. square, over the sternum at the level of the 7th costal cartilage just to the right of the midline. This was covered with a thin parchment-like membrane. There were roughly circular scars in the skin, up to 1 cm. in diameter, in the middle of the volar surface of the distal phalanges of the fingers of both hands. There was a linear scar, 10 cm. long, in the left thigh, antero-lateral aspect, lower third. There was a healed semi-lunar scar in the antero-medial aspect, calf of the left leg. There was a wound, such as a bullet wound of entrance and exit would make, the former at the junction of the middle and lower thirds antero-lateral aspect, the latter in the postero-lateral aspect, slightly above the wound of entrance, in the left thigh. There was a healed wound in the neck, roughly circular in outline, 1 cm. in diameter, posterior aspect 2 cm. to the left of the midline at the level of the 7th cervical vertebra.

HEAD: The scalp, cranial bones and meninges showed no traumatic changes. The brain, on multiple surfaces made by cutting, was pale. The lower portion of the medulla oblongata and the spinal cord to the level of the 5th cervical segment was studded with petechial and ecchymotic hemorrhages.

NECK: The soft tissues of the neck, including the mucous membrane of the buccal cavity, esophagus, pharynx and larynx, were pale.

CHEST: The lungs were subcrepitant and on surfaces made by cutting covered with pale bloody frothy fluid. The trachea and bronchi contained bloody frothy fluid. The tracheo-bronchial lymph nodes were soft and anthracotic.

HEART: The pericardial sac contained straw colored fluid. The myocardium was thickened, pale, soft. The mitral leaflets were thickened, the commissures partly obliterated. The corda tendinae and papillary muscles were thickened. There were pin point to pin head sized semi-firm warty vegetations on the auricular surface of the free margins of the mitral leaflets. The intima of the aorta and coronary arteries contained a few atheromatous placques.

ABDOMEN: The abdominal surfaces were smooth and dry. The liver, kidneys and spleen were pale, soft, the markings were indistinct. The gall bladder and biliary passages were patent. The adrenals, pancreas and lower genito-urinary tract were not remarkable. The stomach contained a partly digested meal consisting of particles of red peppers, and fragments of meat and vegetables.

Jack the Ripper Victims

In 1888, an unidentified serial killer terrorized the streets of London. He killed at least five women in the Whitechapel section of the city. The names of his known victims are Mary Kelly, Catherine Eddowes, Elizabeth Stride, Mary Anne Nichols, and Annie Chapman. Police were unable to catch the murderer, and his identity is still unknown. Below are the autopsy reports of his victims.

Mary Anne "Polly" Nichols

Five teeth were missing, and there was a slight laceration of the tongue. There was a bruise running along the lower part of the jaw on the right side of the face. That might have been caused by a blow from a fist or pressure from a thumb. There was a circular bruise on the left side of the face which also might have been inflicted by the pressure of the fingers. On the left side of the neck, about 1 in. below the jaw, there was an incision about 4 in. in length, and ran from a point immediately below the ear. On the same side, but an inch below, and commencing about 1 in. in front of it, was a circular incision, which terminated at a point about 3 in. below the right jaw. That incision completely severed all the tissues down to the vertebrae. The large vessels of the neck on both sides were severed. The incision was about 8 in. in length. The cuts must have been caused by a long-bladed knife, moderately sharp, and used with great violence. No blood was found on the breast, either of the body or the clothes. There were no injuries about the body until just about the lower part of the abdomen. Two or three inches from the left side was a wound running in a jagged manner. The wound was a very deep one, and the tissues were cut through. There were several incisions running across the abdomen. There were three or four similar cuts running downwards, on the right side, all of which had been caused by a knife which had been used violently and downwards, the injuries were form left to right and might have been done by a left handed person. All the injuries had been caused by the same instrument.

Annie Chapman

The left arm was placed across the left breast. The legs were drawn up, the feet resting on the ground, and the knees turned outwards. The face was swollen and turned on the right side. The tongue protruded between the front teeth, but not beyond the lips. The tongue was evidently much swollen. The front teeth were perfect as far as the first molar, top and bottom and very fine teeth they were. The body was terribly mutilated...the stiffness of the limbs was not marked, but was evidently commencing. He noticed that the throat was dissevered deeply; that the incision through the skin were jagged and reached right round the neck... On the wooden paling between the yard in question and the next, smears of blood, corresponding to where the head of the deceased lay, were to be seen. These were about 14 inches from the ground, and immediately above the part where the blood from the neck lay. He should say that the instrument used at the throat and abdomen was the same. It must have been a very sharp knife with a thin narrow blade, and must have been at least 6 in. to 8 in. in length, probably longer. He should say that the injuries could not have been inflicted by a

bayonet or a sword bayonet. They could have been done by such an instrument as a medical man used for post-mortem purposes, but the ordinary surgical cases might not contain such an instrument. Those used by the slaughtermen, well ground down, might have caused them. He thought the knives used by those in the leather trade would not be long enough in the blade. There were indications of anatomical knowledge...he should say that the deceased had been dead at least two hours, and probably more, when he first saw her; but it was right to mention that it was a fairly cool morning, and that the body would be more apt to cool rapidly from its having lost a great quantity of blood. There was no evidence...of a struggle having taken place. He was positive the deceased entered the yard alive....

A handkerchief was round the throat of the deceased when he saw it early in the morning. He should say it was not tied on after the throat was cut.

Report following the post mortem examination:
He noticed the same protrusion of the tongue. There was a bruise over the right temple. On the upper eyelid there was a bruise, and there were two distinct bruises, each the size of a man's thumb, on the forepart of the top of the chest, The stiffness of the limbs was now well marked. There was a bruise over the middle part of the bone of the right hand. There was an old scar on the left of the frontal bone. The stiffness was more noticeable on the left side, especially in the fingers, which were partly closed. There was an abrasion over the ring finger, with distinct markings of a ring or rings. The throat had been severed as before described. the incisions into the skin indicated that they had been made from the left side of the neck. There were two distinct clean cuts on the left side of the spine. They were parallel with each other and separated by about half an inch. The muscular structures appeared as though an attempt had made to separate the bones of the neck. There were various other mutilations to the body, but he was of the opinion that they occurred subsequent to the death of the woman, and to the large escape of blood from the division of the neck.

The deceased was far advanced in disease of the lungs and membranes of the brain, but they had nothing to do with the cause of death. The stomach contained little food, but there was not any sign of fluid. There was no appearance of the deceased having taken alcohol, but there were signs of great deprivation and he should say she had been badly fed. He was convinced she had not taken any strong alcohol for some hours before her death. The injuries were certainly not self-inflicted. The bruises on the face were evidently recent, especially about the chin and side of the jaw, but the bruises in front of the chest and temple were of

longer standing -- probably of days. He was of the opinion that the person who cut the deceased throat took hold of her by the chin, and then commenced the incision from left to right. He thought it was highly probable that a person could call out, but with regard to an idea that she might have been gagged he could only point to the swollen face and the protruding tongue, both of which were signs of suffocation.

The abdomen had been entirely laid open: the intestines, severed from their mesenteric attachments, had been lifted out of the body and placed on the shoulder of the corpse; whilst from the pelvis, the uterus and its appendages with the upper portion of the vagina and the posterior two thirds of the bladder, had been entirely removed. No trace of these parts could be found and the incisions were cleanly cut, avoiding the rectum, and dividing the vagina low enough to avoid injury to the cervix uteri. Obviously the work was that of an expert -- of one, at least, who had such knowledge of anatomical or pathological examinations as to be enabled to secure the pelvic organs with one sweep of the knife, which must therefore must have at least 5 or 6 inches in length, probably more. The appearance of the cuts confirmed him in the opinion that the instrument, like the one which divided the neck, had been of a very sharp character. The mode in which the knife had been used seemed to indicate great anatomical knowledge.

Elizabeth Stride

Dr. George Baxter Phillips, who also handled the Chapman and Kelly murders, performed the post mortem on Stride. He was also present at the scene and, after examining the body, asserts the deceased had not eaten any grapes. His report is as follows:

The body was lying on the near side, with the face turned toward the wall, the head up the yard and the feet toward the street. The left arm was extended and there was a packet of cachous in the left hand.

The right arm was over the belly, the back of the hand and wrist had on it clotted blood. The legs were drawn up with the feet close to the wall. The body and face were warm and the hand cold. The legs were quite warm.

Deceased had a silk handkerchief round her neck, and it appeared to be slightly torn. I have since ascertained it was cut. This corresponded with the right angle of the jaw. The throat was deeply gashed and there was an abrasion of the skin about one and a half inches in diameter, apparently stained with blood, under her right arm.

At three o'clock p.m. on Monday at St. George's Mortuary, Dr. Blackwell and I made a post mortem examination. Rigor mortis was still thoroughly marked. There was mud on the left side of the face and it was matted in the head.

The body was fairly nourished. Over both shoulders, especially the right, and under the collarbone and in front of the chest there was a bluish discoloration, which I have watched and have seen on two occasions since.

There was a clear-cut incision on the neck. It was six inches in length and commenced two and a half inches in a straight line below the angle of the jaw, one half inch in over an undivided muscle, and then becoming deeper, dividing the sheath. The cut was very clean and deviated a little downwards. The arteries and other vessels contained in the sheath were all cut through.

The cut through the tissues on the right side was more superficial, and tailed off to about two inches below the right angle of the jaw. The deep vessels on that side were uninjured. From this is was evident that the hemorrhage was caused through the partial severance of the left cartoid artery.

Decomposition had commenced in the skin. Dark brown spots were on the anterior surface of the left chin. There was a deformity in the bones of the right leg, which was not straight, but bowed forwards. There was no recent external injury save to the neck. The body being washed more thoroughly I could see some healing sores. The lobe of the left ear was torn as if from the removal or wearing through of an earring, but it was thoroughly healed. On removing the scalp there was no sign of extravasation of blood.

The heart was small, the left ventricle firmly contracted, and the right slightly so. There was no clot in the pulmonary artery, but the right ventricle was full of dark clot. The left was firmly contracted as to be absolutely empty. The stomach was large and the mucous membrane only congested. It contained partly digested food, apparently consisting of cheese, potato, and farinaceous powder. All the teeth on the lower left jaw were absent.

Catherine Eddowes

The body was on its back, the head turned to left shoulder. The arms by the side of the body as if they had fallen there. Both palms upwards, the fingers slightly bent. The left leg extended in a line with the body. The abdomen was exposed. Right leg bent at the thigh and knee. The throat cut across.

The intestines were drawn out to a large extent and placed over the right shoulder -- they were smeared over with some feculent matter. A piece of about two feet

was quite detached from the body and placed between the body and the left arm, apparently by design. The lobe and auricle of the right ear were cut obliquely through.

There was a quantity of clotted blood on the pavement on the left side of the neck round the shoulder and upper part of arm, and fluid blood-coloured serum which had flowed under the neck to the right shoulder, the pavement sloping in that direction.

Body was quite warm. No death stiffening had taken place. She must have been dead most likely within the half hour. We looked for superficial bruises and saw none. No blood on the skin of the abdomen or secretion of any kind on the thighs. No spurting of blood on the bricks or pavement around. No marks of blood below the middle of the body. Several buttons were found in the clotted blood after the body was removed. There was no blood on the front of the clothes. There were no traces of recent connexion.

When the body arrived at Golden Lane, some of the blood was dispersed through the removal of the body to the mortuary. The clothes were taken off carefully from the body. A piece of deceased's ear dropped from the clothing.

I made a post mortem examination at half past two on Sunday afternoon. Rigor mortis was well marked; body not quite cold. Green discoloration over the abdomen. After washing the left hand carefully, a bruise the size of a sixpence, recent and red, was discovered on the back of the left hand between the thumb and first finger. A few small bruises on right shin of older date. The hands and arms were bronzed. No bruises on the scalp, the back of the body, or the elbows.

The face was very much mutilated. There was a cut about a quarter of an inch through the lower left eyelid, dividing the structures completely through. The upper eyelid on that side, there was a scratch through the skin on the left upper eyelid, near to the angle of the nose. The right eyelid was cut through to about half an inch.

There was a deep cut over the bridge of the nose, extending from the left border of the nasal bone down near the angle of the jaw on the right side of the cheek. This cut went into the bone and divided all the structures of the cheek except the mucuous membrane of the mouth.

The tip of the nose was quite detached by an oblique cut from the bottom of the nasal bone to where the wings of the nose join on to the face. A cut from this divided the upper lip and extended through the substance of the gum over the right upper lateral incisor tooth.

About half an inch from the top of the nose was another oblique cut. There was a cut on the right angle of the mouth as if the cut of a point of a knife. The cut extended an inch and a half, parallel with the lower lip.

There was on each side of cheek a cut which peeled up the skin, forming a triangular flap about an inch and a half. On the left cheek there were two abrasions of the epithelium under the left ear. The throat was cut across to the extent of about six or seven inches. A superficial cut commenced about an inch and a half below the lobe below, and about two and a half inches behind the left ear, and extended across the throat to about three inches below the lobe of the right ear.

The big muscle across the throat was divided through on the left side. The large vessels on the left side of the neck were severed. The larynx was severed below the vocal chord. All the deep structures were severed to the bone, the knife marking intervertebral cartilages. The sheath of the vessels on the right side was just opened.

The cartoid artery had a fine hole opening, the internal jugular vein was opened about an inch and a half -- not divided. The blood vessels contained clot. All these injuries were performed by a sharp instrument like a knife, and pointed.

The cause of death was hemorrhage from the left common cartoid artery. The death was immediate and the mutilations were inflicted after death.

We examined the abdomen. The front walls were laid open from the breast bones to the pubes. The cut commenced opposite the ensiform cartilage. The incision went upwards, not penetrating the skin that was over the sternum. It then divided the ensiform cartilage. The knife must have cut obliquely at the expense of that cartilage.

Behind this, the liver was stabbed as if by the point of a sharp instrument. Below this was another incision into the liver of about two and a half inches, and below this the left lobe of the liver was slit through by a vertical cut. Two cuts were shewn by a jagging of the skin on the left side.

The abdominal walls were divided in the middle line to within a quarter of an inch of the navel. The cut then took a horizontal course for two inches and a half towards the right side. It then divided round the navel on the left side, and made a parallel incision to the former horizontal incision, leaving the navel on a tongue of skin. Attached to the navel was two and a half inches of the lower part of the rectus muscle on the left side of the abdomen. The incision then took an oblique direction to the right and was shelving. The incision went down the right side of the vagina and rectum for half an inch behind the rectum.

There was a stab of about an inch on the left groin. This was done by a pointed instrument. Below this was a cut of three inches going through all tissues making a wound of the peritoneum about the same extent.

An inch below the crease of the thigh was a cut extending from the anterior spine of the ilium obliquely down the inner side of the left thigh and separating the left labium, forming a flap of skin up to the groin. The left rectus muscle was not detached.

There was a flap of skin formed by the right thigh, attaching the right labium, and extending up to the spine of the ilium. The muscles on the right side inserted into the frontal ligaments were cut through.

The skin was retracted through the whole of the cut through the abdomen, but the vessels were not clotted. Nor had there been any appreciable bleeding from the vessels. I draw the conclusion that the act was made after death, and there would not have been much blood on the murderer. The cut was made by someone on the right side of the body, kneeling below the middle of the body.

I removed the content of the stomach and placed it in a jar for further examination. There seemed very little in it in the way of food or fluid, but from the cut end partly digested farinaceous food escaped.

The intestines had been detached to a large extent from the mesentery. About two feet of the colon was cut away. The signoid flexure was invaginated into the rectum very tightly.

Right kidney was pale, bloodless with slight congestion of the base of the pyramids.

There was a cut from the upper part of the slit on the under surface of the liver to the left side, and another cut at right angles to this, which were about an inch and a half deep and two and a half inches long. Liver itself was healthy.

The gall bladder contained bile. The pancreas was cut, but not through, on the left side of the spinal column. Three and a half inches of the lower border of the spleen by half an inch was attached only to the peritoneum.

The peritoneal lining was cut through on the left side and the left kidney carefully taken out and removed. The left renal artery was cut through. I would say that someone who knew the position of the kidney must have done it.

The lining membrane over the uterus was cut through. The womb was cut through horizontally, leaving a stump of three quarters of an inch. The rest of the womb had been taken away with some of the ligaments. The vagina and cervix of the womb was uninjured.

The bladder was healthy and uninjured, and contained three or four ounces of water. There was a tongue-like cut through the anterior wall of the abdominal aorta. The other organs were healthy. There were no indications of connexion.

I believe the wound in the throat was first inflicted. I believe she must have been lying on the ground.

The wounds on the face and abdomen prove that they were inflicted by a sharp, pointed knife, and that in the abdomen by one six inches or longer.

I believe the perpetrator of the act must have had considerable knowledge of the position of the organs in the abdominal cavity and the way of removing them. It required a great deal of medical knowledge to have removed the kidney and to know where it was placed. The parts removed would be of no use for any professional purpose.

I think the perpetrator of this act had sufficient time, or he would not have nicked the lower eyelids. It would take at least five minutes.

I cannot assign any reason for the parts being taken away. I feel sure that there was no struggle, and believe it was the act of one person.

The throat had been so instantly severed that no noise could have been emitted. I should not expect much blood to have been found on the person who had inflicted these wounds. The wounds could not have been self-inflicted.

My attention was called to the apron, particularly the corner of the apron with a string attached. The blood spots were of recent origin. I have seen the portion of an apron produced by Dr. Phillips and stated to have been found in Goulston Street. It is impossible to say that it is human blood on the apron. I fitted the piece of apron, which had a new piece of material on it (which had evidently been sewn on to the piece I have), the seams of the borders of the two actually corresponding. Some blood and apparently faecal matter was found on the portion that was found in Goulston Street.

Mary Kelly

The body was lying naked in the middle of the bed, the shoulders flat but the axis of the body inclined to the left side of the bed. The head was turned on the left cheek. The left arm was close to the body with the forearm flexed at a right angle and lying across the abdomen.

The right arm was slightly abducted from the body and rested on the mattress. The elbow was bent, the forearm supine with the fingers clenched. The legs were

wide apart, the left thigh at right angles to the trunk and the right forming an obtuse angle with the pubes.

The whole of the surface of the abdomen and thighs was removed and the abdominal cavity emptied of its viscera. The breasts were cut off, the arms mutilated by several jagged wounds and the face hacked beyond recognition of the features. The tissues of the neck were severed all round down to the bone.

The viscera were found in various parts viz: the uterus and kidneys with one breast under the head, the other breast by the right foot the liver between the feet, the intestines by the right side and the spleen by the left side of the body. The flaps removed from the abdomen and thighs were on a table.

The bed clothing at the right corner was saturated with blood, and on the floor beneath was a pool of blood covering about two feet square. The wall by the right side of the bed and in a line with the neck was marked by blood which had struck it in a number of separate splashes.

The face was gashed in all directions, the nose, cheeks, eyebrows, and ears being partly removed. The lips were blanched and cut by several incisions running obliquely down to the chin. There were also numerous cuts extending irregularly across all the features.

The neck was cut through the skin and other tissues right down to the vertebrae, the fifth and sixth being deeply notched. The skin cuts in the front of the neck showed distinct ecchymosis. The air passage was cut at the lower part of the larynx through the cricoid cartilage.

Both breasts were more or less removed by circular incisions, the muscle down to the ribs being attached to the breasts. The intercostals between the fourth, fifth, and sixth ribs were cut through and the contents of the thorax visible through the openings.

Mary Kelly as she was found in her bed at 13 Miller's Court. The skin and tissues of the abdomen from the costal arch to the pubes were removed in three large flaps. The right thigh was denuded in front to the bone, the flap of skin, including the external organs of generation, and part of the right buttock. The left thigh was stripped of skin fascia, and muscles as far as the knee.

The left calf showed a long gash through skin and tissues to the deep muscles and reaching from the knee to five inches above the ankle. Both arms and forearms had extensive jagged wounds.

The right thumb showed a small superficial incision about one inch long, with extravasation of blood in the skin, and there were several abrasions on the back of the hand moreover showing the same condition.

On opening the thorax it was found that the right lung was minimally adherent by old firm adhesions. The lower part of the lung was broken and torn away. The left lung was intact. It was adherent at the apex and there were a few adhesions over the side. In the substances of the lung there were several nodules of consolidation.

The pericardium was open below and the heart absent. In the abdominal cavity there was some partly digested food of fish and potatoes, and similar food was found in the remains of the stomach attached to the intestines.

Dr. George Bagster Phillips was also present at the scene, and gave the following testimony at the inquest:

The mutilated remains of a female were lying two-thirds over towards the edge of the bedstead nearest the door. She had only her chemise on, or some under linen garment. I am sure that the body had been removed subsequent to the injury which caused her death from that side of the bedstead that was nearest the wooden partition, because of the large quantity of blood under the bedstead and the saturated condition of the sheet and the palliasse at the corner nearest the partition.

The blood was produced by the severance of the cartoid artery, which was the cause of death. The injury was inflicted while the deceased was lying at the right side of the bedstead.

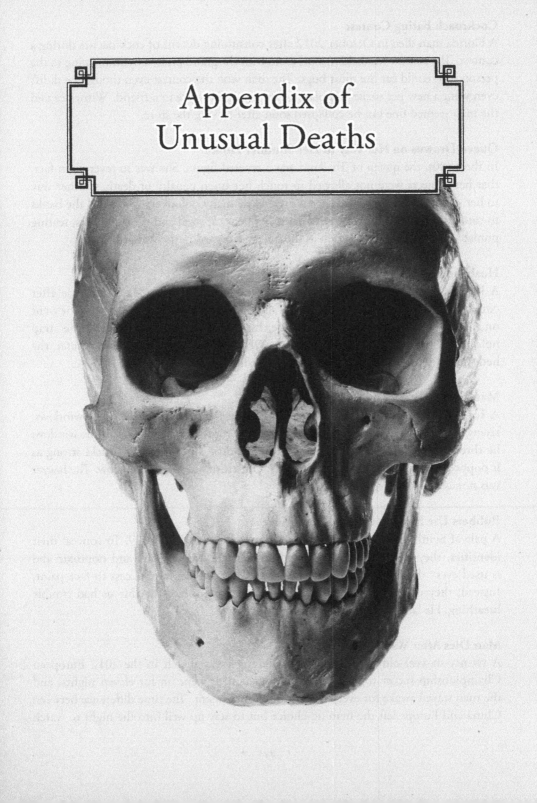

Appendix of
Unusual Deaths

Cockroach Eating Contest

A Florida man died in October 2012 after consuming dozens of cockroaches during a contest. The contest was held in a pet store with the grand prize, a python, going to the person who could eat the most bugs. The man won the contest even though he didn't even want a new pet snake. He planned on giving his prize to a friend. Witnesses said the man seemed fine but he collapsed soon after leaving the store.

Queen Drowns on Her Way to Her Summer Home

In the 1880s, the queen of Thailand was a revered figure. She was so revered, in fact, that her subjects were not allowed to touch her upon penalty of death. On her way to her summer home, the queen was greeted by many onlookers who lined the banks to catch a glimpse of the monarch. Then her boat capsized and the onlookers, fearing punishment, continued to watch as the queen drowned in the waters below.

Husband Sleeps on Couch

A Russian man came home drunk and argued with his wife. As is the case after couples fight, he slept on the fold-out wall bed in the living room. As the night went on, the fight continued. The man's wife, furious at her husband, kicked the strap holding the bed down and left the room. When she returned three hours later, the bed was folded up and her husband was crushed to death inside.

Man Tries to Break Unbreakable Window

A Toronto lawyer was giving a demonstration on the strength of his office windows, trying to prove they were unbreakable. Instead of throwing a chair against the window, he threw himself. The lawyer was right, the window did not break. It held strong as it popped out of the frame and fell twenty-four stories to the street below. The lawyer was not as lucky.

Robbers Use Paint to Conceal Identities

A pair of South Carolina thieves robbed a cell phone store in 2009. To conceal their identities, they painted their faces gold. While face paint is safe and nontoxic and is used every day at children's parties, the robbers did not have access to face paint. Instead, they used spray paint. During the getaway, one of the thieves had trouble breathing. He later died from inhaling paint fumes.

Man Dies After Watching Soccer

A twenty-six-year-old man died after watching every match in the 2012 European Championship soccer tournament. The tournament went on for eleven nights, and the man stayed awake for every night of the tournament. The time difference between China and Europe left the man no choice but to stay up well into the night to watch

the matches. After the championship match, the man took a shower, finally went to sleep, and did not wake up.

Australian Man Dies After Planking

A man from Brisbane, Australia died after trying to "plank" off a balcony. The idea of planking is to lie face down in an unusual setting. Some people plank across a set of chairs or on top of a car; others are more courageous and lie across train tracks and rooftops. The man that fell tried to plank across the safety railing of a balcony before falling to his death.

Women Uses Chimney to Enter Home

A California woman died in September, 2010, when she fell into a chimney and could not get out. The woman was trying to enter her on-again, off-again boyfriend's house but was unsuccessful when she tried the doors and windows. That was when she thought about using the chimney. She climbed onto the roof, removed the chimney cap, and slid down like Santa Claus. Then she got stuck. The next day, she was nowhere to be found and was reported missing. Three days later, she was discovered after a house sitter reported a bad smell inside the house.

Thai Woman Recreates Death of Sister

In 1991, a woman was killed on her farm when she slipped and accidentally grabbed a live wire to steady herself. After the funeral, her sister recreated the death for family members. During the reenactment, the woman slipped and grabbed the same live wire that killed her sister—she was killed outright.

Hungry Sheep Kill Farmer

A farmer in England went out to feed her sheep one day by putting a bale of hay on her motorcycle and bringing it to the pasture where her sheep roamed during the day. On this day, the sheep were especially hungry, and when they saw the hay, they rushed towards the farmer. Forty sheep ran towards the woman, ultimately pushing the farmer off a cliff along with her motorcycle.

Writer Dies Trying to Hug the Moon

Chinese poet Li Po was regarded as the greatest poet of his time and one of the best of the Tang Dynasty. He composed poems for Emperors and their court. He acted as an advisor to the crown prince. Along with his skills as a poet, Li Po also lived a hard lifestyle. He wandered the Chinese countryside from time to time and he liked to imbibe heavily in alcohol. One day, Li Po was on his boat when he saw the moon reflected in the water. Li Po had never seen the moon this close to him and he wanted to embrace it. Li Po fell into the water trying to hug the moon and drowned.

Hiker Climbs up Mountain, Forgets How to Get Down

A hiker in Oregon climbed to the Summit of Saddle Mountain, three thousand feet above sea level. When he reached the top, he decided he didn't want to walk anymore, told his friends he would meet them in the parking lot, and slid down the face of the mountain. One thousand feet later, his body came to a rest in a ravine.

Man Dies on Merry-Go-Round

During a stunt in Germany, a man was duct taped to a merry go round. A rope was attached to the merry go round on one end and a BMW on the other. The idea was, as the BMW sped around, the ride would spin quickly and cause the man to get dizzy. The man survived the spin, but after the duct tape broke, he didn't survive the fall.